Herbal Medicine: Back to the Future
(Volume 3)

(Cancer Therapy)

Edited by

Ferid Murad, (*Nobel Laureate*)
Palo Alto Veterans Hospital, California, USA

Atta-ur-Rahman, *FRS*
Honorary Life Fellow,
Kings College, University of Cambridge, Cambridge, UK

&

Ka Bian
George Washington University, School of Medicine, Washington, USA

Herbal Medicine: Back to the Future

Volume # 3

Cancer Therapy

Editors: Ferid Murad, Atta-ur-Rahman and Ka Bian

ISSN (Online): 2542-999X

ISSN (Print): 2542-9981

ISBN (Online): 978-981-14-1120-5

ISBN (Print): 978-981-14-1119-9

need for a court order if at any point you breach any terms of this License Agreement. In no event will any delay or failure by Bentham Science Publishers in enforcing your compliance with this License Agreement constitute a waiver of any of its rights.

3. You acknowledge that you have read this License Agreement, and agree to be bound by its terms and conditions. To the extent that any other terms and conditions presented on any website of Bentham Science Publishers conflict with, or are inconsistent with, the terms and conditions set out in this License Agreement, you acknowledge that the terms and conditions set out in this License Agreement shall prevail.

Bentham Science Publishers Pte. Ltd.
80 Robinson Road #02-00
Singapore 068898
Singapore
Email: subscriptions@benthamscience.net

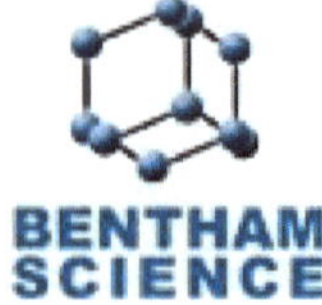

CONTENTS

PREFACE

Herbal Medicine: Back to the Future presents expert reviews on the applications of herbal medicines (including Ayurveda, Chinese traditional medicines and alternative therapies). This volume demonstrates the use of sophisticated methods to explore traditional medicine, while providing readers a glimpse into the future of herbal medicine. The book is a valuable resource for pharmaceutical scientists and postgraduate students seeking updated and critically important information in natural product chemistry and pharmacology. The chapters are written by authorities in the field. The contents of this volume represent exciting recent researches on ROS in Cancer Cell Lines, Natural Antimutagens, Encapsulated Plant-Derived Polyphenols, Cancer-related Fatigue, Indirubins, Plants Used in Ayurveda, Plant Based Bioactive Compounds, and Melanocyte Regeneration. I hope that the readers involved in cancer care will find these reviews valuable and thought provoking so that they may trigger further research in herbal medicine and alternative therapies against cancer.

I am grateful for the timely efforts made by the editorial personnel, especially Mr. Mahmood Alam (Director Publications), and Mr. Shehzad Iqbal Naqvi (Editorial Manager Publications) at Bentham Science Publishers.

Ferid Murad (Nobel Laureate)
Palo Alto Veterans Hospital,
California, USA

Atta-ur-Rahman, *FRS*
Kings College, University of Cambridge,
Cambridge, UK

Ka Bian
George Washington University, School of Medicine,
Washington, USA

List of Contributors

Ayesha S. Ali
Postgraduate Department of Biotechnology and Zoology, Saifia College of Science, Bhopal, India

Aleksandra Tarasiuk
Department of Biochemistry, Faculty of Medicine, Medical University of Lodz, Lodz, Poland

Aleksandra Sobolewska-Włodarczyk
Department of Biochemistry, Faculty of Medicine, Medical University of Lodz, Lodz, Poland

Ana Pontoriero
Instituto de Química Rosario (IQUIR), Facultad de Ciencias Bioquímicas y Farmacéuticas, Universidad Nacional de Rosario, Argentina

Dharmik Joshi
Department of Pharmaceutical Sciences and Technology, Birla Institute of Technology, Mesra, Ranchi, India

Elisa Panzarini
Department of Biological Sciences and Technologies (Di.S.Te.B.A.), University of Salento, 73100 Lecce, Italy

Guangqi Song
Department of Gastroenterology, Zhongshan Hospital, Fudan University, Building 19, Fenglin Road 179, Shanghai Institute of Liver Disease, Shanghai, China

Jakub Włodarczyk
Department of Biochemistry, Faculty of Medicine, Medical University of Lodz, Lodz, Poland

Luciana Dini
Sapienza University of Rome, Department of Biology and Biotechnology "Charles Darwin", 00185 Rome, Italy
CNR-Nanotec, Lecce, Italy

Marcela Rizzotto
Instituto de Química Rosario (IQUIR), Facultad de Ciencias Bioquímicas y Farmacéuticas, Universidad Nacional de Rosario, Argentina

Marcin Włodarczyk
Department of General and Colorectal Surgery, Universidad Nacional de Rosario, Argentina

Merve Deniz Kose
Ege University, Department of Chemical Engineering, Faculty of Engineering, Bornova, İzmir, Turkey

Nikita Sharma
Department of Biotechnology, School of Life Sciences, Central University of Rajasthan, Ajmer 305817, Rajasthan, India

Nidhi Gupta
Department of Biotechnology, The IIS University, Jaipur 302020, Rajasthan, India

Naima Parveen
Postgraduate Department of Biotechnology and Zoology, Saifia College of Science, Bhopal, India

Oguz Bayraktar
Ege University, Department of Chemical Engineering, Faculty of Engineering, Bornova, İzmir, Turkey

Paweł Siwiński
Department of General and Colorectal Surgery, Faculty of Military Medicine, Medical University of Lodz, Lodz, Poland

R. Mankamna Kumari
Department of Biotechnology, School of Life Sciences, Central University of Rajasthan, Ajmer 305817, Rajasthan, India

Stefania Mariano — Department of Biological Sciences and Technologies (Di.S.Te.B.A.), University of Salento, 73100 Lecce, Italy

Surendra Nimesh — Department of Biotechnology, School of Life Sciences, Central University of Rajasthan, Ajmer 305817, Rajasthan, India

Sugato Banerjee — Department of Pharmaceutical Sciences and Technology, Birla Institute of Technology, Mesra, Ranchi, India

Sharique A. Ali — Postgraduate Department of Biotechnology and Zoology, Saifia College of Science, Bhopal, India

Uma Ranjan Lal — Department of Pharmaceutical Sciences and Technology, Birla Institute of Technology, Mesra, Ranchi, India

Xinlai Cheng — Institute of Pharmacy and Molecular Biotechnology, Pharmaceutical Biology, Heidelberg University, Im Neuenheimer Feld 364, Heidelberg, Germany

Yasamin Dabiri — Institute of Pharmacy and Molecular Biotechnology, Pharmaceutical Biology, Heidelberg University, Im Neuenheimer Feld 364, Heidelberg, Germany

CHAPTER 1

Herbal Extracts from *Carica papaya* and *Azadirachta indica*: What Role for ROS in Cancer Cell Lines?

Luciana Dini[1,2,*], **Stefania Mariano**[3] and **Elisa Panzarini**[3]

[1] *Sapienza University of Rome, Department of Biology and Biotechnology "Charles Darwin", 00185 Rome, Italy*

[2] *CNR-Nanotec, Lecce, Italy*

[3] *Department of Biological Sciences and Technologies (Di.S.Te.B.A.), University of Salento, 73100 Lecce, Italy*

Abstract: The use of plant-derived medications in the treatment and prevention of diseases, *i.e.*, phytotherapy, comprises the traditional knowledge of therapeutic advantages deriving from the use of herbal parts to prevent, protect against and cure several pathologic conditions, such as cancerous, metabolic and inflammatory diseases. Herbal medications are prevalent in countries with limited resources, but, recently, increasing attention is devoted to their exploitation in cancer management on the basis of their low cost and side effects absence compared to conventional radiation or chemotherapic cancer approach. Currently, about 114,000 herbal extracts have screened for anticancer activity and 60% of the commercially available and clinically used cancer drugs, such as vinblastine and vincristine, paclitaxel, campothecin and its derivatives, are from natural sources. These compounds are active against a number of cancer types (ovarian, breast, lung, colon, liver, blood, prostate cancer). There are many types of cancer elicited by several factors that still render this disease a major public health problem, almost everywhere in the world.

The human body is constantly exposed to free radicals arising from exogenous and endogenous origins, which cause oxidative stress. Oxidative stress is closely related to various diseases, including cancer. There are many evidences that ROS are pivotal in cancer progression (*via* damage of DNA leading to genomic instability) and regression (*via* cell death induction through oxidative stress burst). Antioxidants stabilize free radicals and, in turn, prevent the oxidative stress, playing a key role in protection of the body, In this context, natural plants-derived antioxidants are universally considered very important for the prevention and treatment of oxidative stress and cancer. However, a dual role of plants in ROS generation or scavenging is recognized as plants extracts can also increase ROS production in the cells. Consequently, the role of plant

* **Corresponding author Luciana Dini**: Sapienza University of Rome, Department of Biology and Biotechnology "Charles Darwin", 00185 Rome, Italy; Tel/Fax: +390649912306; E-mail: luciana.dini@uniroma1.it

Ferid Murad, Atta-ur-Rahman and Ka Bian (Eds.)

extracts in ROS balancing inside cancer cells is a very fascinating feature in phytotherapy.

Among the plants reported in traditional medicine as a very panacea in active compounds, *Carica papaya* and *Azadiracta indica* (also known as Neem) extracts from different parts (leaves, seeds, fruits, *etc.*) are scientifically validated in the treatment of several diseases, including cancer. In this context, the two plants have different impact on cancer cell lines. In particular hydro-alcoolic extract of Neem leaves shows a pro-oxidant activity in hepatoma HepG2 cells, whereas water extract of *C. papaya* seeds exerts an anti-oxidant activity in leukemia HL-60 cells. Neem extract is unable to quench oxidative stress induced on HepG2 and synergizes with hydrogen peroxide (H_2O_2) in inducing cell death. Conversely, *C. papaya* extract quenches ROS induced by H_2O_2 in HL-60 cells but at the same time negatively affects cell viability.

These evidences corroborate the idea that the extracts from plants could act in patients with cancer to modulate oxidative homeostasis and obtain benefit during cancer therapy.

Keywords: Azadirachta indica, Carica papaya, HepG2 cells, HL-60 cells, Neem, Reactive Oxygen Species (ROS).

1. CELLULAR SOURCES OF ROS

Reactive oxygen species (ROS) are a group of molecules including both oxygen radicals, such as hydroxyl ($\bullet OH$), superoxide anion ($\bullet O_2^-$), perossilic radical ($ROO\bullet$) and certain non-radical molecules like hydrogen peroxide (H_2O_2), hypochlorous acid (HOCl) and peroxynitrite ($ONOO^-$) [1].

A free radical can be defined as a molecule, or a part of it, containing one or more unpaired electrons in an atomic or molecular orbital that make the compound highly reactive. The main mechanism through which ROS are produced starts with the reduction of an O_2 molecule to $\bullet O_2^-$. $\bullet O_2^-$ is the first ROS produced in the cell that react with other molecules to generate "secondary" ROS, through enzyme- or metal-catalysed processes [2] depending on the cell type or cellular compartment. Because of anionic charge, electrophilic activity of $\bullet O_2^-$ toward electron-rich molecules is inhibited. $\bullet O_2^-$, that escapes the antioxidant mechanisms of the cell, is involved in the oxidation of enzymes containing the [4Fe-4S] clusters (aconitase or dehydratase as examples) [3] and the reduction of cytochrome C [4]. Furthermore, $\bullet O_2^-$ can accept one electron and two protons to generate H_2O_2. This reaction can occur either nonenzymatically or by Superoxide Dismutase (SOD) catalyzed reaction:

$$2O_2^{\bullet -} + 2H^+ \rightarrow H_2O_2 + O_2$$

$$2O_2^{\bullet -} + 2H^+ \xrightarrow{\text{SOD}} H_2O_2 + O_2$$

The amount of not degraded superoxide may have different destinies: it can be reduced to the highly reactive species ($\bullet$OH) by Haber-Weiss and Fenton reactions to generate $\bullet$OH from $H_2O_2 + O_2$ or it can be rapidly degraded to hydroperoxide ($HO_2\bullet$).

Apparently ROS do not seem to derive from a single source because of their site-specific and function-specific role. In fact, exogenous and endogenous sources have the same contribution in the intracellular generation of ROS. Exogenous sources include irradiation and various chemical compounds including atmospheric pollutants, tobacco and drugs.

Endogenous sources include mitochondria, in which ROS are produced because of the loss of electrons (between complex I and III) along the mitochondrial electron transport chain (ETC), the cytochrome P450, endoplasmic reticulum, peroxisomes [5]. The ETC represents the main source of ROS into the cells, in particular of $\bullet O_2^-$. The flavoprotein region of NADH dehydrogenase segment (complex I) of the respiratory chain is the site where oxygen is directly reduced in $\bullet O2-$. When substrates linked to NAD+ are scarce for complex I, an electron transport from complex II to complex I (reverse electron flow (RET)) can occur. Different electrons escape sites from Complex I have been proposed: i) Fe-S centre; ii) N1a centre; iii) ubisemiquinone; iv) flavin mononucleotide (FMN).

There are many other endogenous sources of ROS, for example the membrane-bound enzyme NADPH oxidase, which is responsible of the production of ROS in response to different ligands, working with other enzymes such as xanthine oxidase, cyclooxygenases, and nitric oxide synthase.

Phagocytic cells, neutrophils, macrophages and dendritic cells merit special attention, as they possess high levels of the NADPH oxidase (Nox) enzyme on their plasma membrane. This enzyme is able to catalyze the reduction of molecular oxygen, using the NADPH compound as an electron donor and thus generating large amounts of superoxide on the membrane surface. This radical acts as a toxic agent against microbial organisms, that are in contact with phagocytic cells at the sites of infection. Other main proteins producing ROS as co-products of their normal functions are listed in Table **1**.

Table 1. Main ROS-producing enzymes.

Enzyme	Catalyzed Reaction	E.C. Number*
Lipoxygenase	Fatty acid + O_2 → Fatty acid Idroperoxide	1.13.11.12
Nitric oxide synthase	L-arginine + O_2 → L-citrulline + NO + H_2O	1.1.4.13.39
Xantine oxidase	Xantine + O_2 → Uric acid + H_2O	1.17.3.2
Peroxidase	Electron donor + H_2O_2 → Oxidated donor + $2H_2O$	1.11.1.7
Galactose oxidase	D-Galactose + O_2 → D-galacto-Hexodialdose + H_2O	1.1.3.9
Nitropropane dioxygenase	Nitropropane + O_2 → Acetone + Nitrite	1.13.11.32
Cytochrome p450	$RH + O_2 + 2H^+ + 2e^- → ROH + H_2O$	1.14.14.1
NAD(P)H oxidase	$NADPH + O_2 ↔ NAD(P)^+ + H_2O_2$	1.6.3.1

*The Enzyme Commission number (E.C. number) is a number that refers to specific name of enzymes, based on the chemical reaction they catalyse.

2. CONVERSION AND CLEARANCE OF ROS

The balance between production and scavenging of ROS is pivotal as they have been linked to numerous biological processes and disease conditions. The relationship between ROS and cancer is based on the different species of ROS and their properties, such as reactivity, chemical structure, specificity for a target molecule and ability to cross subcellular compartments but also to influence biological functions. Furthermore, every aerobic cell have a balance between the normal production of ROS and the presence of biochemical antioxidants.

Cellular redox balance is generally ensured by copious antioxidant systems present in different cellular compartments. These antioxidant compounds can be divided in: i) enzymatic (such as catalase, SOD, glutathione peroxidase, *etc.*, and ii) non-enzymatic (lipoic acid, ascorbic acid, *etc.*).

SODs are metalloenzymes involved in the dismutation of superoxide anion to oxygen and hydrogen peroxide (Fig. **1**), utilizing metal ions as cofactors (*i.e.*, copper, manganese, iron or zinc). There are different SODs that are located in various cell compartments and each one is involved in regulating linked biological processes [6].

Catalases catalyze the demolition of a highly reactive product, hydrogen peroxide (Fig. **1**), which is an intermediate in the oxygen-reducing reaction to H_2O, essential in the biological use of oxygen itself, especially for the purpose of energy production. Catalases are present in almost all aerobic cells because of need of oxygen for their metabolism. The have evolved enzymatic systems to neutralize the risk of potentially damaging byproducts of this adaptation (ROS).

In the Eukaryotes, catalase is localized in a particular class of subcellular organelles, peroxisomes, because they are involved in the demolition of long chain fatty acids by the action of oxidases that produce large amounts of hydrogen peroxide. The presence of catalase in the same cell compartment appears to be clearly functional in defending the cell against this metabolic process. The protective function of catalase is confirmed by its complete absence in oxygen-tolerant bacteria (anaerobes), although the lack of enzyme in humans (acatalasemia) due to a rare genetic defect does not produce many symptoms, probably due to the presence of substitute defense systems (*e.g.*, peroxidase, glutathione and other antioxidants).

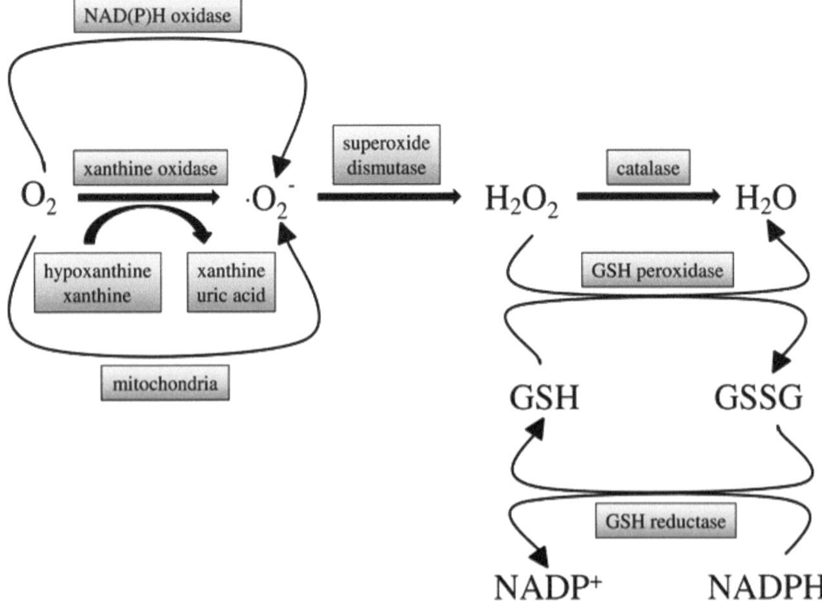

Fig. (1). Pathways of ROS conversion and clearance.

Another antioxidant enzymatic compound is glutathione system that include glutathione (GSH), glutathione reductase, glutathione peroxidases (GPXs) and glutathione S-transferases (GST). Glutathione peroxidases are selenium-dependent enzymes that convert H_2O_2 or water-or-alcohol organic hydroperoxides (ROHs), respectively, through reduced glutathione oxidation. Although all GPXs apparently catalyze the same reaction, each enzyme differs both for cellular localization (cytosol, mitochondria, *etc.*) and for substrate specificity [7]. GST catalyzes the direct link of GSH to oxidized substrates subsequently eliminated from the body. In mammals a family of cytosolic soluble enzymes including seven GST classes have been identified and characterized, and recently two other mitochondrial and microsomal enzymes have been identified.

Among glutathione system, GSH is one of the most effective antioxidant produced at the intracellular level. It is very abundant in the cytosolic (1-11 mM), nuclei (3-15 mM) and mitochondria (5-11 mM) and it is considered the largest soluble antioxidant in these cell compartments [8]. GSH is a tripeptide formed of cysteine, glycine and glutamate. It is involved in the protection of cells from oxidative stress by reducing disulfide bonds of cytoplasmic proteins to cysteines. At the same time, GSH is oxidized to glutathione disulfide (GSSG), then glutathione reductase reduces GSSG refilling GSH pool. GSSG is accumulated within the cells and the GSH/GSSG ratio is a possible index to evaluate the level of oxidative stress of an organism.

Besides glutathione, non-enzymatic antioxidants include different types of molecules, *e.g.*, vitamin E, ascorbic acid (or vitamin C) and α-lipoic acid (ALA). Vitamin E is a powerful liposoluble antioxidant present in humans in different forms. It plays an important role in preventing the oxidation of polyunsaturated fatty acids, which is pivotal in the development of the lipid peroxidation process. Since the development of lipid peroxidation can lead to modifications of cell membranes, the role of vitamin E is recognized as an important part in maintaining tissue structures [8]. Vitamin C is well known as a powerful antioxidant [8]. In occidental countries, it is often introduced in daily diets as a beneficial additive. The use in different fields of ascorbic acid derives from study about the evidence that a several severe diseases can be caused by a vitamin C deficient diet. In fact, the easily oxidizable compounds, donors of H atoms or radical scavengers (vitamins C, E, Q, glutathione, *etc.*), eliminate ROS to avoid damage in surrounding cells and tissues. However, other studies have shown that under certain circumstances, vitamin C may not play the role of beneficial antioxidant, but could act as a pro-oxidant, *i.e.*, promotes oxidative stress.

ALA is an octanoic acid derivative, it can be both fat-soluble and water-soluble and it is largely present in cell membranes and cytosol, both eukaryotic and prokaryotic. ALA is quickly absorbed from the diet and converted into its reduced form, dihydrolipoic acid (DHLA) [8]. Both forms are powerful antioxidants against free radicals, chelate metal ions, recycle antioxidants, and repair proteins damaged by oxidative stress. DHLA has a strong antioxidant action and can act in synergy with other antioxidants such as glutathione, ascorbic acid and tocopherol. It may also have pro-oxidizing properties; for example, it is able to reduce the iron ion and generate sulfur containing radicals that can damage the proteins.

3. FUNCTION OF ROS IN CANCER

ROS production is strictly connected with cancer, ageing, obesity, neurodegenerative and chronic inflammatory diseases. How can ROS contribute to these different clinical pathologies? In recent years, a lot of information has been produced about this topic. Interestingly, the information derives from the study of the role of ROS along the tumorigenesis [9].

If considered as harmful waste products of metabolic processes, ROS were thought to be very toxic and associated only with pathological conditions. Afterward, a noteworthy amount of papers have been published linking ROS to various biological processes and to cell signaling (including apoptosis, gene expression and the activation of cell signaling cascades) [10]. In this way, the biological role of ROS is rather complex and paradoxical. Under normal conditions, free radical production is low and is balanced by the action of the antioxidant defense systems described above. However, in different pathophysiological conditions, the rate of production of free radicals exceeds the capacity of cell defense systems, a condition known as oxidative stress. Then, oxidative stress occurs when an excess of ROS or other cellular events alter the critical balance. In this way ROS concentration, which depend on the ratio between production and detoxification, is an important variable in ROS/cancer relationship.

3.1. Tumor Promoting Function of ROS

3.1.1. Effect on Tumorigenesis

The influence of oxidative stress in tumor promoting is closely linked to induction of tumor promotion and progression phases, causing instability in the activation of specific signaling pathways which are the basis of cellular proliferation, angiogenesis and metastasis. In fact, the exposure to a certain concentration of ROS can induce damage of proteins, lipids and DNA, leading to activation of various signaling cascades related to tumorigenesis [11]. For example, chronic inflammatory diseases deriving from non-infectious disorders such as smoking and asbestosis represent a cause of oxidative damage that can conduce to tumor in lung or in other organs.

It is known that tumor promotion is connected with permanent chromosomal aberrations and the activation of oncogenes, both caused by the action of radicals. The oxidative damage produces a multitude of changes in the DNA structures, *i.e.*, disulfide bridges breakage, crosslink between DNA and proteins in sites missing in nitrogenous bases. DNA is the genetic material of cell and, if damaged, can lead to changes in protein encoding, causing malfunctions or inactivation of encoded proteins. DNA damage due to oxygen-free radicals often causes mutations connected with initiation and progression of human tumors. However, it has been difficult to prove this relationship due to the high amount of reactive oxygen species that have the potential to damage DNA. These highly reactive chemical molecules include •OH, •O_2^-, ROO•, *etc.*, and while each has its own distinct chemistry and cellular distribution, all of them have the potential to alter nucleotide residues. As a result of the reaction with DNA, oxygen radicals generate more than 30 different adducts, in addition to protein and lipid addition products as well as inter- and intra-strand cross-links [12]. Therefore, oxygen free radicals can induce hundreds of different types of chemical changes in DNA that could create mutagenic lesions involved in the etiology of cancer. Other oxidative consequences on DNA are strand breakage, removal of nucleotides and several modification in the organic bases of the nucleotides.

Furthermore, molecules like •O_2^- are produced especially by activated macrophages, the most representative immune cells within tumour microenvironment. Here, they induce the DNA oxidation in the same tumour cells. The oxidation at C8 position of guanine leads to the formation of 8-hydroxy-2'-deoxyguanosine (8-OHdG). ROS can be react directly with guanine free nucleotides, leading to formation of substrates that will be incorporated in the DNA as 8-OHdG. This molecule promotes mutagenesis both in bacterial and mammalian cells. It causes spontaneous and heritable guanine to timine transversion mutations, detectable in mutated oncogenes and tumour suppressor genes. 8-OHdG can be considered a biomarker of the oxidative stress levels of an organism and a potential biomarker of tumorigenesis [13].

In addition to significant genetic changes, ROS may induce tumorigenesis by mediating various epigenetic alterations. Radicals, in particular ROS, affect another process involved in carcinogenesis, *i.e.*, DNA methylation. In normal conditions, DNA is methylated (it has methyl groups on nitrogenous bases) symmetrically on both filaments by DNA methyltransferases. During carcinogenesis the alteration of methylation process can lead to a hypermethylation or hypomethylation of DNA. Since the gene methylation is closely associated to gene expression, hypermethylation can inhibit tumor suppressor gene transcription, leading to silencing of the gene.

For example, H_2O_2 has been shown to downregulate the E-cadherin tumor suppressor (a molecule involved in cell-cell adhesion) expression in hepatocarcinoma cells after hypermethylation of E-cadherin promoter region. This decreased expression is associated to an increased metastasis and poor prognosis in hepatocellular carcinoma [14]. However, further studies are pivotal to understand the biochemical mechanisms involved in ROS-mediated epigenetic regulation of several proliferative and tumor suppressor genes. Effects of ROS on tumorigenesis promotion are shown in Fig. (**2**).

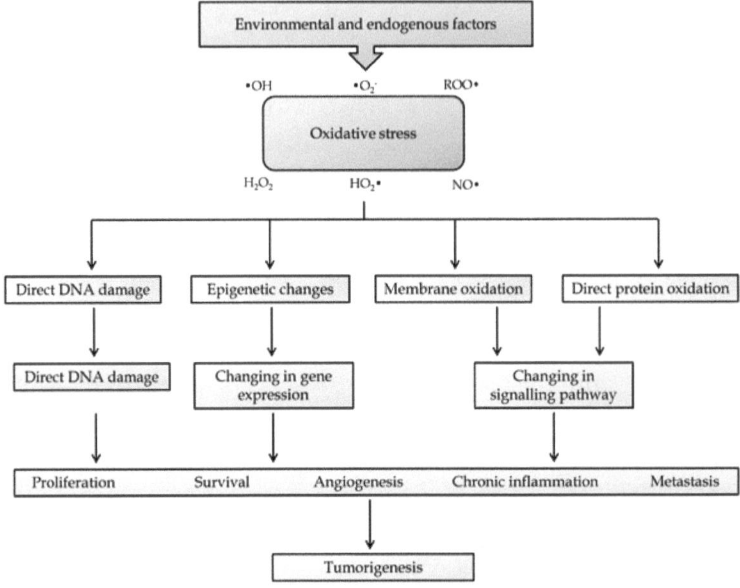

Fig. (2). Effects of ROS on tumorigenesis.

3.1.2. Angiogenesis, Cell Invasion and Metastasis

Tumor cell invasion, angiogenesis and metastasis are correlated processes representing the final stage of cancer. There are several processes involved in malignancy, *i.e.*, cell proliferation, adhesion, migration, degradation of tissue barriers and new blood vessels formation [15]. In particular, angiogenesis is regulated by a network of pro-angiogenic and anti-angiogenic components in the tumor microenvironment (proteolytic enzymes, endothelial growth factor (VEGF) and its receptors, fibroblast growth factor, ephrins, integrins, cadherins, endothelins and transcription factors). VEGF is one of the most powerful pro-angiogenic factors and its action is mediated by the interaction with the VEGFR-2 tyrosine kinase receptor, expressed almost a level of endothelial cells and overexpressed in many solid tumors. VEGF signalling is involved in normal vascular development and homeostasis, but also in tumor progression by promoting growth of tumor vasculature. Of note, ROS have a fundamental role in angiogenesis. ROS, in fact, trigger the secretion of VEGF, inducing proliferation, migration, cytoskeletal reorganization and vascular tube formation.

The direct and indirect inhibition of the angiogenic process, achieved through the blockade of the signalling pathway regulated by VEGFR2 and the removal of

ROS, represents an effective anticancer strategy as it allows to suppress the supply to the tumor cells thus inhibiting the growth and metastasis of the neoplastic mass. Thus, this is reciprocity between oxidative stress and angiogenesis based on the VEGF signalling pathway. Several studies have shown this positive interrelationship. ROS-mediated angiogenesis has been found in several pathologies, for example diabetic retinopathy and injured arteries [16, 17]. Furthermore, VEGF influences ROS production by activating NADPH oxidase in endothelial cells [18]. Production of superoxide anion induced by VEGF is regulated by constituents of NADPH oxidase, such as Rac1, Nox1, and Nox2.

Generally, physiological angiogenesis is pivotal in adult organisms to repair tissue and for remodeling processes, such as wound healing [19], skeletal remodeling, and female reproduction. In particular, in wound healing, angiogenesis induced by tissue hypoxia and ROS, can induce stimulation of VEGF production by macrophages, fibroblasts, endothelial cells, and keratinocytes, or operate in a VEGF-independent manner [20].

In pathological conditions, such as cancer, the balance between factors promoting and inhibiting angiogenesis fails. Tumor cells that have developed an angiogenic phenotype overexpress pro-angiogenic factors and the new network of vessels, penetrating the tumor mass, provides oxygen and nutrients necessary for growth and, secondly, removes metabolic waste from the tumor site. The microenvironment of solid tumors is also characterized by heterogeneity in the distribution of oxygenation and hypoxia is one of the main *stimuli* able to promote pathological angiogenesis and to induce the overexpression of the growth factor VEGF.

Metastasis is a complex event characterized by invasion, migration, intravasation in the blood, survival in the circulation, extravasation in far organs and proliferation [21]. The processes of invasion and metastasis are based on a complex network of molecular signalling pathways that control cytoskeletal dynamics and its interaction with the extracellular matrix (ECM), followed by its invasion of the adjacent tissue. Numerous evidence suggests that ROS, particularly H_2O_2, actively influence various events that are essential for cancer cell invasion and metastasis. For instance, it has been demonstrated that increase of H_2O_2 levels is sufficient and necessary to drive promigratory signalling in human bladder cancer cells [22]. Furthermore, also the increased expression of SOD2 is commonly associated with the invasiveness in different cancers [23, 24]. Elevated SOD levels can increase H_2O_2 levels, indicating that H_2O_2 may be responsible for the invasive/metastatic phenotype in cancer cells. In addition, •OH has also been involved in invasiveness and metastasis in lung cancer cells [25].

The role of ROS in regulation of the tumor growth and survival are closely connected to the control of mechanisms involved in the formation of tumor metastases. A reduced cell adhesion to the basal lamina and an increase in the migratory and invasive potential allowing cancer cells to enter the vascular system, are the events underlying this function. In this context, hypoxia and reoxygenation can induce an increased blood vessel growth and enhance the possibility that the metastasis spreads through the blood. Moreover, detached cells escape from detachment-induced cell death leading to the metastatic phenotype. With the increase of oxidative stress, some tumor cells show a reduced adhesion to the basal lamina [26]. This aspect suggests that tumor cells that are affected by oxidative stress could detach more easily and enter quickly the blood vessels.

3.2. Tumor Suppressive Function of ROS

As above stated, ROS, known for their role in cell signaling, show a dual role in cancer. ROS can be beneficial or harmful to cells and tissues: on one side, ROS can activate protumorigenic signaling, promoting cancer cell proliferation, survival, and adaptation to hypoxia; on the other hand, ROS can promote antitumorigenic signaling and trigger oxidative stress–induced cancer cell death.

3.2.1. Apoptosis

Apoptosis is well known as type I programmed cell death. ROS are regulators of apoptosis, as they induce the opening of the pores on the mitochondrial membrane, cause the release of pro-apoptotic factors and also induce the activation of various cascades of signals, including stimulation of the production of ceramides, activation of JNK [27], activation of p53 [28]. Also, the apoptosis induced by TNF-α begins with a production of ROS: this type of response occurs mainly in T lymphocytes, in monocytes and macrophages following the binding to specific membrane receptors.

The relationship between oxidants and apoptosis is complex and not yet well defined. In fact, while most data indicate that ROS stimulate cell death, other data suggest that ROS are protective in respect of apoptosis. The mechanisms that allow cells to take a decision between death and life are finely regulated, in many cases the same *stimulus* that induces apoptosis also activate an antiapoptotic program [29]. Probably ROS can control both apoptosis and cell survival through a communication network between apoptotic mechanisms and signal transduction systems (such as the protein Serina/tyrosine kinase PI3K/AKT) that activate cell survival. This ROS-induced survival effect seems to be mediated by some redox-sensitive proteins, including NFk-B. As already discussed, an intracellular ROS exposure may lead to apoptosis or cellular senescence. However, some cells can escape these controls and their continuous exposure to ROS can induce DNA mutations with genomic instability that is the basis of neoplastic transformation [30]. It is of note that transformed cells produce high levels of ROS, especially H_2O_2. Such exposure to ROS can induce in malignant cells various responses, *i.e.*, increased cell proliferation, accumulation of oxidative DNA damage with mutations, increased expression of antioxidant genes. These consequences could lead to alterations in the resistance of such cells to anticancer agents.

An explanation of how the ROS participate in such different processes is that their effect depends on quantity and duration of the oxidative stress, even if it is unknown how cell operates a control on the quality and quantity of ROS. Certainly, the production and level of ROS in the cell is under strict control because, as already mentioned, their excessive production involves cytotoxic effects, but specific ROS at low concentrations can have a role as second messengers.

3.2.2. Autophagy

Recent evidence has shown that autophagy has an important role during tumorigenesis. On one hand, autophagy plays a role of protection against the presence of ROS in cells and therefore prevents their harmful consequences on DNA mutation, which could induce tumorigenesis [31]. For this reason, autophagy plays a pivotal role as a tumor suppressor process by inhibiting ROS accumulation through removal of damaged mitochondria, known as the major source of ROS.

ROS levels are able to regulate the induction of autophagy in the cells. In particular, induction of autophagy due to nutrient starvation implies the H_2O_2 production that oxidizes autophagy related gene 4 (ATG4), an enzyme involved in autophagy related gene 8 (ATG8) protein maturation and delipidation. This oxidation modification mainly prevents the delipidation of ATG4, thus generating a greater formation of autophagosomes associated with light chain 3 (LC3) protein [32]. Furthermore, ROS can control autophagy through AMP-activated protein kinase (AMPK). Indeed, the oxygen production and starvation induce AMP generation; in this way ATP accumulation and activation of AMPK lead to the inhibition of mammalian target of rapamycin complex (mTORC1) and to autophagy activation [33]. Another way of regulation of autophagy is the phosphorylation of ULK1/ATG1, which activation is necessary to induce autophagy upon starvation [34]. AMPK is sensitive to oxidative stress and can be phosphorylated by the upstream kinase AMPK kinase (AMPKK) after H_2O_2 accumulation. This condition leads to its activation and to an indirect induction of autophagy. ROS can also regulate autophagy mechanism through the regulation of transcription factor activity such as NF-κB causing the activation of autophagy gene expression *(BECLIN1/ATG6 or SQSTM1/p62)* in cancer cells.

4. CANCER AND PHYTOTHERAPY

As discuss earlier, the production of free radicals within the body can induce several effects, including DNA damage, that lead to cancer development. Neutralization of radicals through antioxidants can be a way to prevent cancer. Numerous evidence have demonstrated that plant-derived antioxidants remove free radicals and regulate oxidative stress. The use of plants as medicines dates back to the Middle Palaeolithic period, approximately 60,000 years ago [35]. Subsequently, an increase of the use of traditional medicines occurred in many parts of the world, especially in developing countries. Medicinal plants are used in many countries as a primary medical treatment due to accessibility and low cost.

Moreover, in many developed countries, the use of medicinal plants as alternative treatment to drugs is becoming more and more common. The National Cancer Institute collected about 35,000 plants samples from 20 different countries. The percentage of the population that has used medicinal plants at least once comprises 48% in Australia, 70% in Canada, 42% in the United States (US), 38% in Belgium and 75% in France (World Health Organization, 2003).

Most of plant extracts contain phenolic and flavonoid components with antioxidant activity and, thus, prevent oxidative stress and cancer. The use of plants in medicine includes crude preparations or extracts, to refined extracts and individual bioactive compounds. Some isolated compounds are used as such (digoxin, digitoxin, morphine, reserpine, taxol, vinblastine and vincristine), other substances derived from plants can be used for the design, semi-synthesis and synthesis of new substances of higher activity and/or less toxicity, such as metformin, nabilone, oxycodone (and other narcotic analgesics), taxotere, teniposide, verapamil and amiodarone [35].

The research on antitumor agents extracted from plants began in 1957 by the US National Cancer Institute (NCI) with the discovery of vinca alkaloids (vinblastine and vincristine) from *Catharanthus roseus* [36], which was used for the treatment of diabetes. These anticancer agents introduced a new era of the medicinal plants as medical treatment. They are used in combination with other drugs to treat different types of cancer, such as leukemia, lymphoma, breast and lung cancer. As a result, from 1960 to 1982, the NCI studied about 114,000 extracts from about 35,000 samples of plants for anti-tumor purposes [37]. Subsequently, in 1987 the studies were performed *in vitro* on human tumor cell lines. Until the end of 1991, 28,800 plant samples were examined from over 20 countries to be screened for chemotherapy [38].

Also, the isolation of paclitaxel (Paxene®, Anzatax®, Taxol®) has been a pivotal discover in the field of natural product drug. Discovered in 1967 by Monroe Wall and Mansukh Wani, who isolated it from the Pacific-rate bark (*Taxus brevifolia*), it was commercially developed by Bristol-Myers Squibb, which changed its name to paclitaxel, marketing it as Taxol. In this formulation, the molecule is dissolved in Cremophor EL and ethanol. Paclitaxel mechanism of action is linked to the ability to interact with microtubules, altering the polymerization/depolymerization balance. This causes the formation of highly stable microtubular structures, with consequent inhibition of the mitosis of the cell (which requires the dissolution of the microtubules for the subsequent formation of the mitotic spindle).

Of particular interest is *Curcuma Longa*, an herbaceous plant belonging to the Zingiberaceae family, from whose rhizome is obtained turmeric, an ocher yellow crystalline powder. For the first time, curcumin was isolated and described by Vogel and Pelletier in 1842. Tumeric is an important part of the medicine and phytotherapy of many countries of Southeast Asia, it is commonly used to treat biliary disorders, jaundice, anorexia, cough, diabetic ulcers, liver disorders, rheumatism, inflammation, sinusitis, menstrual disorders, haematuria, and hemorrhage. Curcumin is also widely used in Ayurvedic medicine for the variety of its therapeutic effects including antioxidant, analgesic, anti-inflammatory, anti-inflammatory, antibacterial and antiviral. The main therapeutic effects of curcumin are mainly due to its direct antioxidant and anti-radical action; it is also able to modulate transcription and activity of numerous molecules (enzymes, second messengers, transcription factors), involved in different cell signal transmission pathways, which are altered in some pathological conditions [39].

Recent studies show that there is an inverse relationship between food intake rich in antioxidants and the incidence of human pathologies [40]. Furthermore, it has been demonstrated that synthetic antioxidants, such as butylated hydroxytoluene (BHT) and butylated hydroxyanisole (BHA), used as additive in food industry, may cause liver damage and carcinogenesis [41]. For this reason, there is a marked propensity towards the use of natural compounds. The use of natural antioxidants in the food, cosmetic and therapeutic fields would be a valid alternative to low-cost synthetic antioxidants, because of their high compatibility with food intake and without harmful effects for the human body.

5. *AZADIRACHTA INDICA* AND *CARICA PAPAYA* EXTRACTS AS MODERN TOOL FOR CANCER TREATMENT WITH ANCIENT ROOTS

Medicinal plants are used in several countries for the treatment of many diseases and for centuries they have been the primary form of medicines. Actually, more than 50% of the worldwide population utilizes plants for their healthcare and more than 70% of the current drugs derives from plants. An imbalance in ROS generation inside the cells causes damage leading to the development of cancer, atherosclerosis, diabetes, neurodegenerative disorders and aging. Also, for these diseases plant derived antioxidants by scavenging free radicals and modulating oxidative stress are indicated as a very *panacea*. Several experimental and clinical studies have proved that antioxidant rich diet is associated with decreased risk of cardiovascular diseases and cancer. In particular, plants could be used in the treatment of cancer: the National Cancer Institute collected about 35,000 plant samples from 20 different countries, and has screened around 114,000 extracts for anticancer activity. Several *in vitro* or *in vivo* studies have proved the anticancer potential of various medicinal plants extracts, mainly due to phenolic and flavonoid compounds, which have antioxidant activities [42]. For example, aqueous extract from willow (*Salix sp.*) prevents proliferation of human acute myeloid leukemia cells [43]; *Ganoderma lucidum* methanolic and Bu-Zhong-Yi-Qi-Tang (a mixture of ten herbs) aqueous extracts induce apoptosis in human breast cancer MCF-7 cells [44] and human hepatoma cell lines (Hep3B, HepG2 and HA22T) [45], respectively. Also, aqueous extract of *Paeoniae lactiflora* triggers apoptotic cell death in HepG2 and Hep3B hepatoma cells [46]. Yano *et al.* stated that aqueous extract of Sho-Saiko-To causes apoptosis and G0/G1 arrest of KIM-1 human hepatoma cells [47]. The seeds extract of *Luffa aegyptiaca* destroys the human metastatic melanoma [48]. Finally, PE-SPES (mixture of eight herbs) has cytotoxic activity against LNCaP prostate carcinoma cells by modulating expression of cell cycle genes [49]. It is important to highlight that the data concord in suggesting herbal medicines advantageous over single purified chemicals [50] as they are the mixtures of more components, and so might have more activity than single products alone.

Among the plants reported in traditional medicine as a very *panacea* in active compounds, *Azadirachta indica (A. indica)* and *Carica papaya (C. papaya)* extracts are scientifically validated in the treatment of several diseases, including cancer.

5.1. *A. indica* for Cancer Prevention and Treatment

A. indica, also known as Neem, is a fast-growing, resistant to drought and high temperature tree typical of semi-tropical and tropical countries. United Nations has declared Neem as the "Tree of the 21st century", "Village pharmacy" and "A tree for solving global problems" as it is able to cure multiple human diseases and illnesses [51 - 53]. The components of Neem extracted from all major parts of the tree including leaves, flowers, fruits, and seeds, possess antifungal, anthelmintic, antibacterial, anti-diabetic, contraceptive, sedative and anticancer effects [54]. To date, over 300 phytochemicals have been isolated from Neem. On the basis of the presence or absence of isoprene units, they can be grouped in two major classes: isoprenoids, including diterpenoids, triterpenoids, vilasinins and limonoids, and non-isoprenoids, including proteins, polysaccharides, sulphur compounds, polyphenolics, dihydrochalcone, coumarin, tannins, flavonoids and aliphatic compounds [52, 55]. Other phytochemicals derived from Neem are nimbolide, nimbin, azadirachtin, azadiradione and geduin. Neem extracts are prepared by using different solvents such as ether, petrol ether, ethyl acetate, and alcohol, and the type and the amount of molecules present in the extracts strictly depend on the procedure of extraction. Unfortunately, the literature data are obtained by using a mixture of neem components and the involvement of individual components and their respective functions are not well understood. Among bioactive components of neem, only nimbin (derived from the neem oil), nimbolide (derived from the leaves and flowers) and azadirachtin (derived from the seeds) have been extensively studied. Neem and its constituents modulate several cell signaling pathways regulating cancer, diabete, parkinson's disease, atherosclerosis, and hypertension.

Accumulating studies suggest the effects of Neem extracts on cancer. In particular, it has been demonstrated that the Neem components are effective against breast, gastrointestinal, gynecological, hematological, prostatic, skin and connective tissue cancers [56]. The effects depend on the expression of several targets (transcription factors, enzymes, growth factors, cytokines, kinases, receptors and proteins involved in cell survival, apoptosis and metastasis) that cause inhibition of survival, proliferation, invasion, angiogenesis and metastasis of cancer cells [57]. A wide number of hallmarks characterizes cancer cells: excessive and uncontrolled cell growth, resistance to cell death and suppression of immune response against tumor cells. In addition, tumor cells modulate surrounding microenvironment to induce angiogenesis, ability to invade and metastatize to distant size and to boorst inflammation. Therefore, tumor microenvironment plays a pivotal role in the onset and progression of cancer [58]. More and more literature data suggest that Neem extracts show selective cytotoxicity towards cancer cells compared to normal cells by inducing proliferation inhibition, cell death induction and reduction of cellular oxidative stress. Moreover, neem components attenuate angiogenesis and inhibit inflammation by modulating tumor microenvironment.

Neem extracts and their phytochemicals modulate various cancer related pathways both *in vitro* (as reported in Table **2**) and *in vivo* (as reported in Table **3**).

Table 2. Effects *in vitro* of different neem components/extracts on cancer related pathways.

Cancer Related Pathways	Neem Components/Extract	Cell Line	Targets	Effects	References
Cell proliferation	Azadirachtin	HeLa	Cyclin B Cyclin D1 p21, p53 PCNA	G0/G1 cell cycle arrest	[59]
	Leaves and seeds aqueous extract	Ehrlich ascites	Unclear	Unclear	[60]
	Nimbolide	HeLa	Cyclin B Cyclin D1 p21, p53 PCNA	G0/G1 cell cycle arrest	[59]
	Ethanolic leaves extract	MCF-7, MDA-MB-231, HeLa, PC-3, LNCaP	Cyclin D1, p21	G0/G1 cell cycle arrest	[61, 62]
	Aqueous leaves extract	KB, K562	Cyclin D1	G0/G1 cell cycle arrest	[63]
	Ethyl acetate leaves extract	HT-29	Unclear	Unclear	[64]
	Nimbolide	WiDr, KBM-5, U937	Cyclin D1	G0/G1 cell cycle arrest	[65]
	Nimbolide	OVCAR-5, U937, HL-60, THP1, PC-3, B16, A-549	Unclear	Unclear	[66 - 70]
Cell death	Ethanolic leaves extract	MCF-7, MDA-MB-231, HeLa, PC-3, LNCaP	Bcl-2,Bax, Cyt c, Bcl-xL, caspase 3, Ras, Raf, p-Akt, p-Erk, CYP, 1A1, CYP 1A2	Apoptosis	[71 - 73]
	Nimbolide	MCF-7, MDA-MB-231, HepG2, KBM-5, U937, PC-3	Bax, Bad, Fas-L, TRAIL, FADDR, cyt c, Bcl-2, Bcl-xL, Mcl-1, XIAP-1, NF-kB, Smac, c-Myc, IAP-1, IAP-2	Apoptosis	[61, 74, 75]

(Table 2) cont.....

Cancer Related Pathways	Neem Components/Extract	Cell Line	Targets	Effects	References
Cell death	Limonoids, Nimbolide	SK-BR-3, HT-29, SW-620, A-549, B16	Unclear	Cytotoxicity	[67, 74, 76]
	Nimbinene	MCF-7, MDA-MB-231	ROS, pJNK, p38	Apoptosis	[77]
	Aqueous leaves extract	KB	Bcl-2, caspase-3	Apoptosis	[78]
	Ethanolic and aqueous leaves extract	HT-29, E6-1	ROS	Apoptosis	[76]
	Nimbolide	HCT116, HT-29, DU145	ROS, DR5, DR4, I-FLICE, cIAP-1, cIAP-2, Bcl-2, Bcl-xL, p53, Bax	Sensitization of cancer cells to TRAIL-induced apoptosis	[77, 78]
	Limonoids	HCT16, HT29, LNCaP, PPC1	Caspases, AIF, ROS LC3-II	Apoptosis Autophagy	[79]
	Azadirachtin, Nimbolide	HeLa	P53, p21, Bax, Bcl-2, ROS	Apoptosis	[80]
	Liminoids	HL-60	Caspase-3, caspase-8, caspase-9	Apoptosis	[81]
	Nimonol	HL-60	Bax, Bcl-2	Apoptosis	[74]
	Supercritical extract of leaves	LNCaO-luc-2, PC-3	Calreticulin, FAK	Apoptosis	[82]
	Leaves glicoprotein	B16	Perforin, granzyme B	Cytotoxicity	[83]
Microenvironment tumor modulation	Leaf glycoprotein	KB, COLO25	CD83, CD80, CD86, CD40, MHCs, IL-10, IL-12, CD28, IL-4, IFN-γ Perforin, granzyme B, CTLA4, CTLA4, HLA-ABC	Optimized anti-tumor T cell functions Created anti-tumor immune environment	[84, 85]

(Table 2) cont.....

Cancer Related Pathways	Neem Components/Extract	Cell Line	Targets	Effects	References
Microenvironment tumor modulation	Nimbolide	WiDr, DU145	MMP-2, MMP-9, VEGF-A, NF-kB ROS	Retardet cell migration Suppressed invasion and migration	[78]
	Leaf glycoprotein	DCs	2,3-dioxygenase, IDO, CTLA4, CD40, CD83, CD80, CD86, MHC II, IL-10, IL-2	Reduced tolerogenecity of DCs	[86]

Table 3. Effects of neem components/extracts on cancer animal models.

Neem Components/extract	Animal Model	Targets	Effects	References
Freeze-dried flowers	DMBA-induced mammary gland carcinogenesis in female Sprague Dawley rats	Unclear	Reduced tumor incidence and multiplicity	[87]
	AFB1-induced hepatocarcinogenesis in male Wistar rats	GGT	Reduced incidence of tumor	[88]
Ethyl acetate and methanolic leaf fraction	DMBA-induced mammary gland carcinogenesis in female Sprague Dawley rats	PCNA, Bcl-2, caspase-3, estradiol, GSH, SOD, CAT, NF-kB	Suppressed tumor incidence	[88]
Ethanolic leaves extract	NMU-induced mammary carcinogenesis in female Sprague Dawley rats	P53, Bax, Bad, Bcl-2, caspases, cyclin D1, MAPK1, Cdk2, Cdk4	Reduced tumor burden and suppressed tumor progression	[89]
	4T1 xenograft in female Balb/c mice	c-Myc	Suppressed tumor progression	[90]
	DMBA-induced buccal pouch carcinogenesis in maleSyrian hamsters	Bim, Bcl-2, caspase-8, caspase-3, PCNA, p53, cytocheratin	Reduced tumor burden and progression	[91]
	MNNG-induced gastric carcinogenesis in male Wistar rats	GSH, GST, lipid peroxidation	Reduced incidence of tumor	[92]

(Table 3) cont.....

Neem Components/extract	Animal Model	Targets	Effects	References
Ethanolic leaves extract	B(a)P-induced forestomach tumorigenesis in Swiss albino mice	GST, SOD, CAT, GSH	Inhibited tumnor burden and reduced tumor incidence	[93]
	C4-2B and PC-3M-luc2 xenografts in nu/nu mice	Apoptosis pathways	Suppressed tumor growth	[94]
	DMBA-induced skin papillomagenesis in Swiss albino mice	GST, GPX, SOD, CAT, GSH	Inhibited tumnor burden and reduced tumor incidence	[93]
Aqueous leaves extract	Erlich carcinoma in female Swiss mice	Unclear	Immunomodulation	[95]
		CD4, CD8	Restricted growth of carcinoma	[95]
		Splenic neutrophil production Leukopenia Neutropenia	Inhibited tumor growth	[96]
		Leukocyte apoptosis T cells, NK cells	Restricted tumor growth	[97]
	Swiss mice, Balb/c mice, Spregue Dawley rats exposed to BTAA	Th1, IFN-γ, IL10	Enhanced immune responses to tumor vaccines	[98]
	DBMA-induced buccal pouch carcinogenesis of male Syrian hamsters	Lipid peroxidation, GSH, GST	Reduced incidence and volume of oral tumors	[98]
	MNNG-induced gastric carcinogenesis in male Wistar rats	GSH, GST, GPX, vitamin C	Suppressed cancer development	[99]
	B(a)P-induced forestomach tumorigenesis in Swiss albino mice	Unclear	Decreased tumor burden and multiplicity	[100]
	DEN/2-AAF-mediated hepatocarcinogenesis in male Sprague Dawley rats	AFP, GST, GPx	Repaired carcinogenic damage	[101]
		AFP, apoptosis	Reduced incidence of neoplasma	[102]
	DMH-induced colon carcinogenesis in male Wistar rats	TSA	Suppressed tumor incidence	[103]
	HT-29xenografts in CD-1 nu/nu mice	Unclear	Inhibited tumor growth	[76]

(Table 3) cont.....

Neem Components/extract	Animal Model	Targets	Effects	References
Aqueous leaves extract	DMBA/TPA-induced skin carcinogenesis in male LACA mice	Bax, Bcl-2, caspase-3, caspase-9	Reduced tumor burden and tumor volume	[105]
		Lipid peroxidation, PCNA, mdm2, p53, p21	Anti-neoplastic activity and regulated cell cycle	[106]
	B16 melanoma tumor in C57BL/6 mice	Immunomodulation	Exerted tumor growth retardation	[95]
Leaf glycoprotein	Erlich carcinoma growth in female Swiss mice	Unclear	Reduced tumor volume	[104]
		CD31, VEGF, VEGFR2	Restricted tumor growth Normalized tumor angiogenesis	[107]
	CT-26 colon carcinoma in athymic nude mice	Immunomodulation	Restricted tumor growth	[108]
	Sarcoma 180 in female Swiss mice	GATA3, IFN-γ	Restricted sarcoma growth	[109]
		IL-2, IL-12, IL-6, IL-10, TGF-β, IFN-γ		[110]
		Perforin, granzyme, IFN-γ, antigen specific T-cell proliferation	Reduced tumor volume	[111]
Leaf fractions	DBMA-induced buccal pouch carcinogenesis of male Syrian hamsters	PCNA, Bcl-2, caspase-3, PARP, VEGF	Suppressed pre-neoplastic lesions	[112]
		PCNA, Bax, Bcl-2, NK-kB, p50, CYP1A1, CYP1B1	Reduced of pre-neoplastic lesions and squamous cell carcinoma	[113]
Azadirachtin and nimbolide	DBMA-induced buccal pouch carcinogenesis of male Syrian hamsters	GST, SOD, GSH, GPX, MMP-2, MMP-9, HIF-1α, VEGF	Reduced incidence of pre-neoplastic and neoplastic lesions	[114]
		Cyclin D1, PCNA, NFkB, IkB, p53, Bcl-2/Bax, Apaf-1, caspase-3, cyt c	Reduced tumor incidence and burden	[115]
Geduin	DBMA-induced buccal pouch carcinogenesis of male Syrian hamsters	PI3K/Akt, NF-kB, miR-21, VEGF, HIF-1α	Prevented progression of tumor	[116]

(Table 3) cont.....

Neem Components/extract	Animal Model	Targets	Effects	References
Nimbolide	HCT1 16 xenografts in athymic nu/nu mice	Bcl-2, Bcl-xL, survivin, Mcl-1, cyclin D1, MMP-9, c-Myc, ICAM-1, VEGF, CXCR4	Inhibited tumor growth	[117]
	TRAMP	Apoptosis, Ki-67, p-STAT	Inhibited tumor growth and metastasis	[78]
Azadirachtin	TPA-promoted skin carcinogenesis in mice	Unclear	Reduced incidence and multiplicity of papillomas	[69]
Supercritical leaf extract	LNCa-luc2 xenografts in nu/nu mice	PSA, AKR1C2	Retarded tumor growth	[82]

5.1.1. Role of ROS in A. indica Treatment

The metabolism of carcinogens and the homeostasis of redox (reduction/oxidation) status are controlled by drug metabolizing enzymes. ROS, produced mainly *via* mitochondrial respiratory chain reactions, are important modulators of cell proliferation and survival. Deregulation of metabolism and mitochondrial function cause the damage of proteins, lipids and DNA by increasing ROS production. This is associated with aging and chronic disease like cancer [118 - 120]. It is noteworthy that neem is able to prevent oxidative stress-induced in several *in vitro* models, such as human choriocarcinoma (BeWo) and cervical (HeLa) cancer cells [59, 121].

In our laboratory a hydro-alcoholic extract of leaves of *A. indica* has been prepared and the effects of this extract on ROS production and oxidative status including the cytotoxicity, has been evaluated by using hepatocarcinoma HepG2 cells.

This extract has been previously tested on diabetic streptozotocin (STZ)-induced Wistar rats (8 weeks old, 150 g) since hyperglycemia is associated with oxidative stress; and the latter one is involved in the etiology of diabetes complications in organs. Diabetic rats showed superficial erosion of ileal mucosa and necrosis of goblet cells, both absent in hyperglycemic rats treated with neem leaves extract [122]. The hepatic microscopic anatomy was ameliorated by treatment with neem extract, and concomitantly the levels of lipid hydroperoxides, aqueous hydroperoxide (hydrogen peroxide), glutathione (GSH), and superoxide dismutase (SOD) in homogenates of the diabetic liver decrease respect to healthy liver [123]. Moreover, the extract ameliorates the damage of Langerhans islets lesions, possibly by enhancing b-cell proliferation, and decreases the amount of oxidative enzymes, such as lipid hydroperoxides, hydrogen peroxide, GSH and SOD in homogenates of the diabetic pancreas [124].

Extraction of A. indica leaves. Fresh leaves of *A. indica* from Nigeria were air-dried and extracted by percolation as described in Chattopadhyay, 1999 [125]. The ethanolic solution of the extract was concentrated under vacuum in a Buchi Rotavapor R-114 (Buchi, Switzerland) at 50°C (bath temperature). The residue was dissolved in bidistilled water and filtered with Whatman paper and then concentrated in the rotavapor at 50°C (bath temperature). The final residue was a dark-brown sticky mass stored at 4°C.

Cell culture. HepG2 cells were cultured in 25 cm^2 flasks (Iwaki, Tokyo, Japan) at the cell density of 5×10^5 cells/ml, in Dulbecco's Modified Eagle Medium (DMEM) medium (Cambrex BioScience,Verviers, Belgium), supplemented with 10% (v/v) inactivated fetal calf serum (Cambrex BioScience), 2 mM L-glutamine (Cambrex BioScience), 100 IU/ml penicillin and streptomycin in a humidified atmosphere of 5% CO^2 at 37 °C.

The cells were treated as follow.

Normal Condition Oxidative Stress Condition

Untreated cells Untreated cells

A. indica 0.005 mg/ml H_2O_2 1 mM 1h +1h recovery

A. indica 0.01 mg/ml vitamin C

A. indica 0.05 mg/ml H_2O_2+vitamic C

A. indica 0.1 mg/ml H_2O_2 + *A. indica* 0.05 mg/ml

A. indica 0.5 mg/ml H_2O_2+ *A. indica* 0.1 mg/ml

A. indica 1 mg/ml H_2O_2 + *A. indica* 0.5 mg/ml

Cell Viability and Morphology. Cell viability was determined by 3-(4,5-dimethylthiazol-2-yl)-2,5-diphenyltetrazolium bromide (MTT) dye mitochondria reduction in living HepG2 cells. Briefly, 5×10^5 cells were incubated with MTT solution (1mg/mL) for 2 h at 37°C and 5% CO_2. MTT formazan crystals were solubilized with DiMethyl SulfOxide (DMSO) (Carlo Erba, Milano, Italy) whose optical density (OD) was read at the spectrophotometer (Ultrospec 4000 UV/Visible Spectrophotometer, Pharmacia Biotech, Stockholm, Sweden) at 570 nm.

Morphological changes of living cells were investigated with an inverted light microscope (LM) Eclipse TS100 (Nikon, Kawasaki, Kanagawa Prefecture, Japan).

NBT Assay. The NBT assay indirectly measures the ROS generation in the cytoplasm of cells. In fact, the oxidase system available in the cytoplasm helps to transfer electrons from NADPH to NBT and reduces NBT into formazan crystals [31]. Briefly, 5×10^5 cells were incubated 2h with NBT solution (335 µg/ml) at 37° C and 5% CO_2 to permit the formation of formazan crystals that are dissolved with freshly prepared 2M KOH (Azienda Chimica E Farmaceutica, Piacenza, Italy)/DMSO solution (460 µl KOH and 540 µl DMSO). The optical density of the solution was measured with a spectrophotometer at 630 nm.

HepG2 cells were treated with different concentrations (0.005, 0.01, 0.05, 0.1, 0.5 and 1 mg/ml) of *A. indica* leaves extract for different periods of time (30 min, 2, 6, 24, 48 and 72h), and the cytotoxicity was evaluated by MTT test. Only the highest concentrations of extract (0.5 and 1 mg/ml) were able to modify the MTT absorbance values with respect to control at 48 and 72h of treatment. The cell viability decreases of about 21% and 40% after 48h and 25% and 43% after 72h of treatment. Concomitantly, cell morphology changes and the cells display necrotic features, such as vacuolization of cytoplasm (Fig. **3**).

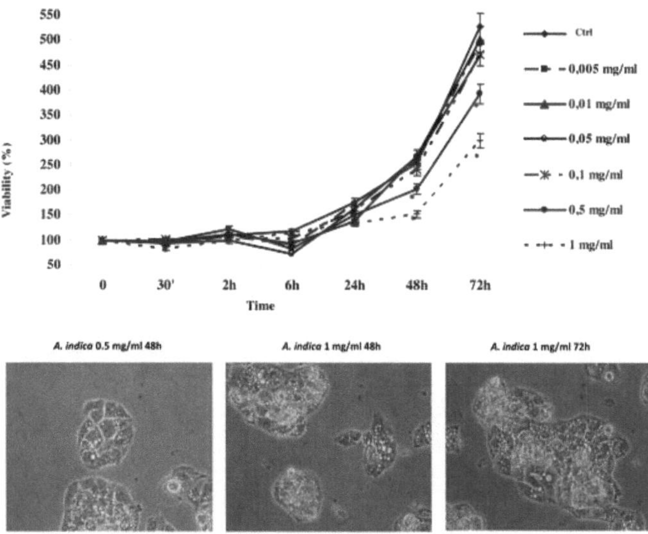

Fig. (3). MTT test of HepG2 cells treated with different concentrations of *A. indica* leaves extract. Micrographs of HepG2 cells were also reported.

To evaluate the effect of Neem on oxidative stress, the generation of ROS after the incubation of HepG2 with leaves extract has been evaluated. Hydrogen peroxide (H_2O_2) was used as inducer of oxidative stress and vitamin C as control of antioxidant activity. The treatment with H_2O_2 significantly reduces cell viability (of about 95%). Only incubation with vitamin C ensures an increment of viability percentage of about 20% and 12% at 4 and 24h respectively. Conversely, any amount of Neem counteracts the cytotoxic effect of H_2O_2 (Fig. **4**).

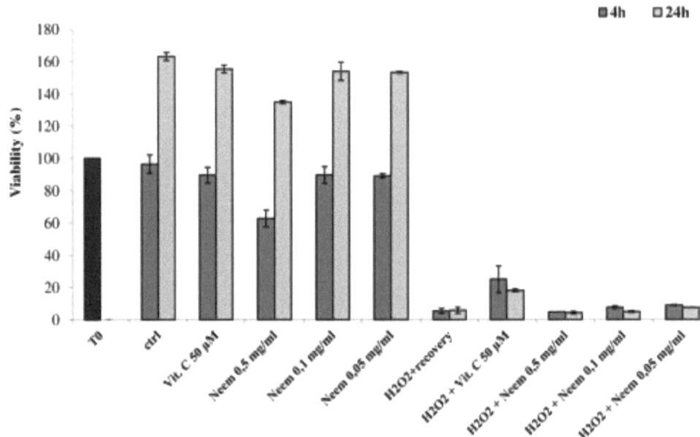

Fig. (4). MTT assay of HepG2 cells treated with different concentrations of *A. indica* leaves extract.

The levels of produced ROS were evaluated by NBT assay. 0.5 mg/ml leaves neem extract induces a significant increment of ROS generation. Moreover, the presence of leaves neem extract during the treatment with H_2O_2 increases the ROS production of about 100% respect to H_2O_2 alone (Fig. **5**).

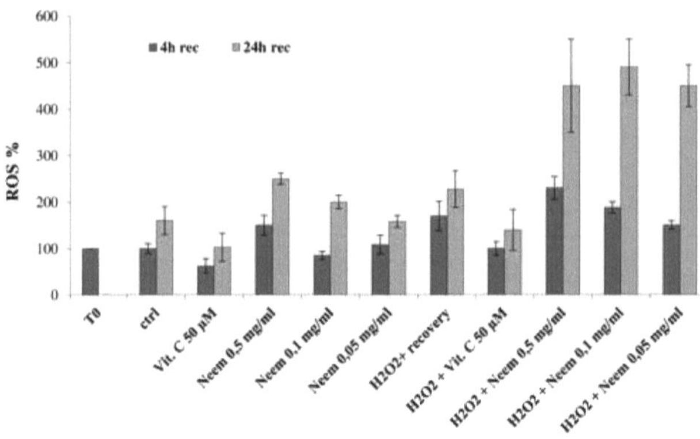

Fig. (5). ROS production evaluated by NBT assay of HepG2 cells treated with different concentrations of *A. indica* leaves extract.

5.2. *C papaya* for Cancer Prevention and Treatment

C. papaya is a tropical fruit tree known with different names depending on regions [126 - 128] and widely cultivated in about 60 countries with over 11.2 million tonnes of fruit produced. It is a fast growing, soft-wooded, herbaceous plant that reaches from 3 to 10 metres in height. Papaya fruit is rich in essential for wellbeing vitamins, including β-carotene, vitamins A, C, B6, E, K, riboflavin, thiamine, folate, niacin, *etc.*, and minerals, including calcium, iron, magnesium, potassium, zinc, and phosphorus (US Department of Agriculture, 2012). All parts of *C. papaya* contain a broad spectrum of phytochemicals: in fruits are present flavonoids, including quercetin, kaempferol, and myricetin, and carotenoids, including β-carotene, lycopene, cryptoxanthin, violaxanthin, and zeaxanthin [129]; milky latex from unripe fruits and other plant parts contain enzymes, such as papain, chymopapain, protease omega, glycyl-endopeptidase and caricain [130 - 133]; leaves are rich in phenolic compounds, such as protocatechuic acid, p-coumaric acid, caffeic acid, chlorogenic acid, 5,7-dimethoxycoumarin, kaempferol, and quercetin, and alkaloids, such as carpaine, pseudocarpaine and dehydrocarpaine I and II [134, 135]; pericarp contains Benzyl glucosinolate (BG) and its enzymatic hydrolysed product, benzyl isothiocyanate [136, 137]; and in seeds are present benzyl glucosinolate and benzyl isothiocyanate, proteins, lipids and crude fibre [138]. Among the molecules present in *C. papaya*, papain displays many important pharmaceutical and industrial applications [139]. It is used in food biotechnology to produce chewing gums and dehydrated pulses and beans, for chill-proofing beer and for tenderising meat, and in the textile industry for degumming silk and softening wool. Moreover, papain is also employed as a component of soap, shampoo, toothpaste and skincare products [140]. In pharmaceutical field, it is approved for topical preparations for necrotic tissue in burns, ulcers and other wounds [141], and in the preparation of vaccines and drugs for various digestive ailments.

In traditional medicine, leaves, bark, roots, latex, fruit, flowers and seeds of *C. papaya* have a wide range of applications. They are used in the treatment of ulcer [142], malaria, hypertension, diabetes mellitus, jaundice and intestinal helminthias treatment [14]; moreover, C. papaya possess a contraceptive action. Further, the leaves have been used to treat asthma, colic, fever, and beriberi (thiamine deficiency) [143, 144], malaria and dengue fever [144 - 146], and cancer [147 - 149]. The milky juice (latex) is employed as a styptic and debridement when applied externally to burns and scalds [14], and to treat eczema and psoriasis [150]. The seeds have been used as a vermifuge, thirst quencher and pain alleviator.

Several scientific studies validate the traditional uses of *C. papaya*. For example, the aqueous extract of *C. papaya* fruit shown the wound-healing activity [151]. Also, *C. papaya* seeds extract administered orally induces a reversible contraceptive effect in male rats, rabbits and langur monkeys [152 - 154], by degeneration of the germinal epithelium and germ cells, and reduction in the number of Leydig cells with the presence of vacuoles in the tubules [155], or by changes in the plasma membrane of the head and mid-piece of human spermatozoa, leading to a total inhibition of *in vitro* motility [156]. Any significant effect on female fertilization has been demonstrated, but the unripe or semi-ripe papaya produces uterine contraction [157] by causing abortifacient effect in female Sprague Dawley rats [158].

100 years ago a book entitled "The Most Wonderful Tree in the World-The Papaw Tree (Carica Papaya)" contained evidences about the cure of breast, liver or rectal cancer upon 'treatment' with *C. papaya* preparations [148]. The number of *in vitro* studies about the effect of *C. papaya* extracts on cancer cells are limited and are reported in Table **4**.

Table 4. Effects *in vitro* of *C. papaya* components/extracts on cancer cell lines.

Carica Papaya components/Extract	Cell Line	Effects	References
Fruit juice	HepG2	Inhibition of viability	[165]
Leaves aqueous extract	H9, Molt, CCRF-CEM, HPB-ALL, Raji, K562, HeLa, PC14, Panc-1, H2452, H226, ARH77, MCF-7, JMN, AGS, T98G, Capan-1, DLD-1, Karpas	Inhibition of proliferation	[147, 166]
Pulp aqueous extract	MCF-7	Inhibition of proliferation	[167]
Pulp ethanolic extract	MCF-7	Inhibition of viability Antioxidant	[168]
Seeds n-hexane extract	HL-60	Antioxidant Inhibition of viability	[168]
Pulp n-hexane extract	HL-60	Antioxidant Inhibition of viability	[168]

Despite these limited data, several studies have claimed the antioxidant properties of papaya extract, but there is still a continuous debate regarding whether high antioxidant activity is a good indicator of high anticancer activity, and no conclusive proof has been attained or presented thus far. Among phytochemicals present in *C. papaya* extracts, three groups of bioactive compounds have attracted considerable interest in anticancer studies: phenolics, carotenoids and gluco-sinolates. These bioactive compounds act *via* multiple mechanisms, such as cancer cell signalling, proliferation, apoptosis, migration and invasion, as well as angiogenesis [169].

5.2.1. Role of ROS in C. papaya Treatment

The studies of the antioxidant nutrients in *C. papaya* have led to the identification of the main compounds related to the different parts. Whole fruit extract contains ferulic, coumaric, and caffeic acid, carotenoids, and vitamin C that collectively protect human cells from oxidative stresses and promote wound healing and skin repair; leaves extract contains folic acid, vitamins B12, A, and C, alkaloids, saponins, glycosides, tannins, and flavonoids with anticancer activity and protection against the alcohol induced oxidative damage to the gastric mucosa; seeds extract contains different phenolic compounds, vanillic acid, and vitamin C with antioxidant and anticancer activities. Thus, *C. papaya* extracts could act as a therapeutic dietary supplement in patients with oxidative stress related diseases or could be added to formulations to promote wound healing. Several studies report the antioxidant effects of extracts of different parts of *C. papaya*.

In our laboratory an aqueous extract of seeds of *C. papaya* has been prepared and the effects of this extract on ROS production and oxidative status, including the cytotoxicity, have been evaluated by using leukemia HL60 cells. The seeds are the less exploited part of *C. papaya* and the aqueous extract has been already tested on human skin Detroit 550 fibroblasts. We have demonstrated that the seeds water extract is potentially useful for protection against oxidative stress. In particular, *C. papaya* seeds water extract is not toxic and acts as a potent free radical scavenger, providing protection to Detroit 550 fibroblasts that underwent H_2O_2 oxidative stress. The maximum protective effect is achieved during the simultaneous administration of the extract with H_2O_2; the extract is more efficient than vitamin C to hamper the oxidative damage; finally, the purified subfractions of the seeds water extract exert the same antioxidant effect of whole extract [170].

C. papaya seeds water extract preparation and fractionation. Seeds were removed from a mature *C. papaya* fruit, washed with water and let to dry. 10 grams of seeds were taken and grinded by pestle and mortar and then soaked in 100 ml of sterile distilled water for 24 h at room temperature (20-25°C). After 24 h the mixture was filtered through a very small pores sieve to eliminate the large particles, then refiltered by using buchner filtration (under vacuum). This solution was sterilized by using millipore filter 0.22 µm, and stored in the freezer at -20°C ready to used. The final concentration of the extract was 100 mg/ mL.

Cell culture and treatment. HL60 cells were cultured in 75cm^2 flasks containing RPMI 1640 supplemented with 10% fetal bovine serum, L-Glutamine (2mM), Penicillin-streptomycin (100 IU/mL), and nystatin (10.000 IU/mL of medium or

0.05 mg/mL of medium). The flasks were incubated at 37 °C in a humidified atmosphere of 5% CO_2.

HL60 cells were treated with different concentrations (weight/volume) of *C. papaya* seeds extract (0.5 mg/mL, 1 mg/mL, 2 mg/mL and 3 mg/mL), for different times (1h, 2h, 4h, 8h, 18h, 24h and 48h) in the presence or absence of oxidative stress.

The general scheme of experiments was as follow:

Normal Condition Oxidative Stress Condition

Untreated cells Untreated cells

C. papaya 0.5 mg/ml H_2O_2 1 mM 1h +1h recovery

C. papaya 1 mg/m H_2O_2+*C. papaya* 0.5 mg/ml

C. papaya 2 mg/ml H_2O_2+*C. papaya* 1 mg/ml

C. papaya 3 mg/ml H_2O_2+ *C. papaya* 2 mg/ml

H_2O_2+*C. papaya* 3 mg/ml

Different concentrations of vitamin C as control of the experiments have been considered both in normal and oxidative stress conditions.

HL60 cells were treated with different concentrations (0.5, 1, 2, 3 mg/mL) of *C. papaya* seeds extract for different periods of time (8, 18, 24 and 48h), and the cytotoxicity was evaluated by MTT test. Only the highest concentration of extract (3 mg/mL) was able to modify the MTT absorbance values with respect to control for all time of treatment; this may be due to the presence of some components in the extracts, that are no toxic to cells at low concentration, but became toxic when concentration increases. The absorbance value significantly increased with the concentration of 1 mg/ml; the maximum value has been measured at 4 h of incubation and then decreased with increasing incubation times (Fig. **6**).

HL-60 cells, treated with different concentrations of *C. papaya* seeds extract, were stained with hematoxylin eosin. About 500 cells in about 10-15 randomly selected fields were counted and the percentages of normal, apoptotic, necrotic and mitotic cells were calculated. The aqueous seeds extract of *C. papaya* decreased the percentage of apoptotic cells. No differences in the percentage of necrotic as well as mitotic cells for all concentrations and all treatment times were observed, thus suggesting that *C. papaya* seeds extract has no effect on both processes (Fig. **7**).

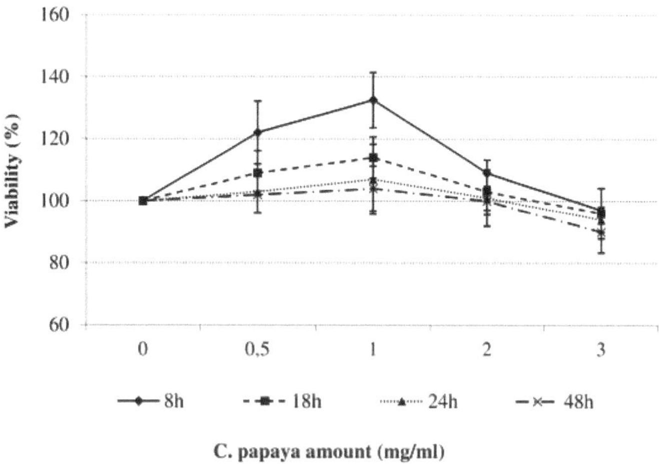

Fig. (6). MTT test of HL60 cells treated with different concentrations of *C. papaya* seeds extract for 8, 18, 24 and 48 h.

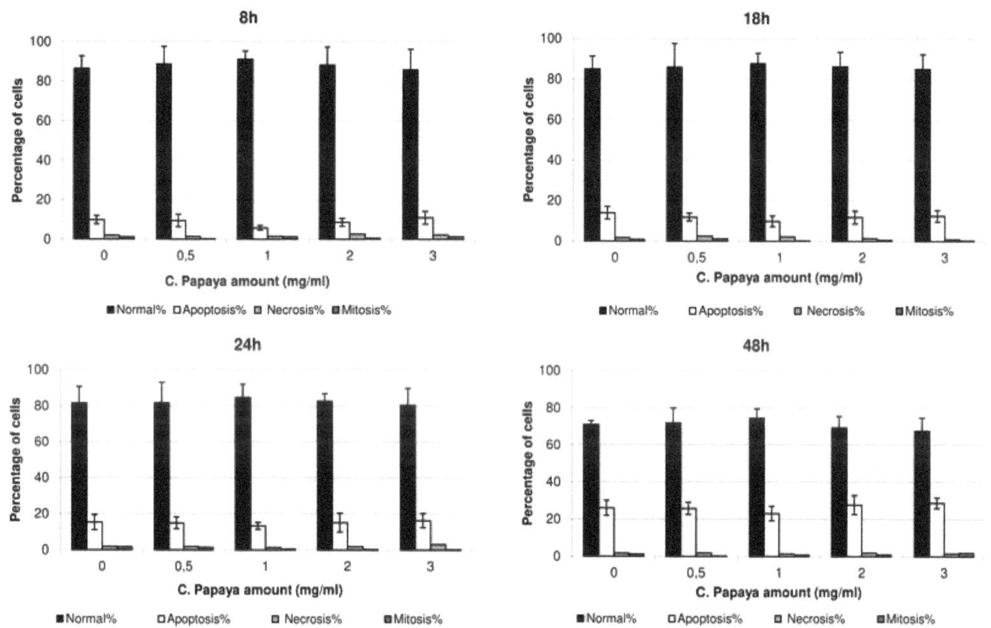

Fig. (7). Percentage of normal, apoptotic, necrotic and mitotic HL60 cells after treatment with different concentrations of *C. papaya* seeds extract for 8h, 18h, 24h and 48h.

The effects of *C. papaya* seeds extract on oxidative stress were studied by using H_2O_2. Our results showed that *C. papaya* seeds extract increased the mitochondrial activity of HL-60 cells treated with hydrogen peroxide. To evaluate if the extract has its major activity when administered during the oxidative stress or during recovery times from oxidative stress, we performed MTT assay by adding *C. papaya* extract concomitantly to treatment with H_2O_2 or during 1h recovery time post H_2O_2 treatment. Cell viability ameliorates when the extract is added simultaneously to oxidative stress. In particular, cell viability increases of about 15% respect to treatment with only H_2O_2 (Fig. **8A**). Moreover, the percentage of apoptotic cells decreased of about 15% respect cells treated with H_2O_2 only. The best activities were achieved with the concentration of 1 mg/ml of extract (Fig. **8B**).

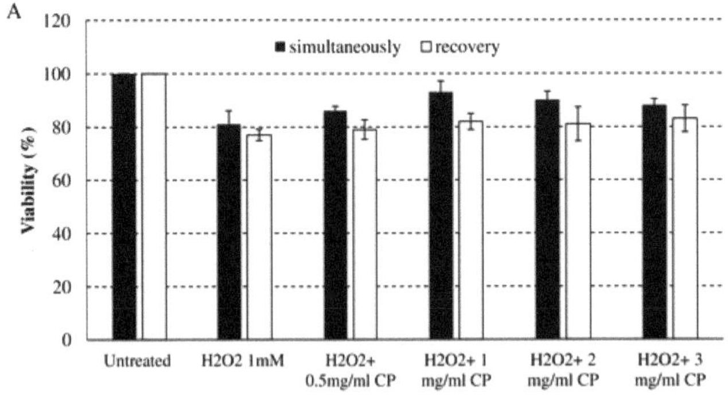

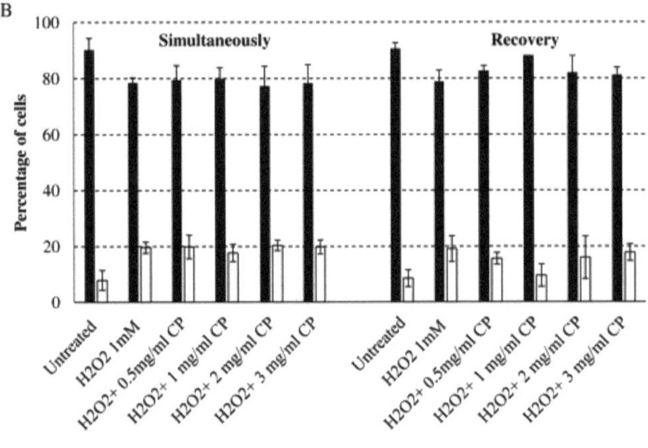

Fig. (8). A: MTT test of HL60 cells incubated with 1mM H_2O_2 for 1 h and different concentrations (0.5, 1, 2, 3 mg/ml) of *C. papaya* (CP) seeds extract added during oxidative stress (simultaneously) or added in recovery after hydrogen peroxide treatment (recovery). B: Percentage of normal and apoptotic HL60 cells after treatment with 1mM H_2O_2 for 1 h and different concentrations (0.5, 1, 2, 3 mg/ml) of *C. papaya* seeds extract added during oxidative stress (simultaneously) or added in recovery after hydrogen peroxide treatment (recovery).

CONCLUSION

Plants extracts and plant derived substances, and their potential usefulness in patients under anticancer therapies are now attracting great attention. However, in Europe and North America the use of herbal medicines still arouses skepticism in standard care of cancer patients. The use of herbal extracts in cancer field is hindered by several drawbacks, such as the lack of data regarding the standard protocols of cultivation of the plants and the standardization of methods of extraction and characterization of active metabolites; the knowledge of tolerable high dosage, minimal effective dosage and specific usage; the lack of preclinical data about the efficacy in cancer conditions. Further, the major drawback in considering herbal extracts as tool in cancer management is the lack of defined intracellular targets upon administration to patients. In fact, both Food and Drug Administration (FDA) and National Institutes of Health (NIH) indicate that the knowledge of the precise target of drugs is fundamental in pharmacology. Unfortunately, herbal extracts prepared on the basis of traditional medicine are a mixture of chemicals with a wide spectrum of action as each of one possess a specific molecular target. This not well defined chemical composition is directly linked to not well understand safety of the extracts, that, in addition, could harmfully interact with other drugs used by cancer patients [171].

Herbal extracts have shown promising effects when oxidative status is considered since many evidences highlight the controversial role of ROS in cancer progression and regression. Thus, the role of plants extracts in ROS generation or scavenging inside cancer cells is a very fascinating feature in phytotherapy. Antioxidant function in biological systems is much more complicated than a simple free radical scavenging process. An antioxidant may affect biological system by suppressing the formation of ROS and reactive nitrogen species (RNS); affecting enzyme activities; inducing *de novo* biosynthesis of defence enzymes and thereby affecting other endogenous antioxidants; preserving NO activity, or sequestering transition metal ions. It is obvious that some compounds use more than one mechanism for their antioxidants effect on biological systems.

Among the plants reported in traditional medicine as a very *panacea* in active compounds, *C. papaya* and *A. indica* (also known as Neem) extracts show their significant impact on oxidative status of cancer cells. Our evidences suggest that *C. papaya* seeds aqueous extract may be a promising source of antioxidants, which may have therapeutic implications. Conversely, alcoholic leaves neem extract possesses pro-oxidant activity that can represent a modality to induce cells death in cancer cells. In conclusions, both *A. indica* and *C. papaya* extracts can potentially be exploited in cancer treatment protocols as death inducers or as adjuvants of conventional molecules.

CONSENT FOR PUBLICATION

Not applicable.

CONFLICT OF INTEREST

The author(s) confirm that this chapter content has no conflict of interest.

ACKNOWLEDGMENT

Declared none.

REFERENCES

[1]   Bayir, H. Reactive oxygen species. *Crit. Care Med.,* **2005,** *33*(12) Suppl., S498-S501.
[http://dx.doi.org/10.1097/01.CCM.0000186787.64500.12] [PMID: 16340433]

[2]   Valko, M.; Morris, H.; Cronin, M.T.D. Metals, toxicity and oxidative stress. *Curr. Med. Chem.,* **2005,**
12(10), 1161-1208.
[http://dx.doi.org/10.2174/0929867053764635] [PMID: 15892631]

[3]   Imlay, J.A. Pathways of oxidative damage. *Annu. Rev. Microbiol.,* **2003,** *57,* 395-418.
[http://dx.doi.org/10.1146/annurev.micro.57.030502.090938] [PMID: 14527285]

[4]   McCord, J.M.; Crapo, J.D.; Fridovich, I. Superoxide dismutase assay. A review of
methodology.*Superoxide and Superoxide Dismutase*; Michelson, A.M.; McCord, J.M.; Fridovich, I.,
Eds.; Academic press: London, UK, **1977,** pp. 11-17.

[5]   Rahman, K. Studies on free radicals, antioxidants, and co-factors. *Clin. Interv. Aging,* **2007,** *2*(2), 219-
236.
[PMID: 18044138]

[6]   Copin, J.C.; Gasche, Y.; Chan, P.H. Overexpression of copper/zinc superoxide dismutase does not
prevent neonatal lethality in mutant mice that lack manganese superoxide dismutase. *Free Radic. Biol.
Med.,* **2000,** *28*(10), 1571-1576.
[http://dx.doi.org/10.1016/S0891-5849(00)00280-X] [PMID: 10927183]

[7]   Brigelius-Flohé, R. Tissue-specific functions of individual glutathione peroxidases. *Free Radic. Biol.
Med.,* **1999,** *27*(9-10), 951-965.
[http://dx.doi.org/10.1016/S0891-5849(99)00173-2] [PMID: 10569628]

[8]   Valko, M.; Rhodes, C.J.; Moncol, J.; Izakovic, M.; Mazur, M. Free radicals, metals and antioxidants in
oxidative stress-induced cancer. *Chem. Biol. Interact.,* **2006,** *160*(1), 1-40.
[http://dx.doi.org/10.1016/j.cbi.2005.12.009] [PMID: 16430879]

[9]   Sabharwal, S.S.; Schumacker, P.T. Mitochondrial ROS in cancer: initiators, amplifiers or an Achilles'
heel? *Nat. Rev. Cancer,* **2014,** *14*(11), 709-721.
[http://dx.doi.org/10.1038/nrc3803] [PMID: 25342630]

[10]   Hancock, J.T.; Desikan, R.; Neill, S.J. Role of reactive oxygen species in cell signalling pathways.
Biochem. Soc. Trans., **2001,** *29*(Pt 2), 345-350.
[http://dx.doi.org/10.1042/bst0290345] [PMID: 11356180]

[11]   Tafani, M.; Sansone, L.; Limana, F.; Arcangeli, T.; De Santis, E.; Polese, M.; Fini, M.; Russo, M.A.
The interplay of reactive oxygen species, hypoxia, inflammation, and sirtuins in cancer initiation and
progression. *Oxid. Med. Cell. Longev.,* **2016,** *2016,* 3907147.
[http://dx.doi.org/10.1155/2016/3907147] [PMID: 26798421]

[12]   Halliwell, B.; Aruoma, O.I. DNA damage by oxygen-derived species. Its mechanism and measurement

in mammalian systems. *FEBS Lett.,* **1991**, *281*(1-2), 9-19.
[http://dx.doi.org/10.1016/0014-5793(91)80347-6] [PMID: 1849843]

[13]   Marnett, L.J. Oxyradicals and DNA damage. *Carcinogenesis,* **2000**, *21*(3), 361-370.
[http://dx.doi.org/10.1093/carcin/21.3.361] [PMID: 10688856]

[14]   Lim, S.O.; Gu, J.M.; Kim, M.S.; Kim, H.S.; Park, Y.N.; Park, C.K.; Cho, J.W.; Park, Y.M.; Jung, G. Epigenetic changes induced by reactive oxygen species in hepatocellular carcinoma: methylation of the E-cadherin promoter. *Gastroenterology,* **2008**, *135*(6), 2128-2140, 2140.e1-2140.e8.
[http://dx.doi.org/10.1053/j.gastro.2008.07.027] [PMID: 18801366]

[15]   Fan, T.P.; Yeh, J.C.; Leung, K.W.; Yue, P.Y.; Wong, R.N. Angiogenesis: from plants to blood vessels. *Trends Pharmacol. Sci.,* **2006**, *27*(6), 297-309.
[http://dx.doi.org/10.1016/j.tips.2006.04.006] [PMID: 16697473]

[16]   Ruef, J.; Hu, Z.Y.; Yin, L.Y.; Wu, Y.; Hanson, S.R.; Kelly, A.B.; Harker, L.A.; Rao, G.N.; Runge, M.S.; Patterson, C. Induction of vascular endothelial growth factor in balloon-injured baboon arteries. A novel role for reactive oxygen species in atherosclerosis. *Circ. Res.,* **1997**, *81*(1), 24-33.
[http://dx.doi.org/10.1161/01.RES.81.1.24] [PMID: 9201024]

[17]   Li, J.; Wang, J.J.; Yu, Q.; Chen, K.; Mahadev, K.; Zhang, S.X. Inhibition of reactive oxygen species by Lovastatin downregulates vascular endothelial growth factor expression and ameliorates blood-retinal barrier breakdown in db/db mice: role of NADPH oxidase 4. *Diabetes,* **2010**, *59*(6), 1528-1538.
[http://dx.doi.org/10.2337/db09-1057] [PMID: 20332345]

[18]   Ushio-Fukai, M.; Alexander, R.W. Reactive oxygen species as mediators of angiogenesis signaling: role of NAD(P)H oxidase. *Mol. Cell. Biochem.,* **2004**, *264*(1-2), 85-97.
[http://dx.doi.org/10.1023/B:MCBI.0000044378.09409.b5] [PMID: 15544038]

[19]   Schreml, S.; Szeimies, R.M.; Prantl, L.; Karrer, S.; Landthaler, M.; Babilas, P. Oxygen in acute and chronic wound healing. *Br. J. Dermatol.,* **2010**, *163*(2), 257-268.
[http://dx.doi.org/10.1111/j.1365-2133.2010.09804.x] [PMID: 20394633]

[20]   West, X.Z.; Malinin, N.L.; Merkulova, A.A.; Tischenko, M.; Kerr, B.A.; Borden, E.C.; Podrez, E.A.; Salomon, R.G.; Byzova, T.V. Oxidative stress induces angiogenesis by activating TLR2 with novel endogenous ligands. *Nature,* **2010**, *467*(7318), 972-976.
[http://dx.doi.org/10.1038/nature09421] [PMID: 20927103]

[21]   Vanharanta, S.; Massagué, J. Origins of metastatic traits. *Cancer Cell,* **2013**, *24*(4), 410-421.
[http://dx.doi.org/10.1016/j.ccr.2013.09.007] [PMID: 24135279]

[22]   Hempel, N.; Bartling, T.R.; Mian, B.; Melendez, J.A. Acquisition of the metastatic phenotype is accompanied by H2O2-dependent activation of the p130Cas signaling complex. *Mol. Cancer Res.,* **2013**, *11*(3), 303-312.
[http://dx.doi.org/10.1158/1541-7786.MCR-12-0478] [PMID: 23345605]

[23]   Hempel, N.; Ye, H.; Abessi, B.; Mian, B.; Melendez, J.A. Altered redox status accompanies progression to metastatic human bladder cancer. *Free Radic. Biol. Med.,* **2009**, *46*(1), 42-50.
[http://dx.doi.org/10.1016/j.freeradbiomed.2008.09.020] [PMID: 18930813]

[24]   Ranganathan, A.C.; Nelson, K.K.; Rodriguez, A.M.; Kim, K.H.; Tower, G.B.; Rutter, J.L.; Brinckerhoff, C.E.; Huang, T.T.; Epstein, C.J.; Jeffrey, J.J.; Melendez, J.A. Manganese superoxide dismutase signals matrix metalloproteinase expression via H2O2-dependent ERK1/2 activation. *J. Biol. Chem.,* **2001**, *276*(17), 14264-14270.
[http://dx.doi.org/10.1074/jbc.M100199200] [PMID: 11297530]

[25]   Luanpitpong, S.; Talbott, S.J.; Rojanasakul, Y.; Nimmannit, U.; Pongrakhananon, V.; Wang, L.; Chanvorachote, P. Regulation of lung cancer cell migration and invasion by reactive oxygen species and caveolin-1. *J. Biol. Chem.,* **2010**, *285*(50), 38832-38840.
[http://dx.doi.org/10.1074/jbc.M110.124958] [PMID: 20923773]

[26]   Chan, D.W.; Liu, V.W.; Tsao, G.S.; Yao, K.M.; Furukawa, T.; Chan, K.K.; Ngan, H.Y. Loss of MKP3

mediated by oxidative stress enhances tumorigenicity and chemoresistance of ovarian cancer cells. *Carcinogenesis,* **2008**, *29*(9), 1742-1750.
[http://dx.doi.org/10.1093/carcin/bgn167] [PMID: 18632752]

[27]   Verheij, M.; Bose, R.; Lin, X.H.; Yao, B.; Jarvis, W.D.; Grant, S.; Birrer, M.J.; Szabo, E.; Zon, L.I.; Kyriakis, J.M.; Haimovitz-Friedman, A.; Fuks, Z.; Kolesnick, R.N. Requirement for ceramide-initiated SAPK/JNK signalling in stress-induced apoptosis. *Nature,* **1996**, *380*(6569), 75-79.
[http://dx.doi.org/10.1038/380075a0] [PMID: 8598911]

[28]   Moll, U.M.; Wolff, S.; Speidel, D.; Deppert, W. Transcription-independent pro-apoptotic functions of p53. *Curr. Opin. Cell Biol.,* **2005**, *17*(6), 631-636.
[http://dx.doi.org/10.1016/j.ceb.2005.09.007] [PMID: 16226451]

[29]   Johnstone, R.W.; Ruefli, A.A.; Lowe, S.W. Apoptosis: a link between cancer genetics and chemotherapy. *Cell,* **2002**, *108*(2), 153-164.
[http://dx.doi.org/10.1016/S0092-8674(02)00625-6] [PMID: 11832206]

[30]   Storz, P. Reactive oxygen species in tumor progression. *Front. Biosci.,* **2005**, *10*, 1881-1896.
[http://dx.doi.org/10.2741/1667] [PMID: 15769673]

[31]   Debnath, J. The multifaceted roles of autophagy in tumors-implications for breast cancer. *J. Mammary Gland Biol. Neoplasia,* **2011**, *16*(3), 173-187.
[http://dx.doi.org/10.1007/s10911-011-9223-3] [PMID: 21779879]

[32]   Scherz-Shouval, R.; Shvets, E.; Fass, E.; Shorer, H.; Gil, L.; Elazar, Z. Reactive oxygen species are essential for autophagy and specifically regulate the activity of Atg4. *EMBO J.,* **2007**, *26*(7), 1749-1760.
[http://dx.doi.org/10.1038/sj.emboj.7601623] [PMID: 17347651]

[33]   Inoki, K.; Zhu, T.; Guan, K.L. TSC2 mediates cellular energy response to control cell growth and survival. *Cell,* **2003**, *115*(5), 577-590.
[http://dx.doi.org/10.1016/S0092-8674(03)00929-2] [PMID: 14651849]

[34]   Kim, J.; Kundu, M.; Viollet, B.; Guan, K.L. AMPK and mTOR regulate autophagy through direct phosphorylation of Ulk1. *Nat. Cell Biol.,* **2011**, *13*(2), 132-141.
[http://dx.doi.org/10.1038/ncb2152] [PMID: 21258367]

[35]   Fabricant, D.S.; Farnsworth, N.R. The value of plants used in traditional medicine for drug discovery. *Environ. Health Perspect.,* **2001**, *109* Suppl. 1, 69-75.
[PMID: 11250806]

[36]   Johnson, I.S.; Armstrong, J.G.; Gorman, M.; Burnett, J.P., Jr The vinca alkaloids: a new class of oncolytic agents. *Cancer Res.,* **1963**, *23*, 1390-1427.
[PMID: 14070392]

[37]   Balunas, M.J.; Kinghorn, A.D. Drug discovery from medicinal plants. *Life Sci.,* **2005**, *78*(5), 431-441.
[http://dx.doi.org/10.1016/j.lfs.2005.09.012] [PMID: 16198377]

[38]   Cragg, G.M.; Boyd, M.R.; Cardellina, J.H., II; Newman, D.J.; Snader, K.M.; McCloud, T.G. Role of plants in the National Cancer Institute drug discovery and development programme.*Human Medicinal Agents from Plants. American Chemical Society*; Kinghorn, A.D.; Balandrin, M.F., Eds.; ACS, **1993**, pp. 80-95.
[http://dx.doi.org/10.1021/bk-1993-0534.ch007]

[39]   Ghosh, S.; Banerjee, S.; Sil, P.C. The beneficial role of curcumin on inflammation, diabetes and neurodegenerative disease: A recent update. *Food Chem. Toxicol.,* **2015**, *83*, 111-124.
[http://dx.doi.org/10.1016/j.fct.2015.05.022] [PMID: 26066364]

[40]   Sies, H. Strategies of antioxidant defense. *Exp. Physiol.,* **1997**, *82*, 291-295.
[http://dx.doi.org/10.1113/expphysiol.1997.sp004024] [PMID: 9129943]

[41]   Papas, A.M. Diet and antioxidant status. *Food Chem. Toxicol.,* **1999**, *37*(9-10), 999-1007.
[http://dx.doi.org/10.1016/S0278-6915(99)00088-5] [PMID: 10541457]

[42]   Ahmed, M.; Khan, M.I.; Khan, M.R.; Muhammad, N.; Khan, R.A. Role of Medicinal Plants in Oxidative Stress and Cancer. *Sci. Rep.,* **2013**, *2*, 641.

[43]   El-Shemy, H.A.; Aboul-Enein, A.M.; Aboul-Enein, M.I.; Issa, S.I.; Fujita, K. The effect of willow leaf extracts on human leukemic cells in vitro. *J. Biochem. Mol. Biol.,* **2003**, *36*(4), 387-389.
[PMID: 12895297]

[44]   Hu, H.; Ahn, N.S.; Yang, X.; Lee, Y.S.; Kang, K.S. *Ganoderma lucidum* extract induces cell cycle arrest and apoptosis in MCF-7 human breast cancer cell. *Int. J. Cancer,* **2002**, *102*(3), 250-253.
[http://dx.doi.org/10.1002/ijc.10707] [PMID: 12397644]

[45]   Kao, S.T.; Yeh, C.C.; Hsieh, C.C.; Yang, M.D.; Lee, M.R.; Liu, H.S.; Lin, J.G. The Chinese medicine Bu-Zhong-Yi-Qi-Tang inhibited proliferation of hepatoma cell lines by inducing apoptosis via G0/G1 arrest. *Life Sci.,* **2001**, *69*(13), 1485-1496.
[http://dx.doi.org/10.1016/S0024-3205(01)01226-7] [PMID: 11554610]

[46]   Meyers, K.J.; Watkins, C.B.; Pritts, M.P.; Liu, R.H. Antioxidant and antiproliferative activities of strawberries. *J. Agric. Food Chem.,* **2003**, *51*(23), 6887-6892.
[http://dx.doi.org/10.1021/jf034506n] [PMID: 14582991]

[47]   Yano, H.; Mizoguchi, A.; Fukuda, K.; Haramaki, M.; Ogasawara, S.; Momosaki, S.; Kojiro, M. The herbal medicine sho-saiko-to inhibits proliferation of cancer cell lines by inducing apoptosis and arrest at the G0/G1 phase. *Cancer Res.,* **1994**, *54*(2), 448-454.
[PMID: 8275481]

[48]   Poma, A.; Miranda, M.; Spanò, L. Differential response of human melanoma and Ehrlich ascites cells in vitro to the ribosome-inactivating protein luffin. *Melanoma Res.,* **1998**, *8*(5), 465-467.
[http://dx.doi.org/10.1097/00008390-199810000-00012] [PMID: 9835461]

[49]   Bonham, M.; Arnold, H.; Montgomery, B.; Nelson, P.S. Molecular effects of the herbal compound PC-SPES: identification of activity pathways in prostate carcinoma. *Cancer Res.,* **2002**, *62*(14), 3920-3924.
[PMID: 12124319]

[50]   Vickers, A. Botanical medicines for the treatment of cancer: rationale, overview of current data, and methodological considerations for phase I and II trials. *Cancer Invest.,* **2002**, *20*(7-8), 1069-1079.
[http://dx.doi.org/10.1081/CNV-120005926] [PMID: 12449740]

[51]   Kumar, V.S.; Navaratnam, V. Neem (Azadirachta indica): prehistory to contemporary medicinal uses to humankind. *Asian Pac. J. Trop. Biomed.,* **2013**, *3*(7), 505-514.
[http://dx.doi.org/10.1016/S2221-1691(13)60105-7] [PMID: 23835719]

[52]   Biswas, K.; Chattopadhyay, I.; Banerjee, R.K.; Bandyopadhyay, U. Biological activities and medicinal properties of Neem (*Azadirachta indica*). *Curr. Sci.,* **2002**, *82*(11), 1136-1345.

[53]   Drabu, S.; Khatri, S.; Babu, S. Neem: healer of all ailments. *Res. J. Pharm. Biol. Chem. Sci.,* **2012**, *3*(1), 120-126.

[54]   Tiwari, R.; Verma, A.K.; Chakraborty, S.; Dhama, K.; Singh, S.V. Neem (Azadirachta indica) and its Potential for Safeguarding Health of Animals and Humans: A Review. *J. Biol. Sci.,* **2014**, *14*, 110-123.
[http://dx.doi.org/10.3923/jbs.2014.110.123]

[55]   Brahmachari, G. Neem--an omnipotent plant: a retrospection. *ChemBioChem,* **2004**, *5*(4), 408-421.
[http://dx.doi.org/10.1002/cbic.200300749] [PMID: 15185362]

[56]   Patel, S.M.; Nagulapalli Venkata, K.C.; Bhattacharyya, P.; Sethi, G.; Bishayee, A. Potential of neem (*Azadirachta indica L.*) for prevention and treatment of oncologic diseases. *Semin. Cancer Biol.,* **2016**, *40-41*, 100-115.
[http://dx.doi.org/10.1016/j.semcancer.2016.03.002] [PMID: 27019417]

[57]   Hao, F.; Kumar, S.; Yadav, N.; Chandra, D. Neem components as potential agents for cancer prevention and treatment. *Biochim. Biophys. Acta,* **2014**, *1846*(1), 247-257.

[PMID: 25016141]

[58]   Hanahan, D.; Weinberg, R.A. Hallmarks of cancer: the next generation. *Cell,* **2011**, *144*(5), 646-674.
[http://dx.doi.org/10.1016/j.cell.2011.02.013] [PMID: 21376230]

[59]   Priyadarsini, R.V.; Murugan, R.S.; Sripriya, P.; Karunagaran, D.; Nagini, S. The neem limonoids azadirachtin and nimbolide induce cell cycle arrest and mitochondria-mediated apoptosis in human cervical cancer (HeLa) cells. *Free Radic. Res.,* **2010**, *44*(6), 624-634.
[http://dx.doi.org/10.3109/10715761003692503] [PMID: 20429769]

[60]   Amer, H.; Helmy, W.A.; Tale, H.A.A. *In vitro* antitumor and antiviral activities of seeds and leaves of neem (*Azadirachta indica*) extracts. *Int. J. Acad. Res.,* **2010**, *2*, 47-52.

[61]   Elumalai, P.; Gunadharini, D.N.; Senthilkumar, K.; Banudevi, S.; Arunkumar, R.; Benson, C.S.; Sharmila, G.; Arunakaran, J. Induction of apoptosis in human breast cancer cells by nimbolide through extrinsic and intrinsic pathway. *Toxicol. Lett.,* **2012**, *215*(2), 131-142.
[http://dx.doi.org/10.1016/j.toxlet.2012.10.008] [PMID: 23089555]

[62]   Sharma, C.; Vas, A.J.; Goala, P.; Gheewala, T.M.; Rizvi, T.A.; Hussain, A. Ethanolic neem (*Azadirachta indica*) leaf extract prevents growth of MCF-7 and HeLa cells and potentiates the therapeutic index of cisplatin. *J. Oncol.,* **2014**, *2014*, 321754.
[http://dx.doi.org/10.1155/2014/321754] [PMID: 24624140]

[63]   Bose, A.; Haque, E.; Baral, R. Neem leaf preparation induces apoptosis of tumor cells by releasing cytotoxic cytokines from human peripheral blood mononuclear cells. *Phytother. Res.,* **2007**, *21*(10), 914-920.
[http://dx.doi.org/10.1002/ptr.2185] [PMID: 17562567]

[64]   Jafari, S.; Saeidnia, S.; Hajimehdipoor, H.; Ardekani, M.R.S.; Faramarzi, M.A.; Hadjiakhoondi, A.; Khanavi, M. Cytotoxic evaluation of Melia azedarach in comparison with, *Azadirachta indica* and its phytochemical investigation. *Daru,* **2013**, *21*(1), 37.
[http://dx.doi.org/10.1186/2008-2231-21-37] [PMID: 23679992]

[65]   Babykutty, S.; S, P.P.; J, N.R.; Kumar, M.A.S.; Nair, M.S.; Srinivas, P.; Gopala, S. Nimbolide retards tumor cell migration, invasion, and angiogenesis by downregulating MMP-2/9 expression via inhibiting ERK1/2 and reducing DNA-binding activity of NF-κB in colon cancer cells. *Mol. Carcinog.,* **2012**, *51*(6), 475-490.
[http://dx.doi.org/10.1002/mc.20812] [PMID: 21678498]

[66]   Sastry, B.S.; Suresh Babu, K.; Hari Babu, T.; Chandrasekhar, S.; Srinivas, P.V.; Saxena, A.K.; Madhusudana Rao, J. Synthesis and biological activity of amide derivatives of nimbolide. *Bioorg. Med. Chem. Lett.,* **2006**, *16*(16), 4391-4394.
[http://dx.doi.org/10.1016/j.bmcl.2006.05.105] [PMID: 16793266]

[67]   Roy, M.K.; Kobori, M.; Takenaka, M.; Nakahara, K.; Shinmoto, H.; Isobe, S.; Tsushida, T. Antiproliferative effect on human cancer cell lines after treatment with nimbolide extracted from an edible part of the neem tree (Azadirachta indica). *Phytother. Res.,* **2007**, *21*(3), 245-250.
[http://dx.doi.org/10.1002/ptr.2058] [PMID: 17163581]

[68]   Raja Singh, P.; Arunkumar, R.; Sivakamasundari, V.; Sharmila, G.; Elumalai, P.; Suganthapriya, E.; Brindha Mercy, A.; Senthilkumar, K.; Arunakaran, J. Anti-proliferative and apoptosis inducing effect of nimbolide by altering molecules involved in apoptosis and IGF signalling via PI3K/Akt in prostate cancer (PC-3) cell line. *Cell Biochem. Funct.,* **2014**, *32*(3), 217-228.
[http://dx.doi.org/10.1002/cbf.2993] [PMID: 23963693]

[69]   Akihisa, T.; Noto, T.; Takahashi, A.; Fujita, Y.; Banno, N.; Tokuda, H.; Koike, K.; Suzuki, T.; Yasukawa, K.; Kimura, Y. Melanogenesis inhibitory, anti-inflammatory, and chemopreventive effects of limonoids from the seeds of Azadirachta indicia A. Juss. (neem). *J. Oleo Sci.,* **2009**, *58*(11), 581-594.
[http://dx.doi.org/10.5650/jos.58.581] [PMID: 19844073]

[70]   Akihisa, T.; Takahashi, A.; Kikuchi, T.; Takagi, M.; Watanabe, K.; Fukatsu, M.; Fujita, Y.; Banno, N.;

Tokuda, H.; Yasukawa, K. The melanogenesis-inhibitory, anti-inflammatory, and chemopreventive effects of limonoids in n-hexane extract of Azadirachta indica A. Juss. (neem) seeds. *J. Oleo Sci.,* **2011**, *60*(2), 53-59.
[http://dx.doi.org/10.5650/jos.60.53] [PMID: 21263200]

[71]   Elumalai, P.; Gunadharini, D.N.; Senthilkumar, K.; Banudevi, S.; Arunakumar, R.; Benson, C.S.; Sharmila, G.; Arunakaran, J. Ethanolic neem (*Azadirachta indica* A. Juss) leaf extract induces apoptosis and inhibits the IGF signaling pathway in breast cancer cell lines. *Biomed. Prev. Nutr.,* **2012**, *2*, 59-68.
[http://dx.doi.org/10.1016/j.bionut.2011.12.008]

[72]   Gunadharini, D.N.; Elumalai, P.; Arunkumar, R.; Senthilkumar, K.; Arunakaran, J. Induction of apoptosis and inhibition of PI3K/Akt pathway in PC-3 and LNCaP prostate cancer cells by ethanolic neem leaf extract. *J. Ethnopharmacol.,* **2011**, *134*(3), 644-650.
[http://dx.doi.org/10.1016/j.jep.2011.01.015] [PMID: 21277364]

[73]   Kavitha, K.; Vidya Priyadarsini, R.; Anitha, P.; Ramalingam, K.; Sakthivel, R.; Purushothaman, G.; Singh, A.K.; Karunagaran, D.; Nagini, S. Nimbolide, a neem limonoid abrogates canonical NF-κB and Wnt signaling to induce caspase-dependent apoptosis in human hepatocarcinoma (HepG2) cells. *Eur. J. Pharmacol.,* **2012**, *681*(1-3), 6-14.
[http://dx.doi.org/10.1016/j.ejphar.2012.01.024] [PMID: 22327045]

[74]   Takagi, M.; Tachi, Y.; Zhang, J.; Shinozaki, T.; Ishii, K.; Kikuchi, T.; Ukiya, M.; Banno, N.; Tokuda, H.; Akihisa, T. Cytotoxic and melanogenesis-inhibitory activities of limonoids from the leaves of *Azadirachta indica* (Neem). *Chem. Biodivers.,* **2014**, *11*(3), 451-468.
[http://dx.doi.org/10.1002/cbdv.201300348] [PMID: 24634075]

[75]   Yadav, N.; Kumar, S.; Kumar, R.; Srivastava, P.; Sun, L.; Rapali, P.; Marlowe, T.; Schneider, A.; Inigo, J.R.; O'Malley, J.; Londonkar, R.; Gogada, R.; Chaudhary, A.K.; Yadava, N.; Chandra, D. Mechanism of neem limonoids-induced cell death in cancer: Role of oxidative phosphorylation. *Free Radic. Biol. Med.,* **2016**, *90*, 261-271.
[http://dx.doi.org/10.1016/j.freeradbiomed.2015.11.028] [PMID: 26627937]

[76]   Roma, A.; Ovadje, P.; Steckle, M.; Nicoletti, L.; Saleem, A.; Pandey, S. Selective induction of apoptosis by Azadirachta indica leaf extract by targeting oxidative vulnerabilities in human cancer cells. *J. Pharm. Pharm. Sci.,* **2015**, *18*(4), 729-746.
[http://dx.doi.org/10.18433/J3VG76] [PMID: 26626256]

[77]   Gupta, S.C.; Reuter, S.; Phromnoi, K.; Park, B.; Hema, P.S.; Nair, M.; Aggarwal, B.B. Nimbolide sensitizes human colon cancer cells to TRAIL through reactive oxygen species- and ERK-dependent up-regulation of death receptors, p53, and Bax. *J. Biol. Chem.,* **2011**, *286*(2), 1134-1146.
[http://dx.doi.org/10.1074/jbc.M110.191379] [PMID: 21078664]

[78]   Zhang, J.; Ahn, K.S.; Kim, C.; Shanmugam, M.K.; Siveen, K.S.; Arfuso, F.; Samym, R.P.; Deivasigamanim, A.; Lim, L.H.; Wang, L.; Goh, B.C.; Kumar, A.P.; Hui, K.M.; Sethi, G. Nimbolide-induced oxidative stress abrogates STAT3 signaling cascade and inhibits tumor growth in transgenic adenocarcinoma of mouse prostate model. *Antioxid. Redox Signal.,* **2016**, *24*(11), 575-589.
[http://dx.doi.org/10.1089/ars.2015.6418] [PMID: 26649526]

[79]   Sastry, B.S.; Suresh Babu, K.; Hari Babu, T.; Chandrasekhar, S.; Srinivas, P.V.; Saxena, A.K.; Madhusudana Rao, J. Synthesis and biological activity of amide derivatives of nimbolide. *Bioorg. Med. Chem. Lett.,* **2006**, *16*(16), 4391-4394.
[http://dx.doi.org/10.1016/j.bmcl.2006.05.105] [PMID: 16793266]

[80]   Priyadarsini, R.V.; Murugan, R.S.; Sripriya, P.; Karunagaran, D.; Nagini, S. The neem limonoids azadirachtin and nimbolide induce cell cycle arrest and mitochondria-mediated apoptosis in human cervical cancer (HeLa) cells. *Free Radic. Res.,* **2010**, *44*(6), 624-634.
[http://dx.doi.org/10.3109/10715761003692503] [PMID: 20429769]

[81]   Kikuchi, T.; Ishii, K.; Noto, T.; Takahashi, A.; Tabata, K.; Suzuki, T.; Akihisa, T. Cytotoxic and apoptosis-inducing activities of limonoids from the seeds of Azadirachta indica (neem). *J. Nat. Prod.,*

2011, *74*(4), 866-870.
[http://dx.doi.org/10.1021/np100783k] [PMID: 21381696]

[82]   Wu, Q.; Kohli, M.; Bergen, H.R., III; Cheville, J.C.; Karnes, R.J.; Cao, H.; Young, C.Y.; Tindall, D.J.; McNiven, M.A.; Donkena, K.V. Preclinical evaluation of the supercritical extract of azadirachta indica (neem) leaves in vitro and in vivo on inhibition of prostate cancer tumor growth. *Mol. Cancer Ther.,* **2014**, *13*(5), 1067-1077.
[http://dx.doi.org/10.1158/1535-7163.MCT-13-0699] [PMID: 24674886]

[83]   Barik, S.; Bhuniya, A.; Banerjee, S.; Das, A.; Sarkar, M.; Paul, T.; Ghosh, T.; Ghosh, S.; Roy, S.; Pal, S.; Bose, A.; Baral, R. Neem leaf glycoprotein is superior than cisplatin and sunitinib malate in restricting melanoma growth by normalization of tumor microenvironment. *Int. Immunopharmacol.,* **2013**, *17*(1), 42-49.
[http://dx.doi.org/10.1016/j.intimp.2013.05.005] [PMID: 23747315]

[84]   Goswami, S.; Bose, A.; Sarkar, K.; Roy, S.; Chakraborty, T.; Sanyal, U.; Baral, R. Neem leaf glycoprotein matures myeloid derived dendritic cells and optimizes anti-tumor T cell functions. *Vaccine,* **2010**, *28*(5), 1241-1252.
[http://dx.doi.org/10.1016/j.vaccine.2009.11.018] [PMID: 19969119]

[85]   Chakraborty, T.; Bose, A.; Goswami, K.K.; Goswami, S.; Chakraborty, K.; Baral, R. Neem leaf glycoprotein suppresses regulatory T cell mediated suppression of monocyte/macrophage functions. *Int. Immunopharmacol.,* **2012**, *12*(2), 326-333.
[http://dx.doi.org/10.1016/j.intimp.2011.12.002] [PMID: 22210373]

[86]   Roy, S.; Barik, S.; Banerjee, S.; Bhuniya, A.; Pal, S.; Basu, P.; Biswas, J.; Goswami, S.; Chakraborty, T.; Bose, A.; Baral, R. Neem leaf glycoprotein overcomes indoleamine 2,3 dioxygenase mediated tolerance in dendritic cells by attenuating hyperactive regulatory T cells in cervical cancer stage IIIB patients. *Hum. Immunol.,* **2013**, *74*(8), 1015-1023.
[http://dx.doi.org/10.1016/j.humimm.2013.04.022] [PMID: 23628394]

[87]   Tepsuwan, A.; Kupradinun, P.; Kusamran, W.R. Chemopreventive potential of neem flowers on carcinogen-induced rat mammary and liver carcinogensis. *Asian Pac. J. Cancer Prev.,* **2002**, *3*(3), 231-238.
[PMID: 12718580]

[88]   Vinothini, G.; Manikandan, P.; Anandan, R.; Nagini, S. Chemoprevention of rat mammary carcinogenesis by Azadirachta indica leaf fractions: modulation of hormone status, xenobiotic-metabolizing enzymes, oxidative stress, cell proliferation and apoptosis. *Food Chem. Toxicol.,* **2009**, *47*(8), 1852-1863.
[http://dx.doi.org/10.1016/j.fct.2009.04.045] [PMID: 19427891]

[89]   Arumugam, A.; Agullo, P.; Boopalan, T.; Nandy, S.; Lopez, R.; Gutierrez, C.; Narayan, M.; Rajkumar, L. Neem leaf extract inhibits mammary carcinogenesis by altering cell proliferation, apoptosis, and angiogenesis. *Cancer Biol. Ther.,* **2014**, *15*(1), 26-34.
[http://dx.doi.org/10.4161/cbt.26604] [PMID: 24146019]

[90]   Othman, F.; Motalleb, G.; Lam Tsuey Peng, S.; Rahmat, A.; Basri, R.; Pei Pei, C. C. Effect of neem leaf extract (*Azadirachta indica*) on c-myc oncogene expression in 4T1 breast cancer cells of Balb/c mice. *Cell J.,* **2012**, *14*(1), 53-60.
[PMID: 23626938]

[91]   Subapriya, R.; Bhuvaneswari, V.; Nagini, S. Ethanolic neem (Azadirachta indica) leaf extract induces apoptosis in the hamster buccal pouch carcinogenesis model by modulation of Bcl-2, Bim, caspase 8 and caspase 3. *Asian Pac. J. Cancer Prev.,* **2005**, *6*(4), 515-520.
[PMID: 16436003]

[92]   Subapriya, R.; Nagini, S. Ethanolic neem leaf extract protects against N-methyl -N'-nitr--N-nitrosoguanidine-induced gastric carcinogenesis in Wistar rats. *Asian Pac. J. Cancer Prev.,* **2003**, *4*(3), 215-223.
[PMID: 14507242]

[93]   Dasgupta, T.; Banerjee, S.; Yadava, P.K.; Rao, A.R. Chemopreventive potential of Azadirachta indica (Neem) leaf extract in murine carcinogenesis model systems. *J. Ethnopharmacol.,* **2004**, *92*(1), 23-36.
[http://dx.doi.org/10.1016/j.jep.2003.12.004] [PMID: 15099843]

[94]   Mahapatra, S.; Karnes, R.J.; Holmes, M.W.; Young, C.Y.F.; Cheville, J.C.; Kohli, M.; Klee, E.W.; Tindall, D.J.; Donkena, K.V. Novel molecular targets of *Azadirachta indica* associated with inhibition of tumor growth in prostate cancer. *AAPS J.,* **2011**, *13*(3), 365-377.
[http://dx.doi.org/10.1208/s12248-011-9279-4] [PMID: 21560017]

[95]   Haque, E.; Mandal, I.; Pal, S.; Baral, R. Prophylactic dose of neem (Azadirachta indica) leaf preparation restricting murine tumor growth is nontoxic, hematostimulatory and immunostimulatory. *Immunopharmacol. Immunotoxicol.,* **2006**, *28*(1), 33-50.
[http://dx.doi.org/10.1080/08923970600623632] [PMID: 16684666]

[96]   Ghosh, D.; Bose, A.; Haque, E.; Baral, R. Pretreatment with neem (*Azadirachta indica*) leaf preparation in Swiss mice diminishes leukopenia and enhances the antitumor activity of cyclophosphamide. *Phytother. Res.,* **2006**, *20*(9), 814-818.
[http://dx.doi.org/10.1002/ptr.1948] [PMID: 16807877]

[97]   Ghosh, D.; Bose, A.; Haque, E.; Baral, R. Neem (Azadirachta indica) leaf preparation prevents leukocyte apoptosis mediated by cisplatin plus 5-fluorouracil treatment in Swiss mice. *Chemotherapy,* **2009**, *55*(3), 137-144.
[http://dx.doi.org/10.1159/000211558] [PMID: 19346744]

[98]   Mandal-Ghosh, I.; Chattopadhyay, U.; Baral, R. Neem leaf preparation enhances Th1 type immune response and anti-tumor immunity against breast tumor associated antigen. *Cancer Immun.,* **2007**, *7*, 8.
[PMID: 17394284]

[99]   Arivazhagan, S.; Velmurugan, B.; Bhuvaneswari, V.; Nagini, S. Effects of aqueous extracts of garlic (Allium sativum) and neem (Azadirachta indica) leaf on hepatic and blood oxidant-antioxidant status during experimental gastric carcinogenesis. *J. Med. Food,* **2004**, *7*(3), 334-339.
[http://dx.doi.org/10.1089/jmf.2004.7.334] [PMID: 15383228]

[100]   Gangar, S.C.; Sandhir, R.; Rai, D.V.; Koul, A. Modulatory effects of *Azadirachta indica* on benzo(a)pyrene-induced forestomach tumorigenesis in mice. *World J. Gastroenterol.,* **2006**, *12*(17), 2749-2755.
[http://dx.doi.org/10.3748/wjg.v12.i17.2749] [PMID: 16718763]

[101]   Manal, M.E.T.; Hanachi, P.; Patimah, I.; Siddig, I.A.; Fauziah, O. The effect of neem (*Azadirachta indica*) leaves extract on alpha-fetoprotein serum concentration, glutathione S-transferase and glutathione peroxidase activity in hepatocarcinogenesis induced rats. *Int. J. Cancer Res.,* **2007**, *3*, 111-118.
[http://dx.doi.org/10.3923/ijcr.2007.111.118]

[102]   Taha, M.M.E.; Wahab, S.I.A.; Othman, F.; Hanachi, P.; Bustamam, A.; Al-Zubairi, A.S. *In vivo* anti-tumor effects of Azadirachta indica in rat liver cancer. *Res. J. Biol. Sci.,* **2009**, *4*, 48-53.

[103]   Ramzanighara, A.; Ezzatighadi, F.; Rai, D.V.; Dhawan, D.K. Effect of Neem (Azadirchta indica) on serum glycoprotein contents of rats administered 1,2 dimethylhydrazine. *Toxicol. Mech. Methods,* **2009**, *19*(4), 298-301.
[http://dx.doi.org/10.1080/15376510802646523] [PMID: 19778220]

[104]   Kundu, P.; Barik, S.; Sarkar, K.; Bose, A.; Baral, R.; Laskar, S. Chemical investigation of neem leaf glycoprotein used as immunoprophylatic agent for tumor growth restriction. *Int. J. Pharm. Pharm. Sci.,* **2015**, *7*, 195-199.

[105]   Arora, N.; Koul, A.; Bansal, M.P. Chemopreventive activity of Azadirachta indica on two-stage skin carcinogenesis in murine model. *Phytother. Res.,* **2011**, *25*(3), 408-416.
[PMID: 20734334]

[106]   Arora, N.; Bansal, M.P.; Koul, A. *Azadirachta indica* acts as a pro-oxidant and modulates cell cycle

associated proteins during DMBA/TPA induced skin carcinogenesis in mice. *Cell Biochem. Funct.,* **2013**, *31*(5), 385-394.
[http://dx.doi.org/10.1002/cbf.2909] [PMID: 23055378]

[107]	Banerjee, S.; Ghosh, T.; Barik, S.; Das, A.; Ghosh, S.; Bhuniya, A.; Bose, A.; Baral, R. Neem leaf glycoprotein prophylaxis transduces immune dependent stop signal for tumor angiogenic switch within tumor microenvironment. *PLoS One,* **2014**, *9*(11), e110040.
[http://dx.doi.org/10.1371/journal.pone.0110040] [PMID: 25391149]

[108]	Das, A.; Barik, S.; Bose, A.; Roy, S.; Biswas, J.; Baral, R.; Pal, S. Pal Murine carcinoma expressing carcinoembryonic antigen-like protein is restricted by antibody against neem leaf glycoprotein. *Immunol. Lett.,* **2014**, *162*(1 PtA), 132-139.

[109]	Mallick, A.; Barik, S.; Goswami, K.K.; Banerjee, S.; Ghosh, S.; Sarkar, K.; Bose, A.; Baral, R. Neem leaf glycoprotein activates CD8(+) T cells to promote therapeutic anti-tumor immunity inhibiting the growth of mouse sarcoma. *PLoS One,* **2013**, *8*(1), e47434.
[http://dx.doi.org/10.1371/journal.pone.0047434] [PMID: 23326300]

[110]	Barik, S.; Banerjee, S.; Mallick, A.; Goswami, K.K.; Roy, S.; Bose, A.; Baral, R. Normalization of tumor microenvironment by neem leaf glycoprotein potentiates effector T cell functions and therapeutically intervenes in the growth of mouse sarcoma. *PLoS One,* **2013**, *8*(6), e66501.
[http://dx.doi.org/10.1371/journal.pone.0066501] [PMID: 23785504]

[111]	Mallick, A.; Barik, S.; Ghosh, S.; Roy, S.; Sarkar, K.; Bose, A.; Baral, R. Immunotherapeutic targeting of established sarcoma in Swiss mice by tumor-derived antigen-pulsed NLGP matured dendritic cells is CD8+ T-cell dependent. *Immunotherapy,* **2014**, *6*(7), 821-831.
[http://dx.doi.org/10.2217/imt.14.53] [PMID: 25290415]

[112]	Manikandan, P.; Letchoumy, P.V.; Gopalakrishnan, M.; Nagini, S. Evaluation of Azadirachta indica leaf fractions for in vitro antioxidant potential and in vivo modulation of biomarkers of chemoprevention in the hamster buccal pouch carcinogenesis model. *Food Chem. Toxicol.,* **2008**, *46*(7), 2332-2343.
[http://dx.doi.org/10.1016/j.fct.2008.03.013] [PMID: 18442880]

[113]	Manikandan, P.; Ramalingam, S.M.; Vinothini, G.; Ramamurthi, V.P.; Singh, I.P.; Anandan, R.; Gopalakrishnan, M.; Nagini, S. Investigation of the chemopreventive potential of neem leaf subfractions in the hamster buccal pouch model and phytochemical characterization. *Eur. J. Med. Chem.,* **2012**, *56*, 271-281.
[http://dx.doi.org/10.1016/j.ejmech.2012.08.008] [PMID: 22939101]

[114]	Harish Kumar, G.; Vidya Priyadarsini, R.; Vinothini, G.; Vidjaya Letchoumy, P.; Nagini, S. The neem limonoids azadirachtin and nimbolide inhibit cell proliferation and induce apoptosis in an animal model of oral oncogenesis. *Invest. New Drugs,* **2010**, *28*(4), 392-401.
[http://dx.doi.org/10.1007/s10637-009-9263-3] [PMID: 19458912]

[115]	Kishore T, K.K.; Ganugula, R.; Gade, D.R.; Reddy, G.B.; Nagini, S. Gedunin abrogates aldose reductase, PI3K/Akt/mToR, and NF-κB signaling pathways to inhibit angiogenesis in a hamster model of oral carcinogenesis. *Tumour Biol.,* **2016**, *37*(2), 2083-2093.
[http://dx.doi.org/10.1007/s13277-015-4003-0] [PMID: 26342697]

[116]	Gupta, S.C.; Prasad, S.; Sethumadhavan, D.R.; Nair, M.S.; Mo, Y.Y.; Aggarwal, B.B. Nimbolide, a limonoid triterpene, inhibits growth of human colorectal cancer xenografts by suppressing the proinflammatory microenvironment. *Clin. Cancer Res.,* **2013**, *19*(16), 4465-4476.
[http://dx.doi.org/10.1158/1078-0432.CCR-13-0080] [PMID: 23766363]

[117]	Sena, L.A.; Chandel, N.S. Physiological roles of mitochondrial reactive oxygen species. *Mol. Cell,* **2012**, *48*(2), 158-167.
[http://dx.doi.org/10.1016/j.molcel.2012.09.025] [PMID: 23102266]

[118]	Fruehauf, J.P.; Meyskens, F.L., Jr Reactive oxygen species: a breath of life or death? *Clin. Cancer Res.,* **2007**, *13*(3), 789-794.

[http://dx.doi.org/10.1158/1078-0432.CCR-06-2082] [PMID: 17289868]

[119]   Nogueira, V.; Hay, N. Molecular pathways: reactive oxygen species homeostasis in cancer cells and implications for cancer therapy. *Clin. Cancer Res.,* **2013**, *19*(16), 4309-4314.
[http://dx.doi.org/10.1158/1078-0432.CCR-12-1424] [PMID: 23719265]

[120]   Priyadarsini, R.V.; Murugan, R.S.; Sripriya, P.; Karunagaran, D.; Nagini, S. The neem limonoids azadirachtin and nimbolide induce cell cycle arrest and mitochondria-mediated apoptosis in human cervical cancer (HeLa) cells. *Free Radic. Res.,* **2010**, *44*(6), 624-634.
[http://dx.doi.org/10.3109/10715761003692503] [PMID: 20429769]

[121]   Harish Kumar, G.; Chandra Mohan, K.V.; Jagannadha Rao, A.; Nagini, S. Nimbolide a limonoid from Azadirachta indica inhibits proliferation and induces apoptosis of human choriocarcinoma (BeWo) cells. *Invest. New Drugs,* **2009**, *27*(3), 246-252.
[http://dx.doi.org/10.1007/s10637-008-9170-z] [PMID: 18719855]

[122]   Akinola, O.B.; Zatta, L.; Dosumu, O.O.; Akinola, O.S.; Adelaja, A.A.; Dini, L.; Caxton-Martins, E.A. Intestinal lesions of streptozotocin-induced diabetes and the effects of *Azadirachta indica* treatment. *Pharmacologyonline,* **2009**, *3*, 872-881.

[123]   Akinola, O.B.; Dosumu, O.O.; Akinola, O.S.; Zatta, L.; Dini, L.; Caxton-Martins, E.A. *Azadirachta indica* leaf extract ameliorates hyperglycemia and hepatic glycogenosis in streptozotocin-induced diabetic wistar rats. *Int. J. Phytomed.,* **2010**, *2*, 320-331.

[124]   Akinola, O.B.; Caxton-Martins, E.A.; Dini, L. Chronic Treatment with Ethanolic Extract of the Leaves of *Azadirachta indica* Ameliorates Lesions of Pancreatic Islets in Streptozotocin Diabetes. *Int. J. Morphol.,* **2010**, *28*(1), 291-302.
[http://dx.doi.org/10.4067/S0717-95022010000100043]

[125]   Chattopadhyay, R.R. Possible mechanism of antihyperglycemic effect of *Azadirachta indica* leaf extract: part V. *J. Ethnopharmacol.,* **1999**, *67*(3), 373-376.
[http://dx.doi.org/10.1016/S0378-8741(99)00094-X] [PMID: 10617075]

[126]   Parle, M. Gurditta. Basketful benefits of Papaya. *Int. Res. J. Pharm.,* **2011**, *2*, 6-12.

[127]   Lim, T.K. Edible Medicinal and Non-Medicinal Plants. **2012**; Vol 1, *Fruits*, Springer.

[128]   Silva, J.A.T.; Rashid, Z.; Nhut, D.T.; Sivakumar, D.; Gera, A.; Souza, M.T.; Tennant, P. Papaya (*Carica papaya L.*) biology and biotechnology. *Tree and Forestry Science and Biotechnology,* **2007**, *1*, 47-73.

[129]   Chandrika, U.G.; Jansz, E.R.; Wickramasinghe, S.N.; Warnasuriya, N.D. Carotenoids in yellow and red fleshed papaya (Carica papaya L). *J. Sci. Food Agric.,* **2003**, *83*, 1279-1282.
[http://dx.doi.org/10.1002/jsfa.1533]

[130]   Dubois, T.; Jacquet, A.; Schnek, A.G.; Looze, Y. The thiol proteinases from the latex of *Carica papaya L. I.* Fractionation, purification and preliminary characterization. *Biol. Chem. Hoppe Seyler,* **1988**, *369*(8), 733-740. a
[http://dx.doi.org/10.1515/bchm3.1988.369.2.733] [PMID: 3214554]

[131]   Azarkan, M.; El Moussaoui, A.; van Wuytswinkel, D.; Dehon, G.; Looze, Y. Fractionation and purification of the enzymes stored in the latex of Carica papaya. *J. Chromatogr. B Analyt. Technol. Biomed. Life Sci.,* **2003**, *790*(1-2), 229-238.
[http://dx.doi.org/10.1016/S1570-0232(03)00084-9] [PMID: 12767335]

[132]   Brocklehurst, K.; Salih, E.; McKee, R.; Smith, H. Fresh non-fruit latex of Carica papaya contains papain, multiple forms of chymopapain A and papaya proteinase omega. *Biochem. J.,* **1985**, *228*(2), 525-527.
[http://dx.doi.org/10.1042/bj2280525] [PMID: 4015629]

[133]   Dubois, T.; Kleinschmidt, T.; Schnek, A.G.; Looze, Y.; Braunitzer, G. The thiol proteinases from the latex of Carica papaya L. II. The primary structure of proteinase omega. *Biol. Chem. Hoppe Seyler,* **1988**, *369*(8), 741-754.

[http://dx.doi.org/10.1515/bchm3.1988.369.2.741] [PMID: 3063283]

[134]   Imaga, N.O.A.; Gbenle, G.O.; Okochi, V.I.; Akanbi, S.O.; Edeoghon, S.O.; Oigbochie, V.; Kehinde, M.O.; Bamiro, S.B. Antisickling property of *Carica papaya* leaf extract. *Afr. J. Biochem. Res.,* **2009**, *3*, 102-106.

[135]   Canini, A.; Alesiani, D.; D'Arcangelo, G.; Tagliatesta, P. Gas chromatography-mass spectrometry analysis of phenolic compounds from *Carica papaya L.* leaf. *J. Food Compos. Anal.,* **2007**, *20*, 584-590.
[http://dx.doi.org/10.1016/j.jfca.2007.03.009]

[136]   Nakamura, Y.; Yoshimoto, M.; Murata, Y.; Shimoishi, Y.; Asai, Y.; Park, E.Y.; Sato, K.; Nakamura, Y. Papaya seed represents a rich source of biologically active isothiocyanate. *J. Agric. Food Chem.,* **2007**, *55*(11), 4407-4413.
[http://dx.doi.org/10.1021/jf070159w] [PMID: 17469845]

[137]   Rossetto, M.R.; Oliveira do Nascimento, J.R.; Purgatto, E.; Fabi, J.P.; Lajolo, F.M.; Cordenunsi, B.R. Benzylglucosinolate, benzylisothiocyanate, and myrosinase activity in papaya fruit during development and ripening. *J. Agric. Food Chem.,* **2008**, *56*(20), 9592-9599.
[http://dx.doi.org/10.1021/jf801934x] [PMID: 18826320]

[138]   Marfo, E.K.; Oke, O.L.; Afolab, O.A. Chemical-composition of papaya (Carica-papaya) seeds. *Food Chem.,* **1986**, *22*, 259-266.
[http://dx.doi.org/10.1016/0308-8146(86)90084-1]

[139]   El Moussaoui, A.; Nijs, M.; Paul, C.; Wintjens, R.; Vincentelli, J.; Azarkan, M.; Looze, Y. Revisiting the enzymes stored in the laticifers of Carica papaya in the context of their possible participation in the plant defence mechanism. *Cell. Mol. Life Sci.,* **2001**, *58*(4), 556-570.
[http://dx.doi.org/10.1007/PL00000881] [PMID: 11361091]

[140]   Morton, J. *Papaya Fruits of warm climates*; Creative Resource Systems, Inc.: Miami, **1987**.

[141]   Ernst, E. Evidence-Based Herbal Medicine. *Eur. J. Clin. Pharmacol.,* **2000**, *56*, 523.
[http://dx.doi.org/10.1007/s002280000194] [PMID: 11151739]

[142]   Hewitt, H.; Whittle, S.; Lopez, S.; Bailey, E.; Weaver, S. Topical use of papaya in chronic skin ulcer therapy in Jamaica. *West Indian Med. J.,* **2000**, *49*(1), 32-33.
[PMID: 10786448]

[143]   Krishna, K.L.; Paridhavi, M.; Patel, J.A.; Krishna, K.L.; Jagruti, A.P. Review on nutritional, medicinal and pharmacological properties of Papaya (*Carica papaya Linn.*). *Nat. Prod. Radiance,* **2008**, *7*, 364-373.

[144]   Gamulle, A.; Ratnasooriya, W.D.; Jayakody, J.R.A.C.; Fernando, C.; Kanatiwela, C.; Udagama, P. Thrombocytosis and anti-inflammatory properties and toxicological evaluation of Carica papaya mature leaf concentrate in a murine model. *Int. J. Med. Plants Res.,* **2012**, *1*, 21-30.

[145]   Ahmad, N.; Fazal, H.; Ayaz, M.; Abbasi, B.H.; Mohammad, I.; Fazal, L. Dengue fever treatment with *Carica papaya* leaves extracts. *Asian Pac. J. Trop. Biomed.,* **2011**, *1*(4), 330-333.
[http://dx.doi.org/10.1016/S2221-1691(11)60055-5] [PMID: 23569787]

[146]   Subenthiran, S.; Choon, T.C.; Cheong, K.C.; Thayan, R.; Teck, M.B.; Muniandy, P.K.; Afzan, A.; Abdullah, N.R.; Ismail, Z. Carica papaya leaves juice significantly accelerates the rate of increase in platelet count among patients with dengue fever and dengue haemorrhagic fever. *Evid. Based Complement. Alternat. Med.,* **2013**, *2013*, 616737.
[http://dx.doi.org/10.1155/2013/616737] [PMID: 23662145]

[147]   Otsuki, N.; Dang, N.H.; Kumagai, E.; Kondo, A.; Iwata, S.; Morimoto, C. Aqueous extract of Carica papaya leaves exhibits anti-tumor activity and immunomodulatory effects. *J. Ethnopharmacol.,* **2010**, *127*(3), 760-767.
[http://dx.doi.org/10.1016/j.jep.2009.11.024] [PMID: 19961915]

[148]   Lucas, T.P. *The most wonderful tree in the world, the papaw tree (Carica papaia)*; Carter-Watson:

Brisbane, **1914**.

[149]   Vien, D.T.H.; Thuy, P.T. Research on Biological Activity of some Extracts from Vietnamese *Carica papaya* Leaves. *ASEAN Journal of Chemical Engineering,* **2013**, *2*, 43-51.

[150]   Amenta, R.; Camarda, L.; Di Stefano, V.; Lentini, F.; Venza, F. Traditional medicine as a source of new therapeutic agents against psoriasis. *Fitoterapia,* **2000**, *71* Suppl. 1, S13-S20.
[http://dx.doi.org/10.1016/S0367-326X(00)00172-6] [PMID: 10930708]

[151]   Nayak, S.B.; Pinto Pereira, L.; Maharaj, D. Wound healing activity of *Carica papaya* L. in experimentally induced diabetic rats. *Indian J. Exp. Biol.,* **2007**, *45*(8), 739-743.
[PMID: 17877152]

[152]   Lohiya, N.K.; Goyal, R.B.; Jayaprakash, D.; Ansari, A.S.; Sharma, S. Antifertility effects of aqueous extract of *Carica papaya* seeds in male rats. *Planta Med.,* **1994**, *60*(5), 400-404.
[http://dx.doi.org/10.1055/s-2006-959518] [PMID: 7997464]

[153]   Lohiya, N.K.; Manivannan, B.; Mishra, P.K.; Pathak, N.; Sriram, S.; Bhande, S.S.; Panneerdoss, S. Chloroform extract of Carica papaya seeds induces long-term reversible azoospermia in langur monkey. *Asian J. Androl.,* **2002**, *4*(1), 17-26.
[PMID: 11907624]

[154]   Lohiya, N.K.; Pathak, N.; Mishra, P.K.; Manivannan, B. Contraceptive evaluation and toxicological study of aqueous extract of the seeds of Carica papaya in male rabbits. *J. Ethnopharmacol.,* **2000**, *70*(1), 17-27. b
[http://dx.doi.org/10.1016/S0378-8741(99)00139-7] [PMID: 10720785]

[155]   Udoh, P.; Kehinde, A. Studies on antifertility effect of pawpaw seeds (Carica papaya) on the gonads of male albino rats. *Phytother. Res.,* **1999**, *13*(3), 226-228.
[http://dx.doi.org/10.1002/(SICI)1099-1573(199905)13:3<226::AID-PTR396>3.0.CO;2-E]   [PMID: 10353163]

[156]   Lohiya, N.K.; Kothari, L.K.; Manivannan, B.; Mishra, P.K.; Pathak, N. Human sperm immobilization effect of *Carica papaya* seed extracts: an in vitro study. *Asian J. Androl.,* **2000**, *2*(2), 103-109. a
[PMID: 11232785]

[157]   Adebiyi, A.; Adaikan, P.G.; Prasad, R.N. Papaya (*Carica papaya*) consumption is unsafe in pregnancy: fact or fable? Scientific evaluation of a common belief in some parts of Asia using a rat model. *Br. J. Nutr.,* **2002**, *88*(2), 199-203.
[http://dx.doi.org/10.1079/BJN2002598] [PMID: 12144723]

[158]   Oderinde, O.; Noronha, C.; Oremosu, A.; Kusemiju, T.; Okanlawon, O.A. Abortifacient properties of aqueous extract of Carica papaya (Linn) seeds on female Sprague-Dawley rats. *Niger. Postgrad. Med. J.,* **2002**, *9*(2), 95-98.
[PMID: 12163882]

[159]   Maisarah, A.M.; Nurul, A.B.; Asmah, R.; Fauziah, O. Antioxidant analysis of different parts of Carica papaya. *Int. Food Res. J.,* **2013**, *20*, 1043-1048.

[160]   Zunjar, V.; Mammen, D.; Trivedi, B.M. Antioxidant activities and phenolics profiling of different parts of Carica papaya by LCMS-MS. *Nat. Prod. Res.,* **2015**, *29*(22), 2097-2099.
[http://dx.doi.org/10.1080/14786419.2014.986658] [PMID: 25495879]

[161]   Huang, S.H.; Wu, L.W.; Huang, A.C.; Yu, C.C.; Lien, J.C.; Huang, Y.P.; Yang, J.S.; Yang, J.H.; Hsiao, Y.P.; Wood, W.G.; Yu, C.S.; Chung, J.G. Benzyl isothiocyanate (BITC) induces G2/M phase arrest and apoptosis in human melanoma A375.S2 cells through reactive oxygen species (ROS) and both mitochondria-dependent and death receptor-mediated multiple signaling pathways. *J. Agric. Food Chem.,* **2012**, *60*(2), 665-675.
[http://dx.doi.org/10.1021/jf204193v] [PMID: 22148415]

[162]   Zhang, A.; Sun, H.; Wang, X. Potentiating therapeutic effects by enhancing synergism based on active constituents from traditional medicine. *Phytother. Res.,* **2014**, *28*(4), 526-533.

[http://dx.doi.org/10.1002/ptr.5032] [PMID: 23913598]

[163]   Navarro, S.L.; Li, F.; Lampe, J.W. Mechanisms of action of isothiocyanates in cancer chemoprevention: an update. *Food Funct.,* **2011**, *2*(10), 579-587.
[http://dx.doi.org/10.1039/c1fo10114e] [PMID: 21935537]

[164]   Tanaka, T.; Shnimizu, M.; Moriwaki, H. Cancer chemoprevention by carotenoids. *Molecules,* **2012**, *17*(3), 3202-3242.
[http://dx.doi.org/10.3390/molecules17033202] [PMID: 22418926]

[165]   Rahmat, A.; Rosli, R.; Wan Nor, I.W.; Endrini, S.; Sani, H.A. Antiproliferative activity of pure lycopene compared to both extracted lycopene and juices from watermelon (*Citrullus vulgaris*) and papaya (*Carica papaya*) on human breast and liver cancer cell lines. *J. Med. Sci.,* **2002**, *2*, 55-58.
[http://dx.doi.org/10.3923/jms.2002.55.58]

[166]   Nguyen, T.T.; Shaw, P.N.; Parat, M.O.; Hewavitharana, A.K. Anticancer activity of Carica papaya: a review. *Mol. Nutr. Food Res.,* **2013**, *57*(1), 153-164.
[http://dx.doi.org/10.1002/mnfr.201200388] [PMID: 23212988]

[167]   Morimoto, C.; Dang, N. H.; Dang, N. YS Therapeutic Co Ltd (YSTH-Non-standard) Toudai Tlo Ltd (TOUDNon-standard) Morimoto C (MORI-Individual) Dang N H (DANG-Individual), Cancer prevention and treating composition for preventing, ameliorating, or treating solid cancers, ss. lung, or blood cancers, *e.g.* lymphoma, comprises components extracted from brewing papaya. Patent number-WO2006004226-A1; EP1778262- A1; JP2008505887-W; US2008069907-A1, **2008**.

[168]   García-Solís, P.; Yahia, E.M.; Morales-Tlalpan, V.; Díaz-Muñoz, M. Screening of antiproliferative effect of aqueous extracts of plant foods consumed in México on the breast cancer cell line MCF-7. *Int. J. Food Sci. Nutr.,* **2009**, *60* Suppl. 6, 32-46.
[http://dx.doi.org/10.1080/09637480802312922] [PMID: 19468947]

[169]   Nakamura, Y.; Miyoshi, N. Cell death induction by isothiocyanates and their underlying molecular mechanisms. *Biofactors,* **2006**, *26*(2), 123-134.
[http://dx.doi.org/10.1002/biof.5520260203] [PMID: 16823098]

[170]   Panzarini, E.; Dwikat, M.; Mariano, S.; Vergallo, C.; Dini, L. Administration Dependent Antioxidant Effect of Carica papaya Seeds Water Extract. *Evid. Based Complement. Alternat. Med.,* **2014**, *2014*, 281508.
[http://dx.doi.org/10.1155/2014/281508] [PMID: 24795765]

[171]   Goldman, P. Herbal medicines today and the roots of modern pharmacology. *Ann. Intern. Med.,* **2001**, *135*(8 Pt 1), 594-600.
[http://dx.doi.org/10.7326/0003-4819-135-8_Part_1-200110160-00010] [PMID: 11601931]

CHAPTER 2

Natural Antimutagens. Chemopreventive Action of L-Ascorbic Acid and Green Tea Infusions on the Acute Toxicity and Mutagenicity of Reaction Mixtures Nitrite-Sulfonamide

Ana Pontoriero and **Marcela Rizzotto**[*]

Instituto de Química Rosario (IQUIR), Facultad de Ciencias Bioquímicas y Farmacéuticas, Universidad Nacional de Rosario, Argentina

Abstract: An agent that causes irreversible and hereditary (mutation) changes in cellular genetic material, deoxyribonucleic acid (DNA) is defined as a mutagen. Changes in DNA caused by mutagens can damage the cells and cause certain diseases, such as cancer. Among the oldest and most recognized tests for the detection of mutagens we can mention those of Ames, which works with bacteria, and the test of the onion or *Allium cepa* test. One of the most effective ways to minimize the harmful effect of mutagenic substances is through the use of natural antimutagens. Natural antimutagenic substances, which may be present in plants, human diet and other sources have protective effects against mutagens. We showed that vitamin C and green tea infusions, in the Ames test, significantly mitigate the mutagenicity of sulfatiazole (a sulfa drug, an antibacterial commonly used) and nitrite (a food preservative and a normal body component) mixtures in acidic medium.

Keywords: Chemoprevention, Mutagen, Natural antimutagens, Nitrite, sulfonamides.

INTRODUCTION

Mutagens and Carcinogens

Genetic information is transmitted from one cell to its successor by the precise duplication of the deoxyribonucleic acid (DNA) chains [1]. A mutagen is an agent capable of interacting chemically or physically with the base sequence of the genetic material or alter its physical structure, increasing the frequency of mutations above baseline.

[*] **Corresponding author Marcela Rizzotto**: Institute of Chemistry Rosario (Instituto de Química Rosario: IQUIR), Faculty of Biochemical and Pharmaceutical Sciences, National University of Rosario, Argentina; Tel/Fax: +54 (0341)4804598; E-mails: mrizzott@fbioyf.unr.edu.ar; marcela.rizzotto@gmail.com

Ferid Murad, Atta-ur-Rahman and Ka Bian (Eds.)

Mutagens may be classified as:

Biological mutagens: are exemplified by very small organisms, such as bacteria, viruses, mushrooms, *etc*.

Chemical mutagens: represented by compounds or chemical elements which can alter rapidly the genetic structure of living organisms, such as drugs, *etc*. Their effects are associated with their chemical structure and pathways of exposure [2].

Physical mutagens: they are among the most harmful, since they cause dangerous mutations in the living beings, such as hereditary diseases and congenital diseases. They include ultraviolet radiation and nuclear radiation [1].

Some mutagens are direct: do not need an activation mechanism to act. Others are indirect: that is, they must be activated (*e.g.* by cytochrome P450) to exert their action. It should be noted that not all mutations are caused by mutagens. There are "Spontaneous mutations", so-called because of errors in DNA recombination and repair.

About carcinogens, we can say that these are chemical, biological, or physical agents that can induce malignant neoplasms [1]. Substances are classified as carcinogenic when they affect a population whose organisms have not been exposed to it previously, suffer a significant increase, according to statistics, of some form of neoplasia [3].

A classification has been established for chemical carcinogens based on their reactivity with DNA:

Genotoxic carcinogens, which cause direct damage to DNA. Many mutagens are in this category and frequently the mutation is the first step in the development of cancer.

Epigenetic carcinogens: do not react with DNA, and exercise their action by increasing the number of DNA replications in a target cell [4].

Biological Tests

In the last 50 years more than 50 test systems have been developed to detect changes induced by agents capable of damaging the genetic material, using the entire spectrum of organisms, from bacteria to whole animals. In general, it is accepted the existence of 4 levels for the evaluation of genetic damage, contemplating *in vitro* as *in vivo* studies:

• Primary level: also known as bacterial or molecular. Allows detection of point mutations, such as base substitutions and framework of reading, using the use of prokaryotes. Among these tests we can mention the Ames test or tests with *Bacillus subtillis* [2]. In general, assays that use bacteria involve changes in genes that encode the synthesis of certain amino acids and also antibiotic resistance [5].

- Secondary level: cell cultures are used, either in monolayer or suspension. (*e.g.*: Micronucleus Test, Sister Chromatid Exchange, Aberration Rate Chromosomal, *etc.*).
- Tertiary level: applied in plants and animals, including humans. They use the whole organism, allowing access to the metabolic products of a compound under study. By working in this level, some authors prefer to use plants (*Allium cepa, Vicia faba*).
- Quaternary level (also called epidemiological level): uses the prospective and/or retrospective study for exposed populations. The cytogenetic techniques mentioned above are employed, with long-term follow-up.

These tests can be applied sequentially or as a battery, working in different evidence of increasing complexity. At present, a battery of assays is often used [2]. Damage or risk assessments using animal models may be long, expensive, low sensitivity and difficult extrapolation. Short-term trials, on the contrary, allow a rapid assessment of the mutagenic character of the substances or complex mixtures, they are economical and in a few days it is possible to obtain results. It is important to remember that when evaluating a complex substance or mixture, it is essential to use a battery of tests, including at least *in vitro* and *in vivo* models.

This allows the study to be extended and obtain more information on the mode of action of the substance. Many substances can be positive in an *in vitro* assay and may be either negative or weakly positive in an *in vivo* system due to some process of inhibition of mutagenicity in some instance of the process metabolic. In the *in vivo* system it is possible to detect substances (called promutagens) that are not detected in the *in vitro* systems [6].

Ames Test

Mutations have been described as important first steps in carcinogenesis; so, an assay as the Ames test have been used with great success for the detection of mutagens as well as for the detection of antimutagens [7].

The Ames test, a bacterial mutation assay that uses *Salmonella typhimurium* as an indicator bacterium has been universally adopted for the detection of mutagens in a simple, rapid and economical way [8]. Strains TA98 and TA100 are considered "reference" because, together, they detect 93% of mutagens [9], including 2-nitrofluorene and nitroso derivatives of aromatic carcinogenic amines (in general, mutagens that cause frameshift) are detected by the TA98 strain; and mutagens that produce substitution of base pairs, as NaN_3 and aflatoxin B1, are detected by the TA100 strain.

In addition, the Ames test is useful not only for testing pure substances, but also for complex mixtures [10] and reaction mixtures such as sulfonamides and nitrite in acidic media [11].

Allium Test

Plants are test organisms that are recommended for their low maintenance costs and due to the possibility of working with meristem and reproductive tissue to analyze effects associated with modifications of the cell cycle or meiosis dynamics. In addition, they allow detecting chromosomal alterations resulting from the direct effect of different agents on the DNA or proteins associated therewith. The results obtained are comparable to those obtained in animals [6]. *Allium cepa* species have been frequently used to determine cytotoxicity, mutagenicity and genotoxic effects of various substances [12]. It has been demonstrated that the Allium test has a similar sensitivity to algae and lymphocytes [13]. The work with *A. cepa* has the advantages of exposing the organism directly to complex mixtures without pretreatment of the sample and, in addition, the presence of an own oxidase system essential for the evaluation of promutagens [14].

On the other hand, *A. cepa* is a favorable organism for evaluation of chromosomal damage and disturbances in mitosis due to their low number of chromosomes (2n = 16), which are also large in size [15]. At the assay, root lengths before and after exposure to the substance are evaluate. Microscopic parameters such as mitotic index, presence of aberrations chromosomes and other cellular abnormalities are evaluated too [6].

NATURAL ANTIMUTAGENIC AGENTS

Substances that diminish or reduce the effects of mutagens are generally called anti-mutagens [16]. In nature it is possible to find antimutagenic substances in plants and other natural sources; there are also dietary components that exhibit protective effects against mutagenic agents. These include flavonoids, phenolics, coumarins, carotenoids, anthraquinones, tannins, saponins and many more [17]. Many plants that have been used for centuries in traditional medicine are currently studied for their possible content of antimutagenic substances [18]. In recent years, the use of medicinal plant extracts for the treatment of human diseases has increased a lot [19]. More than 500 compounds belonging to at least 25 chemical classes have been recognized as possessing antimutagenic and/or protective effects [20], including different spices [21].

A number of basic chemical structures found in antimutagenic compounds are presented, in alphabetical order, in Figs. (**1-9**) and briefly described in the following paragraphs. In these chemical formulas can be observed, in general, the presence of phenolic oxhydrils and quinone-like structures. In relation to each basic chemical formula, particular examples of plants are given, indicating a few macroscopic and/or origin characteristics. The selected plants generally contain a wide variety of useful compounds, therefore the selection is arbitrary and for the sole purpose of giving some examples.

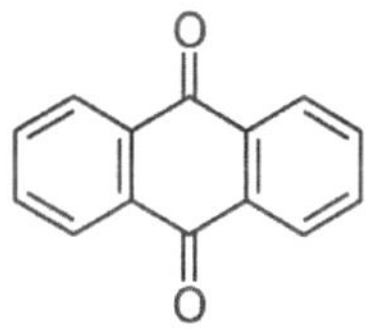

Fig. (1). Anthraquinone.

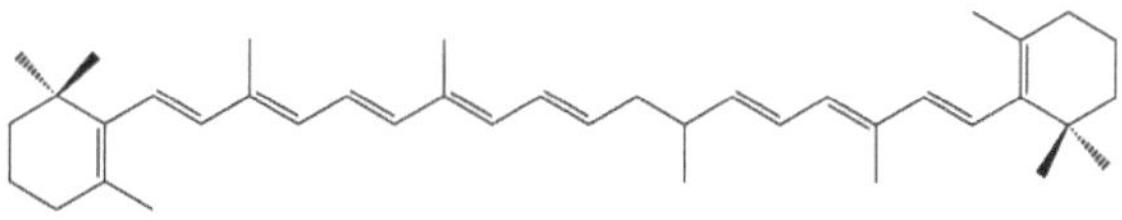

Fig. (2). β-carotene.

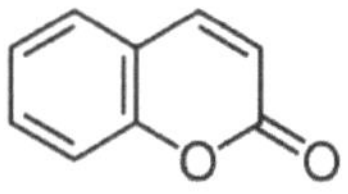

Fig. (3). Coumarin (1-benzopyran-2-one).

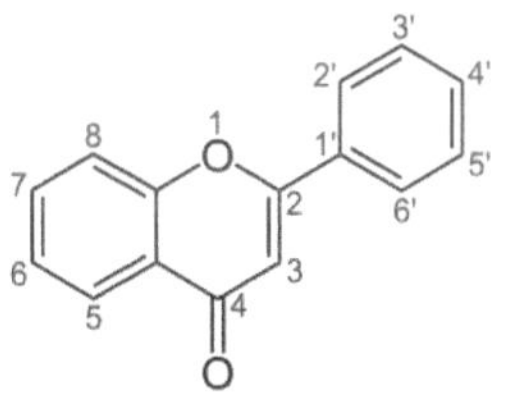

Fig. (4). Flavone.

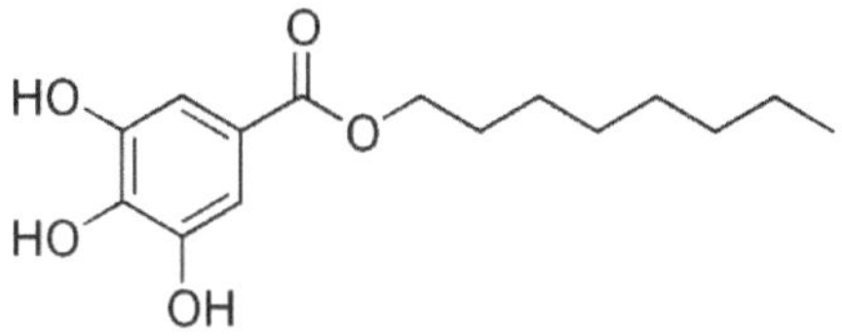

Fig. (5). Octyl gallate.

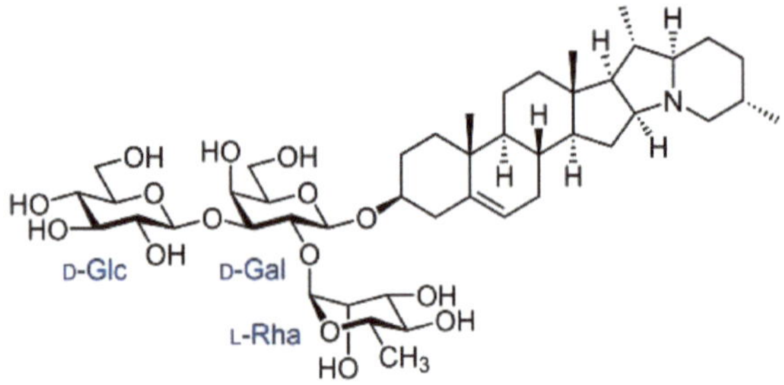

Fig. (6). Solanine (an steroidal saponin).

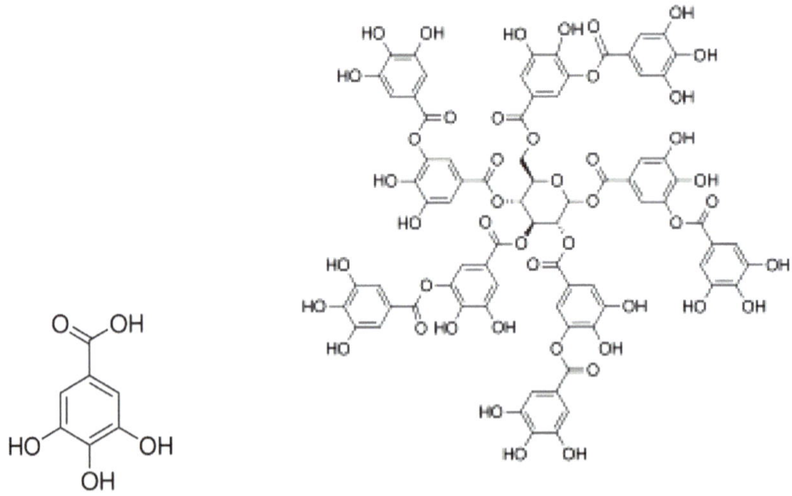

Fig. (7). a) Gallic acid, a tannin b) Tannic acid.

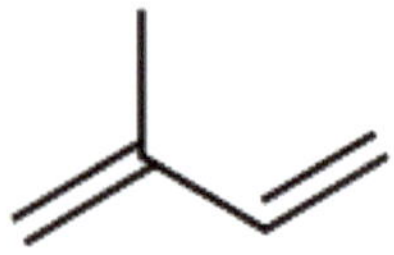

Fig. (8). Molecular structure of isoprene, the chemical unit of terpenes.

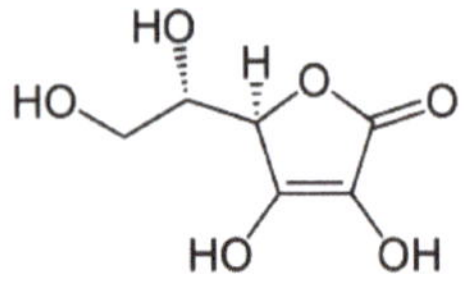

Fig. (9). L-ascorbic acid (vitamin C).

Anthraquinones

Shankel *et al.*, in 2000 [22], reported the antimutagenic activity of anthraquinones (aloe-emodin-anthraquinone isolated from *Aloe barborescence)*. Among compounds structurally related to anthraquinones, anthrone, acridone and xanthone exerted antimutagenecity, anthrone being the most potent one. All naphthaquinones were strong antimutagens, among them, plumbagin (5-hydrox--2-methyl-1,4-naphthoquinone) and 2-methyl-5-hydroxy naphthoquinone showed exceptional antimutagenicity [23].

Aloe Species

These plants, of the Xanthorrhoeaceae family, are widely used in ethnomedicine for treating various ailments [24]. Plants of the genus Aloe have been used for centuries in various cultures around the world. On the African continent, the Arabian Peninsula, Madagascar and the eastern islands of the Indian Ocean there are more than 500 species, from shrubs to trees. Approximately 125 species are native in South Africa [25].

Rhamnus alaternus L.

R. alaternus L. (Rhamnaceae), an indigenous or native species of the Mediterranean region, is commonly found in the North of Tunisia [26]. These plant species contain hydroxyanthraquinone compounds such as emodin, chrysophanol and physcion [27]. Different extracts of *R. alaternus*, particularly the aqueous one, significantly decreased the genotoxicity induced by aflatoxin B1 and nifuroxazide in the *S. typhimurium* assay system. Moreover, the extracts showed no mutagenicity when tested with *Salmonella typhimurium* strains TA1535 and TA1538 either with or without the S9 mix. The results obtained by the Ames test assay confirm those of SOS chromotest [28].

Carotenoids

Several studies showed that the activation of promutagens are affected by carotenoids. Antimutagenicity of carotenoids extracted from five different types of green peppers *(Capsicum* sp.) has been reported on *S. typhimurium* tester strain YG1024, against the mutagenicity of some nitroarenes [29]. Antimutagenic activity of P-carotene, canthaxanthin, P-carotene-8-apo-P-carotenal and 8-apo-P-carotene methyl ester showed a dose dependent decrease in the mutagenicity compared with 1-methyl-3-nitro-1-nitrosoguanidine and benzo[a]pyrene in Ames test [30].

Artocarpus heterophyllus Lam (Jackfruit)

This is an evergreen tree, of 10-15 m tall with a dense crown. It is from the family of Moraceae, original from Indonesia. Jackfruit is a rich source of several high-value compounds [31], with chemoprotective properties to reduce the mutagenicity of aflatoxin B1 [32].

Capsicum spp.

Green pepper, (*Capsicum* spp.), a significant component in the Mexican diet, is one of the main spices and food additives consumed in Latin-American countries. Green pepper juice may cause antimutagenic effect by interfering with the nitrosation process [33].

Moringa Plants

Ficus benghalensis (family: Moraceae), is an important medicinal and widely distributed tree found in different regions of India [34]. *Moringa oleifera* Lam (Moringaceae) is a highly valued plant, distributed in many countries of the tropical and subtropical zone [35]. Both *F. benghalensis* stem bark extract and *M. oleifera* root extract showed strong antimutagenic effect on *S. typhimurium* TA100 strain against sodium azide (NaN_3) [36].

Coumarins

Coumarins are chemically 2H-1-benzopyran-2-ones, widely distributed in the plant kingdom. A wide range of structures with varying complexity occurs in angiosperms. Coumarins have been shown to behave both as antimutagenic as well as anticarcinogen [37]. Non-toxicity and high activity of several coumarins from *Selinum monniere* were observed in the inhibition of mutagenicity of benzo[α]pyrene [38].

Echeveria DC.

Echeveria, since its high endemism, historical–cultural significance and role in the ecosystems of Mexico, is the most representative genus from Crassulaceae of the country [39]. These are frequently used as decorative plants [40]. Some genera of the Crassulaceae family (such as *Rhodiola* and *Kalanchoe*) are used in traditional medicine. Its medical importance was sustained with the characterization of pure compounds (*e.g.*, phenolics, coumarins, terpenes and sterols) with biological activities (*e.g.*, antimicrobial, anti-inflammatory, antimutagenic and antitumoral) [41]. Remarkably, the *Echeveria* samples may be a readily accessible source of natural products for the food and pharmaceutical industries [42].

Prunus mahaleb L.

It is a marginal fruit crop producing cherry-like dark purple drupes with a very bitter taste. A mahaleb fruit concentrated extract (*mfce*) has been assayed for its biological activities, and further studies are required to elucidate the contribution of various chemical compounds identified in *mfce* (anthocyanins, flavonols, flavanols and coumarin) to its biological activities [43].

Flavonoids

Flavonoids are a class of phytochemicals that possess a great potential as antimutagens and anticarcinogens, in addition to a wide range of biological activities. Flavonoids from citrus juice were reported to possess anticarcinogenic and antimutagenic properties [44]. Antimutagenic activity of flavonoids from *Glycyrrhiza glabra,* include glaberene quercetin, myricetin, kaemferol, hesperidin and other flavonoids isolated from *Ocimum jauonica* was tested using *S. typhimurium* against various types of mutagens [37].

Artemisia absinthium L.

The genus *Artemisia* has pharmaceutical interest and is useful in traditional medicines [45]. Among them, *A. absinthium* L. is a species of wormwood, native to temperate regions of Eurasia and Northern Africa [46]. 1,8-Cineole (36.46%), borneol (25.99%) and camphor (10.20%) are the main components of the leaf oil of *A. absinthium* [47]. The oil showed antimutagenic activity against the carcinogen benzo(α) pyrene tested with TA97 and TA98 assay systems [48] and against sodium azide in the TA100 strain without S9 [49].

Aspalathus linearis (rooibos)

This is an indigenous South African herbal. From these plants a traditional drink is prepared, without caffeine, and that has a reputation of being healthy [50]. Aqueous extracts of rooibos also exhibited a high antimutagenic protection against aflatoxin B1 (AFB1) and 2-acetamidofluorene the Ames test (with the TA100 and TA 98 strains respectively) [51]. However, the major rooibos flavonoids (aspalathin and nothofagin), only showed moderate antimutagenic effects against 2-acetamido-fluorene and aflatoxin B1 as mutagens in the presence of metabolic activation [52].

Belamcanda chinensis DC Goldblatt & Mabb

Also called *Iris domestica* L. (family: Iridaceae), is an important species used in traditional Chinese medicine [53], whose isoflavonoids have phytoestrogenic and preventive properties towards the hormonedependent cancers such as the prostate one [54]. The isoflavonoid fractions (from a methanolic extract) of the rhizomes showed antimutagenicity against N-nitroquinoline (direct mutagenesis), and 2-aminofluorene (metabolically activated) in *Salmonella typhimurium* TA98 and TA100 in the Ames test [55].

Cyperus rotundus L.

C. rotundus Linn, a sedge of the family of *Cyperaceae*, which is widely distributed in the Mediterranean areas, is a plant used in traditional oriental medicine (in India, China and Japan) for the treatment of spasms stomach disorder and anti-inflammatory diseases [56]. Aqueous total oligomers flavonoids (TOF), ethyl acetate and methanol extracts from aerial parts of *C. rotundus* showed antimutagenic activity against Aflatoxin B1 (AFB1) in TA100 and TA98 *S. typhimurium* assay system (Ames test), and against sodium azide with TA100 and TA1535 strains. In addition, these extracts demonstrated an important free radical scavenging activity towards the 1,1-diphenyl-2-picrylhydrazyl (DPPH) free radical [57].

Phenolic Compounds

Phenolic compounds are a widely studied group of compounds from natural food and medicinal plants, which are associated with several biological activities too. Some phenolic compounds such as ellagic acid, present in strawberries, raspberries, grapes, walnuts, and so on showed antimutagenic properties. Moreover, compounds such as epicatechin, (-)-epicatechin gallate, (-)-epi-gallocatechins, (-)-epigallocatechin gallate were reported as the liable for the antimutagenic activity of green and black tea [58]. The antimutagenic activity of green tea catechins was demonstrated against oxidative mutagens such as tertiary butyl hydroxide and hydrogen peroxide using *Salmonella typhimurium* 102 tester strains. Antimutagenic effect of green tea against smoke-induced mutations in humans was established by the blockade of cigarette smoking-induced increase in sister chromatid exchange frequency [59]. Phenolics present in turmeric inhibited the mutagenicity produced by direct acting mutagens such as N-methyl-N'-niro-N-nitrosoguanidine in the Ames test with TA100 and TA1535 *S. typhimurium* strains [60]. Alkyl gallates (derivatives of gallic acid, which are phenolic compounds) with side chains varying from five to eight carbons (pentyl, hexyl, heptyl, and octyl gallates) showed evidence of chemopreventive effect against the the mutagenicity of hydrogen peroxide [61].

Carum copticum L. (ajwain)

It is a herbaceous annual plant of the family Apiaceae, which has white flowers and small brownish fruits. It grows in India, Iran, and Egypt. The ajwain is a popular spice traditionally employed in Indian system of medicine [62]. The methanolic fraction showed antimutagenic potential (using the TA97, TA98, TA100, and TA102 tester strains of *S. typhimurium*) against the direct acting mutagens sodium azide (NaN$_3$) and methyl methane sulphonate (MMS), and the indirect acting mutagens 2-aminofluorene (2-AF) and benzo(a)pyrene [63].

Curcuma longa L. (Turmeric)

Curcumin (a polyphenol) is a natural yellow colourant from turmeric. It is used in India for food, medicinal and nutraceutical purposes [64]. Amino acid derivatives of curcumin displayed very high antimutagenic activities against both *S. typhimurium* TA 98 and TA 1531 and with both sodium azide and methyl methanesulfonate (MMS) as mutagens [60]. The unsaturation in the side chain, a methoxy group on the benzene ring and a central β-diketone moiety in the curcumin molecule are the important structural requirements responsible for high antimutagenic potential of curcumin against cooked food heterocyclic amines [65].

Pistachia Vera

Iran is the main producer of pistachio nuts. Pistachio green hull possesses a high content in phenolic compounds [66], which showed antimutagenicity activity against the direct mutagen 2-nitrofluorene [67].

Salvia nemorosa L.

Salvia species are traditionally used as food and medicinal plants all around the world, and several *Salvia* species have economic importance because of their utilization as food, spices, and flavors [68]. Methanolic extract of *S. nemorosa* showed a high total phenolic and flavonoid contents and a strong DPPH radical scavenging activity [69].

Veronica spp.

Veronica (Plantaginaceae) genus, which contains nearly 500 species, is widely distributed in different environments, both in the northern hemisphere and in many areas of the southern hemisphere [70]. These species may be contemplated good sources of phenolic compounds for industrial or pharmacological uses [71]. Tested extracts showed antimutagenic activity against the mutagenicity of nitroquinoline-N-oxide with the Ames test (*S. typhimurium* TA100 strain) [72].

Saponins

Saponins isolated from *Calendula arvensis* and *Hedera helix* showed antimutagenic activity against benzo[a]pyrene with a dose-response relationship in the Ames test [73].

Amaranthaceae Plants

Amaranthaceae is a widespread family of flowering plants that grow in tropical to cool weather. The family comprises about 180 genera and 2500 species, which have different bioactive compounds, including phenolic acids, flavonoids, tannins, saponins and triterpenoids [74].

Amaranthus spinosus L.

A. spinosus (Family: *Amaranthaceae*), is a spinous herb, used in tribal medicine [75]. *A. spinosus* has several active constituents like alkaloids, flavonoids, glycosides, phenolic acids, steroids, terpenoids, saponins, betalains, bsitosterol, stigmasterol, rutin, catechuic tannins, *etc* [76]. The extract of the plant possesses, among others, anticancer properties [77] and chemoprotective activities [78]. The aqueous plant extract of *A. spinosus* inhibited the oxidative damage induced by the direct-acting mutagen of H_2O_2 at 5 mg/L using the *Allium* cepa assay [79].

Tannins

Several tannins have been found to reduce the mutagenic activity of numerous mutagens. Their anticarcinogenic and antimutagenic potential has been related to their antioxidative properties [80]. The antimutagenic effect of tannic acid was observed *in vivo* in the mouse spot test using male PW and female C57BL/10 mice [81]. Tannic acid showed a good binding affinity ($\square$10 to 10 M) towards mammalian serum albumins, enhancing the antioxidant activity of these proteins [82].

Phyllanthus amarus Schum. et Thonn.

This small Euphorbiaceous herb is one of the most important plants in traditional medicine of India and Thailand [83]. The major pharmacological active compounds are gallotannins and the lignans phyllanthin and hypophyllanthin [84]. The mutagenic effect of 2-aminofluorene, 2-aminoanthracene and 4-nitro-quinolone-1-oxide was inhibit by aqueous extract of the entire plant in *S. typhimurium* TA98 and TA100 strains, and in *Escherichia coli* WP2 uvrA/ pKM101. The extract also exhibited activity against 2-nitrofluorene and sodium azide-induced mutagenesis with *S. typhimurium* TA98 and TA100, respectively [85].

Pomegranate (Punica granatum)

Pomegranate trees, from the Punicaceae family [86], which are native of Iran and the Himalayas in north Pakistan and Northern India, today are extensively cultivated in China and recognised for their nutritional and commercial value [87]. Dried pomegranate peels were powdered and extracted with ethyl acetate, acetone, methanol and water. All the extracts decreased sodium azide mutagenicity in *S. typhimurium* TA100 and TA1535 strains [88]. Furthermore, the methanol fraction also showed antimutagenic activity against methyl methane sulphonate, 2-aminofluorene and benzo(a)pyrene (B(a)P) in *S. typhimurium* (TA97a, TA98, TA100 and TA102) tester strains. Phytochemical analysis by HPLC, LC–MS and total phenolic content revealed great content of ellagitannins which could be responsible for the promising antioxidant and antimutagenic activities of *P. granatum* peel extract [89].

Terpenoids

Diterpenoid like erythroxydiol isolated from *Aquillaria agallocha* demonstrated antimutagenic as well as antitumor activity [90]. The natural sesquiterpene β-caryophyllene and its metabolite β-caryophyllene oxide, in the Ames test (TA98 and TA100 strains) and *Escherichia coli* WP2uvrA and WP2uvrA/R inhibited the mutagenicity of a condensate of cigarette smoke [91].

Morina Plants

Morina persica L. has weak rosy smell flowers that together with aerial parts are infused or decocted and used as a functional tea. It is a representative of the Anatolian traditional medicine and is used for the cold treatment [92]. Besides, it has another ingredients for further use in healthful formulations [93]. *M. oleifera* leaf extracts has anticancer properties and can be claimed as a therapeutic target for cancer [94].

Zingiber zerumbet Smith

This is a wild ginger variety, which is also known as medicinal ginger [95]. In several parts of Asia the rhizomes of *Z. zerumbet* are used as a flavouring agent. The compound which is responsible for its bioactivity is a sesquiterpene: zerumbone [96]. It has been a molecule of hight interest because of its capability to inhibit growth of human leukaemia cell lines [97] besides its antiproliferative activity. The chemical potential of zerumbone and its therapeutic applications has recently been reviewed [98]. The activities as antibacterial and antimutagenic exhibited by zerumbone and its analogues establish their potential for use as nutraceuticals and in food preservation [99].

Vitamins

Vitamins have been extensively studied for their antimutagenic potential. Vitamin C (L-ascorbic acid) and vitamin E showed antimutagenic activity against doxorubicin induced chromosomal aberrations [100]. Vitamin A, C and E were found to be antimutagenic towards Methyl Azoxy Methanol (MAM) induced mutagenesis in *S. typhimurium* TA100 strain [101]. When vitamin C was administered concurrently with a pesticide, a significant decrease in the frequency of pesticide-induced mutations was observed [102].

Vitamin B1 (thiamine) showed antimutagenic activity against methyl-N-nitro- N-nitrosoguanidine and ethyl-N-nitro-N-nitrosoguanidine in the Ames test [103].

Actinidia Lindl (kiwifruit)

Actinidia species derived predominantly from south-western China [104]. Only three have been domesticated (in the past century), although more than 50 species are currently recognized [105]. The fruit available commercially are usually of *A. chinensis* Planch., or of *A. deliciosa* (A. Chev.) C.F. Consumption of green kiwifruit contributes by having positive effects on cardiovascular and gut health [106]. The health benefits attributed to vitamin C, which is present in the fruit, include antioxidant, antiatherogenic, anticarcinogenic [107] and chemopreventive properties [108].

We will not discuss here mechanisms of antimutagenicity, but they have been widely described by De Flora *et al.* (1992), and roughly refer to chemical or enzymatic inactivation, prevention of formation of active species, scavenging and antioxidant free radical scavenging [109].

CHEMOPREVENTIVE ACTION OF L-ASCORBIC ACID AND GREEN TEA INFUSIONS ON THE ACUTE TOXICITY AND MUTAGENICITY OF NITRITE-SULFONAMIDE REACTION MIXTURES

Mutagens and Carcinogens

A classification for chemical carcinogens has been established depending on its reactivity with the DNA:

Genotoxic carcinogens, which cause direct DNA damage. Many mutagens are in this category and often the mutation is the first step in the development of cancer.

Epigenetic carcinogens: do not react with DNA; exercise their action by increasing number of DNA replications in a target cell [4].

Nitrites and Nitrosocompounds

Nitrite is a normal component of the organism and can also be found in micromolar concentrations in cured meats, vegetables, fertilizers and drinking contaminated water. High levels of nitrite, in the range of 50-200 µM, are found in the human saliva, and concentrations as 400 µM may be present in gastric juice, after consumption of 100 g of spinach. Nitrite plays an important role in human physiology. In acidic media, or under conditions of oxidative stress, can be converted to a wide range of species reactive molecules, which can modify a large number of molecules, including drugs and xenobiotics, and can modify structurally a large variety of exogenous compounds and endogenous (polyunsaturated fatty acids, tocopherols, catecholamines, furans, retinoids, dietary phenols, *etc.*).

The N-nitrosocompounds can be generated from the nitrosation of amines and amides. Nitrosamines constitute a group of indirect carcinogens; its action depends on activation by the cytochrome P-450 enzyme and are capable of renting the DNA [110]. Nitrosamides do not need metabolic activation [111]. In a study of the carcinogenic capacity of 300 nitrosocompounds, it was found that 90% of them stimulate carcinogenicity in 40 animal species, including higher primates [112]. In humans, there is evidence of the role of these compounds in gastric cancer, esophagus, nasopharynx and colon cancer [113]. The N-nitrosocompounds exert their action through the alkylation of bases in the DNA [112].

Exposure to N-nitrosocompounds (NOCs)

Humans are exposed to preformed NOCs from sources such as tobacco, drugs or diet. With regard to this last item, the consumption of red meats and, in particular, processed or cured meats (*i.e,* meats treated with nitrites, as an additive, *e.g,* Sausages, bacon, salami) have been linked to the incidence of colorectal cancer since 1975. The World Health Organization has recommended in 2003, moderation in the consumption of these cured meats [114]. In addition, we are also exposed to NOCs produced *in vivo*. It is estimated that between 45% and 75% of NOCs are of endogenous synthesis [113]. These N-nitrosocompounds endogenous are mainly synthesized in the stomach [115].

Dietary nitrate, on the other hand, can be converted into nitrite in the oral cavity by bacteria there [110]. Approximately 20% of salivary nitrite passes into the stomach [116]. There, in acid medium, it can be converted into nitrous acid and in species nitrosating agents, including N_2O_3 and NO+. acidic conditions may facilitate the formation of nitrosocompounds, in the presence of amines and amides. The true nitrosation intermediate is pH dependent. For most dialkylamines the nitrosation is optimal at pH between 2.5-3.5 and the nitrosing species is N_2O_3. In contrast, nitrosation of the amides is acid catalyzed without a pH maximum and involves nitrous acid [117].

Sulfa Drugs

A large number of drugs are potentially nitrosable, and many of them are used in high daily doses for long periods of time. From the pioneering studies of Lijinsky *et al.* numerous papers were published on drug-nitrite interactions, but despite this the endogenous nitrosation of drugs is still ignored [118]. This author demonstrated that the nitrite reaction products of a number of drugs -such as methadone, lucanone, disulfiram, *etc.*, included nitrosamines-diethylnitrosamine and dimethylnitrosamine- which have a recognized carcinogenic potential [119].

N-substituted sulfonamides are still widely used antimicrobial agents in the world, mainly because of its low cost, low toxicity and excellent activity against diseases [120]. They exert their antibacterial action through inhibition competitive effect of the enzyme dihydropteroate synthetase (DHPS), due to its structural similarity with substrate of the enzyme (p-aminobenzoic acid), a factor required by bacteria for synthesis of folic acid [121].

Glibenclamide (5-chloro-N- [2- [4- (cyclohexylcarbamoylsulfamoyl) phenyl] ethyl] -2-methoxy-benzamide) is an oral hypoglycemic medication of the sulphonylureas class, indicated in the treatment of diabetes mellitus type 2. By having nitrogenous functions it is susceptible to undergo nitrosation by reaction with nitrite in the acid medium of the stomach [118]. The sulfas drugs have amine and amide functions in their molecules, for which would be potentially nitrosable (Fig. **10**).

Fig. (10). a) sulfathiazole (HStz, as sodium salt: NaStz) b) Glibenclamide (Glyburide).

Reaction mixtures formed by sodium nitrite and selected sulfa-drugs (sulfathiazole, phtalylsulfathiazole, and the complex formed by sulfathiazole and the metal ion cobalt(II) in acidic medium showed mutagenic effects toward the

Ames test [11].

The Concept of Chemoprevention

The impact of the formation of N-nitrosamines in the stomach can vary significantly in function of nitrite levels and the amount and type of dietary components. Various factors present in the diet may modify the levels of N-nitrosocompounds generated endogenously, acting as catalysts or inhibitors [122]. In this sense, research has been directed towards the search for natural compounds capable of neutralizing the danger they represent. Natural compounds that possess activities anticancer, antimutagenic and other beneficial properties are called chemopreventives. The concept of chemoprevention was postulated initially by Watternberg in 1985. This concept is based on the idea that the consumption of exogenous substances can help to prevent certain types of cancer, especially those caused by chemicals [123].

Many of these substances are present in vegetables, fruits, grains and tea. The consumption of fruits and vegetables has been associated with the prevention of cardiovascular and cerebrovascular diseases and cancer, an effect attributed to its vitamin C, β-carotene, chlorophyll and polyphenols [124]. In past decades, the study of interactions between nitrite and key components of the diet, such as antioxidant phenols, has emerged as an area of increasing interest in the design of chemoprevention strategies, especially after the evaluation of the beneficial effects of green tea catechins, hydroxytyrosol and resveratrol, Mediterranean diets, which are seen today as a model for the improvement of health [125].

L-ascorbic acid and green tea infusions were selected by Pontoriero in her PhD Thesis [108] as antimutagens for sulfa-nitrite mixtures. Such substances, besides being recognized as antimutagens, are easily accessible by the population.

L-ascorbic Acid (AA)

L-ascorbic acid (AA) is a necessary nutrient for humans. It is synthesized by plants and by most mammals, though not by humans and non-human primates. Chemically AA is a carbohydrate (Fig. **9**), widely distributed in nature and vital importance for living organisms.

L-ascorbic acid (AA) or vitamin C can react with nitrous acid leading to the formation of an unstable intermediate with the final generation of dehidroascorbic acid (ADA) and nitric oxide [126] (Fig. **11**).

L-ascorbic acid (AA)   **L-dehydroascorbic acid (ADA)**

$+ 2\,e^- + 2\,H^+$

$(HNO_2 \; + 1\,e^- \; + 1\,H^+ \quad \rightarrow \quad NO + H_2O\,)\,\partial\,2$

Fig. (11). Scheme of the reaction between AA and nitrite in acidic medium.

Vitamin C doses as low as 9 mg to 1 g per day have been shown to inhibit formation of N-nitrosoproline in an extent of between 20 and 100% [127]. By on the other hand, supplementation with 250 mg of L-ascorbic acid decreased the excretion of Nitrosodimethylamine [128]. In a study on the inhibition of nitrosation of aminopyrin and oxytetracycline in saliva proved to be a potent inhibitor of the reaction at pH 3.

Although the normal pH of the oral cavity is 7, we must take into account that in certain areas we can more acidic pHs, such as bacterial plaque, where drugs with nitrite would be more feasible [129].

With respect to other properties of vitamin C over its ability to prevent damage gene, it was observed that vitamin supplementation decreased the frequency of aberrations chromosomal in workers with dietary deficiency exposed to mutagens. Besides, the vitamin C correlated with decreased frequency of micronuclei in smokers, a lower prevalence of DNA adducts in groups exposed to high concentrations of polycyclic aromatic hydrocarbons and a lower level of 8-oxoguanine, indicating damage oxidative [130].

Green Tea

The tea, obtained from *Camellia sinensis*, is the world's most consumed beverage after water. Commercial teas are hybrids of two different ecotypes: the Assam type (Var. Assanica) and the Chinese type (var. Sinensis). The sinensis variety is more resistant to heat and cold, although it is inferior in quantity and quality of performance. In Argentina, tea is cultivated in the provinces of Misiones and Corrientes. Approximately 90% of the production is exported, with Argentina representing 2% of world tea production [131].

Green tea and black tea are obtained from the same plant, but in green tea a treatment that inactivates the enzyme polyphenol oxidase prevents the oxidation of its polyphenols. These polyphenols, known as catechins, belong to the family of flavonoids and are characterized by a di- or tri-hydroxyl group on ring B and a 5,7-dihydroxy target on ring A. Most of the polyphenols present in green tea are monomeric catechins (approximately 70%), of (-)-epicatechin, (-)-epicatechin-3-gallate, (-)-epigallocatechin and (-)-epigallocatechin-3-gallate (Fig. **12**).

Gallic acid may also be found and other phenolic acids such as quercetin, kaferol, myceritin and their glycosides, in addition to polyphenols. Epigallocatechin-3-gallate is the main catechin present in green tea, constituting between 50 and 80% of the total catechins present [132].

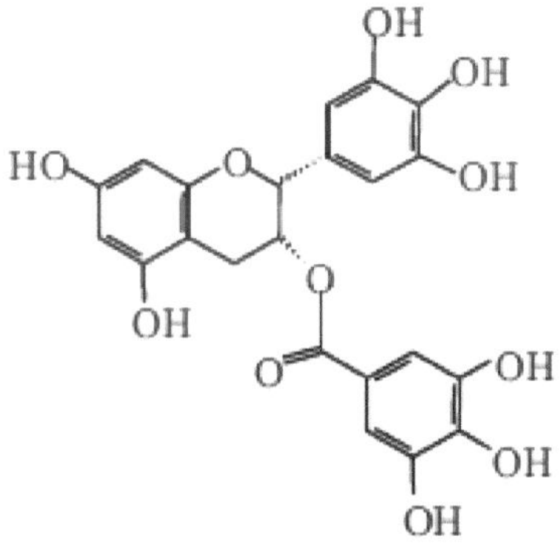

Fig. (12). Tea Polyphenol (−)-Epigallocatechin-3-Gallate.

Historically, tea has been recognized for its beneficial effects on health. It has been shown that epigallocatechin gallate is a powerful antioxidant and can act as an agent antiangiogenic and antitumor. In addition, it is capable of inducing apoptosis and promoting the cell cycle in cancer cells. A number of clinical studies have concluded that the treatment with epigallocatechin-3-gallate inhibits the incidence of tumors in different organs (Lungs, stomach, mammary gland, stomach and skin [133].

Both the monomeric and dimeric epicatechin can act as nitrite scavengers, and that the reaction with nitrous acid leads to the formation of mono- and di-nitroso flavonols. Both the epicatechin and dimer can inhibit the formation of nitrotyrosine and the formation of nitrosodimethylamine.

It was found that the dimer was capable of inhibiting the proliferation of and firing the apoptosis in cancerous cells, presumably through inhibition of a pathway of survival. The dinitroso derivative of the dimer and, to a lesser extent, the epicatechin, also induce apoptosis in cancer cells [134].

BIOLOGICAL TESTS

Ames Test

According to the Ames test, a substance, natural or synthetic, is considered mutagenic when the reversion coefficient: RC (N^o. of revertant colonies per test plate / N^o. of colonies revertants per control plaque - spontaneous) is greater than 2, obtained from the linear part of the curve dose response [9]. Since the mutagenicity criterion is the dose-response relationship, there must be a range in which the number of revertants is increased with the dose [9]. Many mutagens are also toxic, and, consequently, the number of revertants usually decreases with the increase in dose. This problem does not occur in substances of high mutagenic power (aflatoxin B1 for example), since mutagenic power manifests itself at doses much lower than its toxic power. However, there are other substances with low mutagenic power and high toxicity, and it is difficult to find a concentration range in which mutagenic do not be concealed by toxicity.

Experimental

In general terms, in order to evaluate the effect of L-ascorbic acid or green tea on reaction mixtures sulfadrug-nitrite in the Ames test, a constant dose of the mixture was mixed in test tubes reaction, a variable dose of antimutagen and a variable dose of water, in order to bring the tubes to a constant volume. 100 μL of each tube was taken and seeded according to protocol of Ames with strains TA98 and TA100 of *S. typhimurium*. Figs. (**13a** and **b**) shows photos of some made experiences in our laboratory.

In this work we report in the following figures, the results obtained in the Ames test for mixtures of sulfathiazole-nitrite and glibenclamide (antidiabetic, sulfa derivative)-nitrite in the presence and absence of L-ascorbic acid (AA) and green tea aqueous extracts.

In those experiments in which the addition of the antimutagen was made before or after the aggregate of $NaNO_2$, stock solutions of each reagent (NaStz, AA and $NaNO_2$-whose concentrations are indicated in each figure - or an infusion of green tea, and doses of these were mixed in test tubes, with addition of distilled water to bring to constant volume. They were taken 100 μL of each flask and were seeded with TA98 and TA100 strains of *S. typhimurium*, according to Ames Protocol [9, 135].

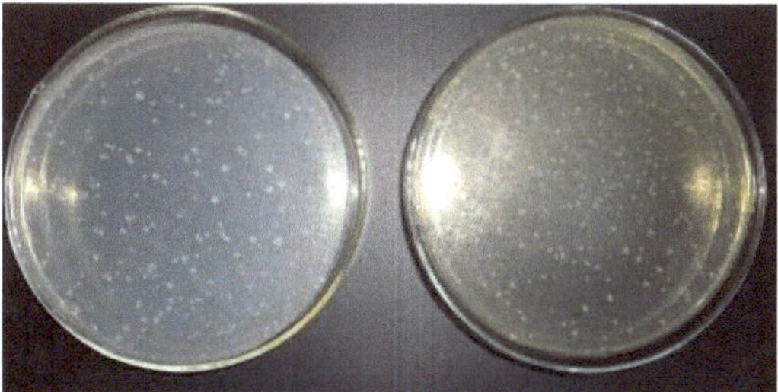

Fig. (13). a) Photo of: (left) spontaneous revertants (TA100 strain) and (right) revertants after treatment with the mixture NaStz-NaNO$_2$ in acidic medium.

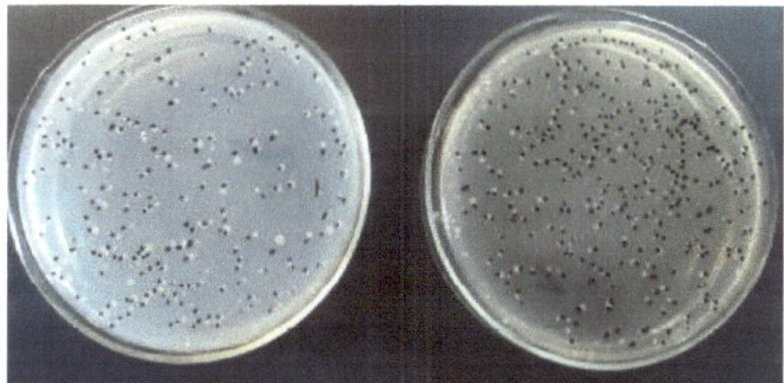

Fig. (13). b) The same previous photo showing the manual counting of revertant colonies.

The percent inhibition of mutagenicity (% Inh.) was calculated according to the following formula:

% Inh. = [(RCwithout AM - RCwith AM) / (RCwithout AM - 1)]·100 [136], where RC: reversion coefficient; AM: antimutagen (AA or green tea)

Previously we had tested the innocuity of the employed antimutagens in the same biological tests (Figs. **14-17**).

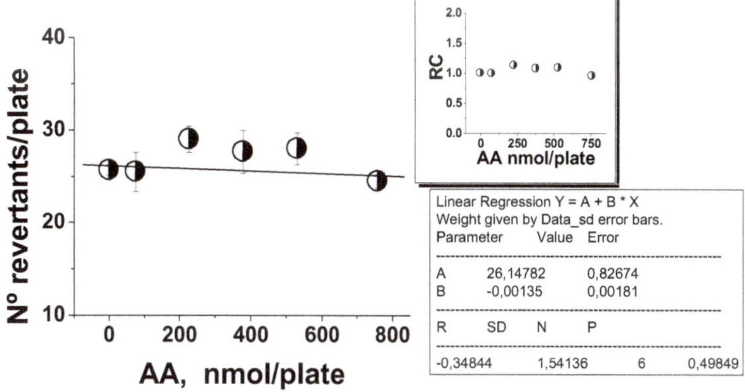

Fig. (14). L-Ascorbic acid did not show mutagenicity in the tested conditions in the Ames test with *S. typhimurium* TA9. y-axis: number of revertant colonies in the petri dish studied.

NaStz-nitrite Mixture

Already in our laboratory we had checked the mutagenicity of sulfatiazol-nitrite mixtures in 1 M HCl [11]. This initial concentration of acid produced a measured pH of about 1 due to the various bases present (NaStz, NO_2^-).

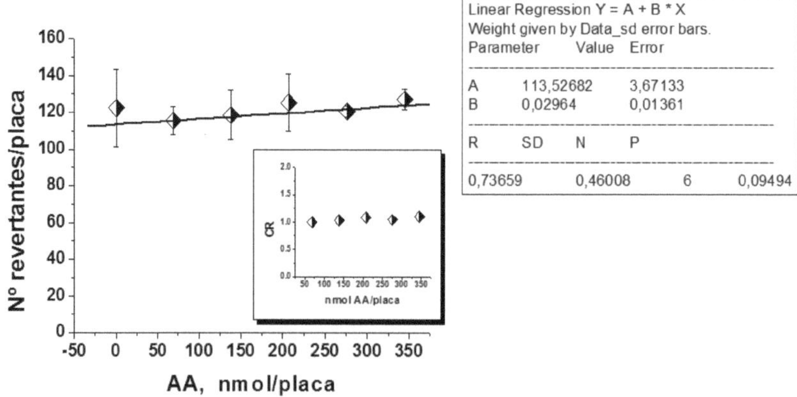

Fig. (15). L-Ascorbic acid did not show mutagenicity in the in the tested conditions in the Ames test with *S. typhimurium* TA100 strain.

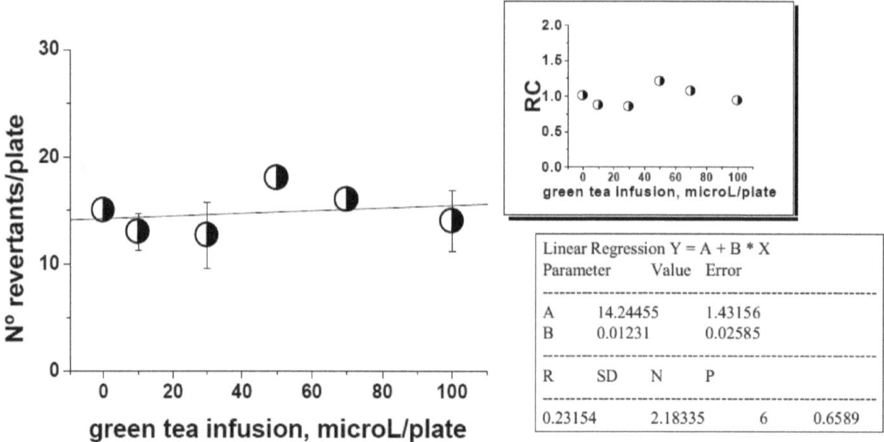

Fig. (16). Green tea extract (μL infusion/plate) did not show mutagenicity in the tested conditions in the Ames test with *S. typhimurium* TA98 strain. y-axis: number of revertant colonies in the petri dish studied.

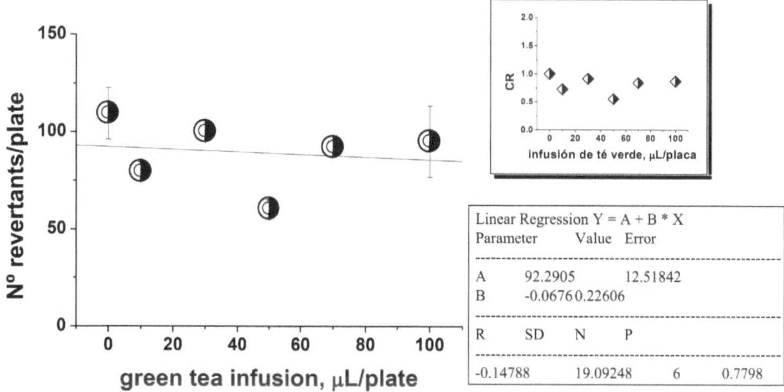

Fig. (17). Green tea extract (μL infusion/plate) did not show mutagenicity in the tested conditions in the Ames test with *S. typhimurium* TA100 strain.

Attempts to work at a pH close to that of the stomach were made at pHs between 2 and 3 (generally titrated as pH $\geq$ 2). First, it was verified if there was mutagenicity due to the mixture that was studied in such conditions. The dose response curves for the NaStz-nitrite mixture in 1/3 molar ratio are presented in Figs. (**18** and **19**) with the TA98 and TA100 strains of *S. typhimurium* respectively. It was graphed in all the cases with respect to the initial concentration of NaStz in the mixture, expressed in nmol/plate.

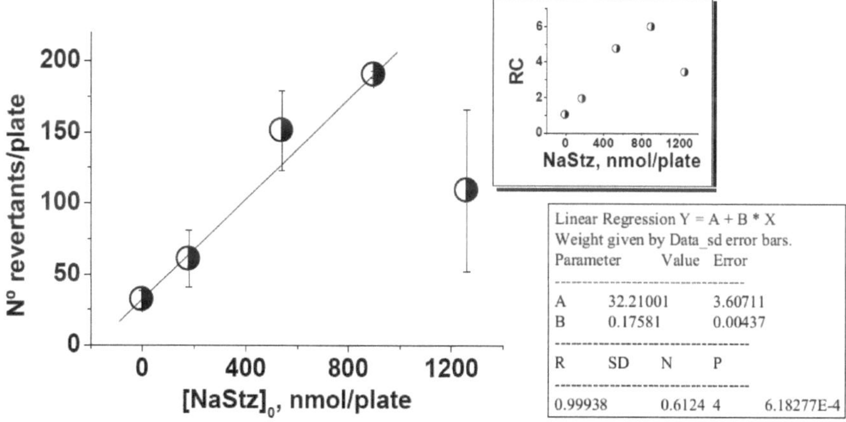

Fig. (18). Reaction mixture sulfathiazole-nitrite showed mutagenicity in the Ames test with *S. typhimurium* TA98 strain. pH 2.0.

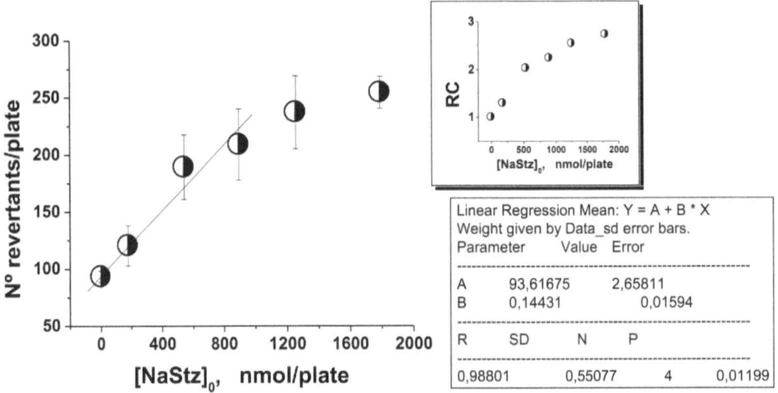

Fig. (19). Reaction mixture sulfathiazole-nitrite showed mutagenicity in the Ames test with *S. typhimurium* TA100 strain. pH 2.4.

A considerable fraction of drugs are theoretically nitrosable due to the presence of amines, amides or other groups which may react with nitrites in the stomach, or even elsewhere, giving N-nitroso compound or other reactive species, potentially mutagenic and/or carcinogenic [118]. In addition to our own experience on the mutagenicity of sulfa-nitrite mixtures in strongly acid medium [137], there are other data in the literature on nitrosation of sulfonamides at higher pHs. Thus, the incubation of sulfanilamide and sodium nitrite in human gastric juice led to the production of genotoxic 1,3-di (4-sulfamoylphenyl) triacene, which was also obtained *in vivo*. The reaction had place in a wide range of conditions (pH 1-4, between 0 and 37 °C) [138].

Linear dose-response curves and CRs greater than 2 were observed for the NaStz-nitrite mixtures at pH 2, (Figs. **10** and **11**) whereby we also found that at pH close to the stomach the mixture NaStz-nitrite is mutagenic. As on other occasions, the points of greatest concentration show RC that do not follow the linear curve, evidencing indications of toxicity.

EFFECT OF L-ASCORBIC ACID (AA) ON THE MUTAGENICITY OF THE NASTZ-NITRITE MIX

It is known that AA exerts effective protection in the case of nitrosable drugs (such as sulfonamides) by reacting with nitrite, reducing or even eliminating the risk of nitrosation [139]. The following figures shown the results of some experiments in which we evaluate the effect of the AA on the NaStz-NaNO$_2$ mixture.

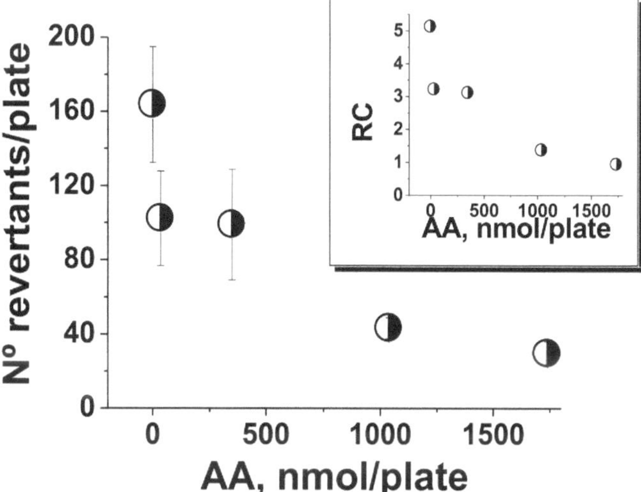

Fig. (20). AA added before nitrite to the reaction mixture inhibited the mutagenic activity of the mixture. strain TA98; [AA max]/[NaNO$_2$]: 1
AA was added before nitrite, *i.e.*: NaStz + HCl + AA + NaNO$_2$
NaStz: 539 nmol/plate NaNO$_2$: 1740 nmol/plate. Control with 1740 nmol AA/plate: 21 ± 3 revertants/plate

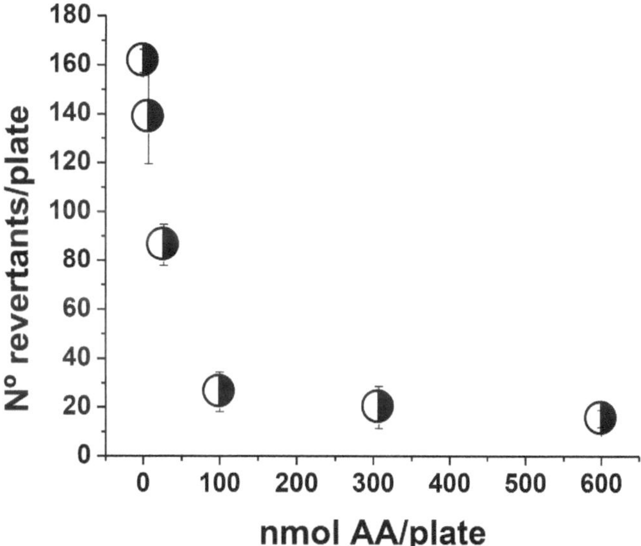

Fig. (21). AA added to the reaction mixture sulfathiazole-nitrite previously formed inhibited the mutagenic activity of the mixture. strain TA98; [AA max]/[NaNO$_2$]:1
AA was added after nitrite, *i.e.*: NaStz + HCl + NaNO$_2$ + AA. AA added after nitrite inhibited mutagenicity
NaStz: 179 nmol/plate NaNO$_2$: 579 nmol/plate. Control with 1740 nmol AA/plate: 21 ± 3 revertants/plate.

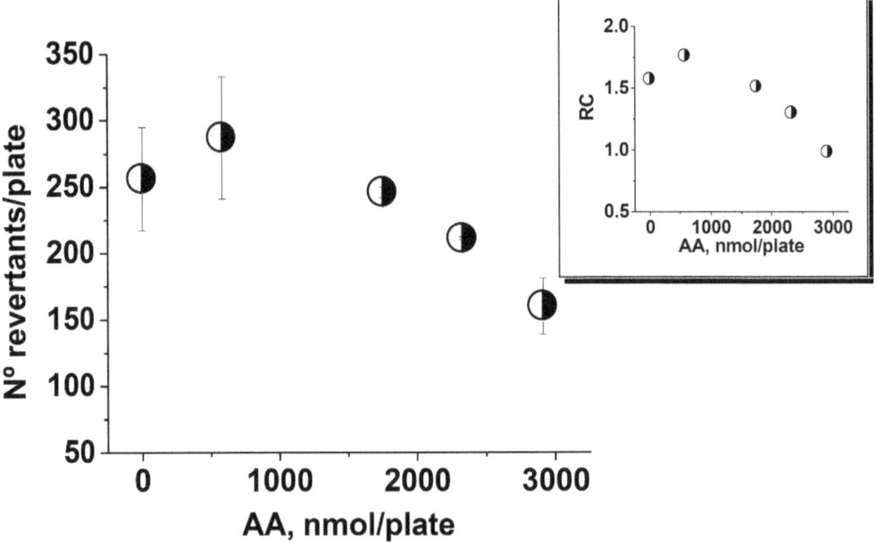

Fig. (22). AA added before nitrite to the reaction mixture inhibited the mutagenic activity of the mixture. Strain TA100; [AA max]/[NaNO2]:1.5. AA was added before nitrite, *i.e.*: NaStz + HCl + AA + $NaNO_2$. AA added before nitrite inhibited mutagenicity. NaStz: 539 nmol/plate $NaNO_2$: 1740 nmol/plate. Control with 1740 nmol AA/plate: 163 ± 9 revertants/plate

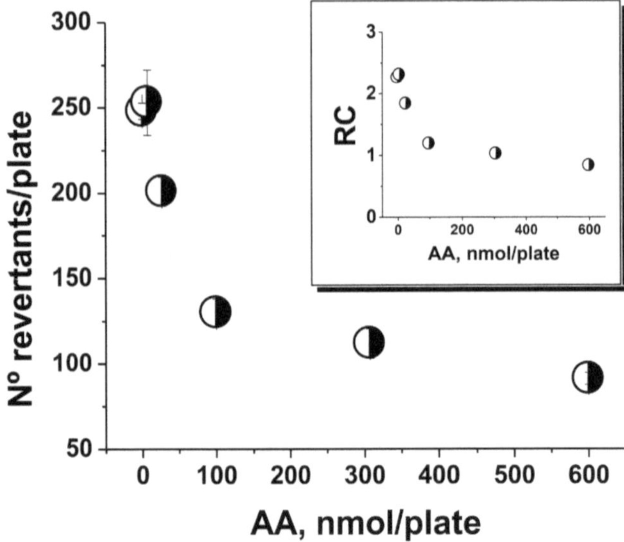

Fig. (23). AA added to the reaction mixture sulfathiazole-nitrite previously formed inhibited the mutagenic activity of the mixture. strain TA100; [AA max]/[NaNO2]:1. AA was added after nitrite, *i.e.*: NaStz + HCl + $NaNO_2$ + AA. AA added after nitrite inhibited mutagenicity. NaStz: 179 nmol/plate $NaNO_2$: 579 nmol/plate. Control with 1740 nmol AA/plate: 106 ± 10 revertants/plate.

EFFECT OF GREEN TEA INFUSION (GT) ON THE MUTAGENICITY OF THE NASTZ-NITRITE MIX

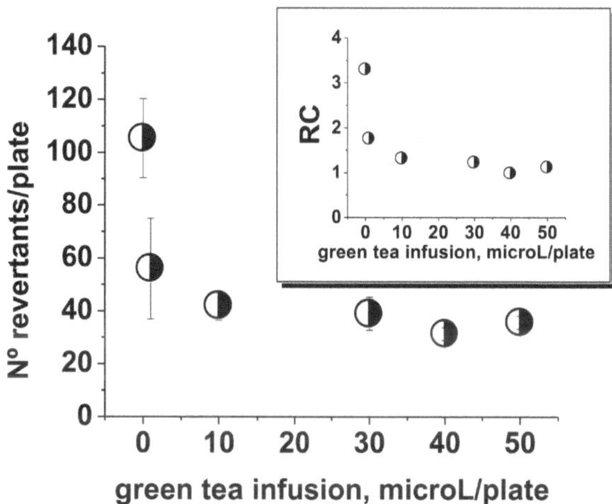

Fig. (24). Green tea infusion, without dilution, added before nitrite to the reaction mixture inhibited the mutagenic activity of the mixture from 10 µL/plate (the first added); strain TA98.

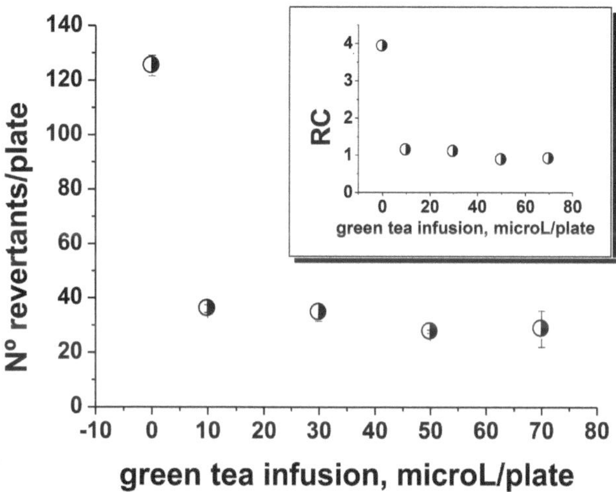

Fig. (25). Green tea infusion, without dilution, added to the reaction mixture sulfathiazole-nitrite previously formed inhibited the mutagenic activity of the mixture from 10 µL/plate (the first added); strain TA98.
GT was added after nitrite, *i.e.*: NaStz + HCl + NaNO$_2$ + GT
GT added after nitrite inhibited mutagenicity. NaStz: 539 nmol/plate NaNO$_2$: 1740 nmol/plate.

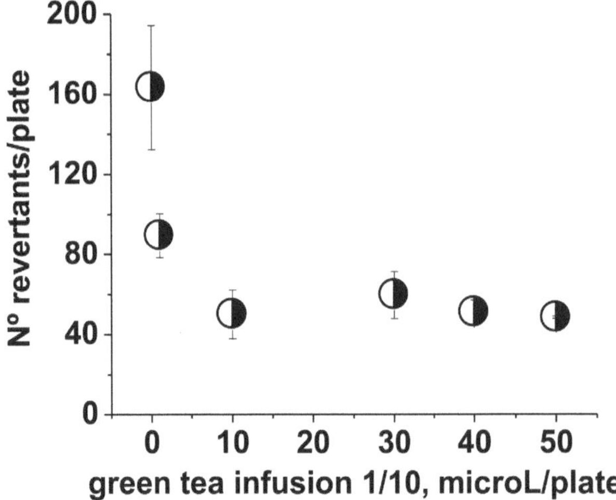

Fig. (26). Green tea infusion, diluted 1/10, added before nitrite to the reaction mixture inhibited the mutagenic activity of the mixture. Strain TA98.
GT was added before nitrite, *i.e.*: NaStz + HCl + GT + NaNO$_2$
GT 1/10 added before nitrite inhibited mutagenicity. NaStz: 539 nmol/plate NaNO$_2$: 1740 nmol/plate.
Spontaneous revertants: 32.00 ± 8.00.

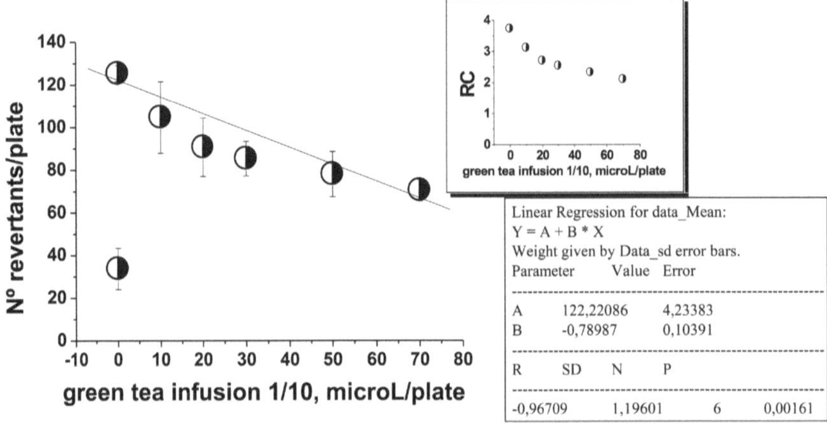

Fig. (27). Green tea infusion, diluted 1/10, added to the reaction mixture sulfathiazole-nitrite previously formed inhibited the mutagenic activity of the mixture following a dose-response curve; strain TA98.
GT was added after nitrite, *i.e.*: NaStz + HCl + NaNO$_2$ + GT
GT 1/10 added after nitrite inhibited mutagenicity. NaStz: 539 nmol/plate NaNO$_2$: 1740 nmol/plate

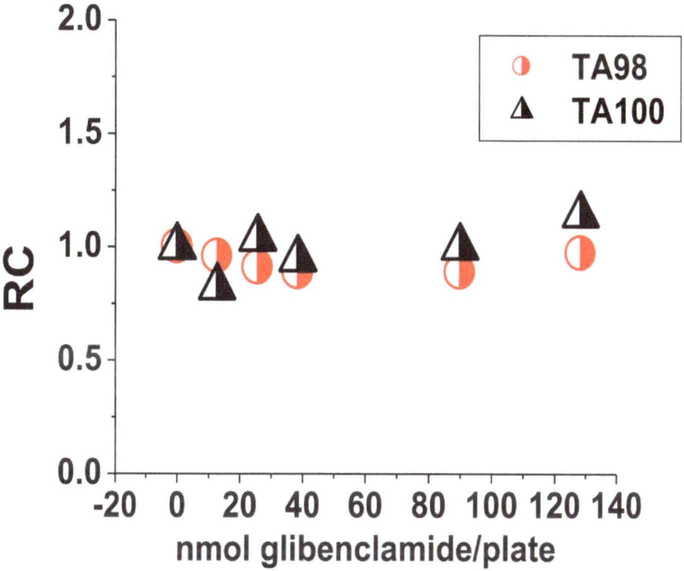

Fig. (28). Increasing concentrations of glibenclamide did not influence the coefficient of reversion of *S. typhimurium* strains TA98 and TA100: glibenclamide did not show mutagenicity in the Ames test in the tested conditions.

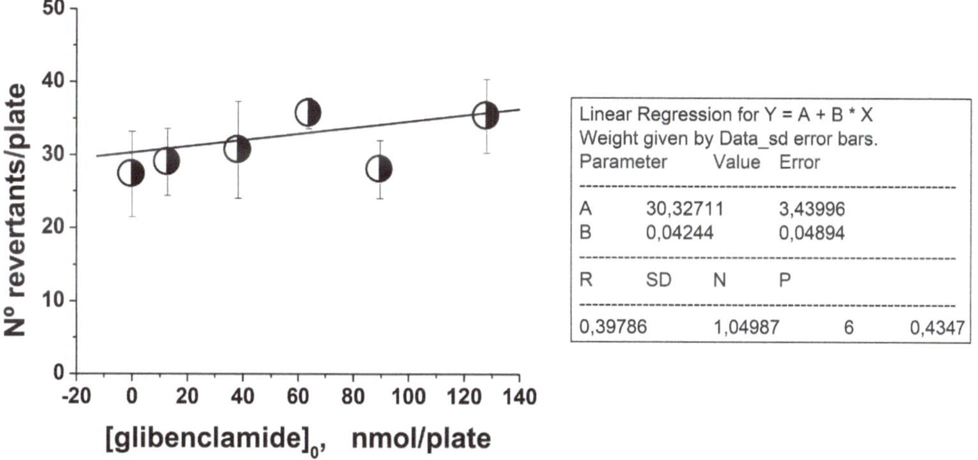

Fig. (29). Glibenclamide-nitrite reaction mixture did not show mutagenicity in the Ames test with *S. typhimurium* TA98 strain in the tested conditions.

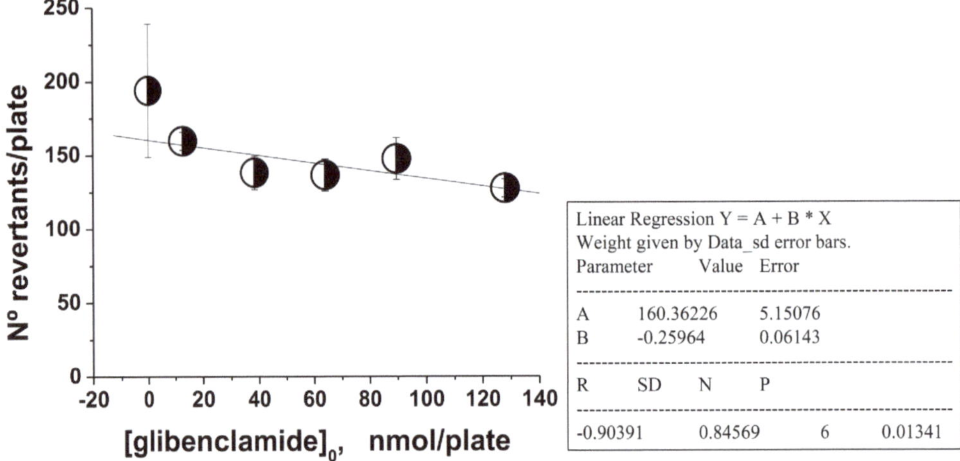

Fig. (30). Glibenclamide-nitrite reaction mixture did not show mutagenicity in the Ames test with *S. typhimurium* TA100 strain in the tested conditions. The negative slope would indicate the toxicity of the mixture on the bacterial strain.

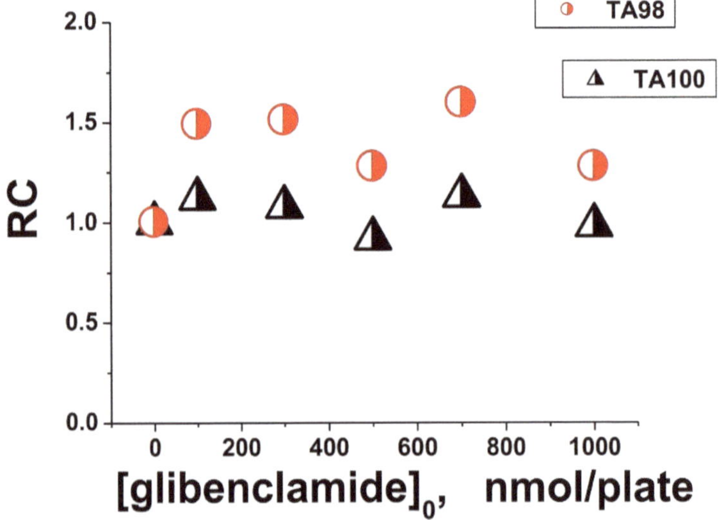

Fig. (31). Glibenclamide-nitrite reaction mixture prepared according to the conditions suggested by the World Health Organization for the study of a drug nitrosabilidad did not show mutagenicity in the Ames test with *S. typhimurium* TA98 and TA100 strain (RC < 2).
NaNO$_2$/glibenclamide: 4/1; [glibenclamide]$_0$: 10 mM; [NaNO$_2$]$_0$: 40 mM; pH: 4

UV-VIS SPECTRA

L-ascorbic Acid (AA)

As it was said, the reaction between AA and nitrite is very rapid, making it very difficult to follow kinetic. Therefore, spectra of a fixed amount of nitrite (500 μL 1.15 x 10^{-3} M) were performed on the addition of increasing amounts of equimolar AA and nitrite solution. The use of UV-Vis spectroscopy for the determination of AA is widely used in food research [140], since this acid presents strong electronic transitions in the UV region, facilitating its identification and quantification by this technique. The molar absorptivity of AA depends on the pH, given the dissociable protons. Taking the peak of maximum absorbance at 242 nm, the measured ε was 1.05×10^{4} $M^{-1} \cdot cm^{-1}$, which is within the values reported in the literature (1.42×10^{4} dm^{3} mol^{-1} cm^{-1} at 266 nm; Beer's law is obeyed in the concentration range of 0.857 - 12.0 μg AA / mL [141].

NaStz-nitrite System

AA

Upon the addition of increasing amounts of AA to the sulfathiazole-nitrite reaction mixture in 0.01 M HCl, the gradual (but instantaneous disappearance in time) disappearance of a peak at 357 nm, present in the reaction mixture without AA, as the antimutagen dose increased (Fig. **32**). The aggregates of AA (in μL) were made 5 min after the start of the reaction NaStz-nitrite.

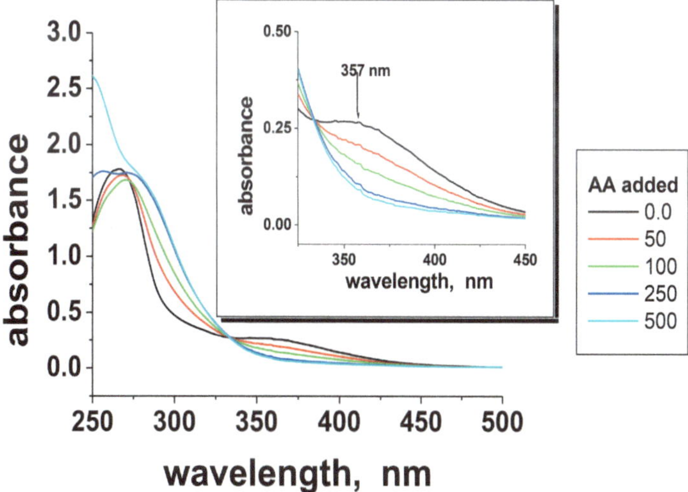

Fig. (32). Spectral pattern of sulfathiazole-nitrite mixture plus AA was the same both AA (μL) being added before or after the nitrite. As the concentration of AA increases, the absorbance at 357 nm decreases.

The same spectra were observed when the nitrite was added before or after nitrite, that is, if the order of reagent addition was: NaStz + HCl + AA + NaNO$_2$ or: NaStz + HCl + NaNO$_2$ + AA the observed spectra were the same. [AA]$_0$ = [NaNO$_2$]$_0$.

NaStz /nitrite molar ratio = 1/3. Medium: 0.01 M HCl

Similar results were observed with green tea.

Green Tea

Fig. (**33**) shows the spectra obtained by dosing total polyphenols in a green tea infusion, by the Folin-Ciocalteu method, in the presence and absence of NaStz-

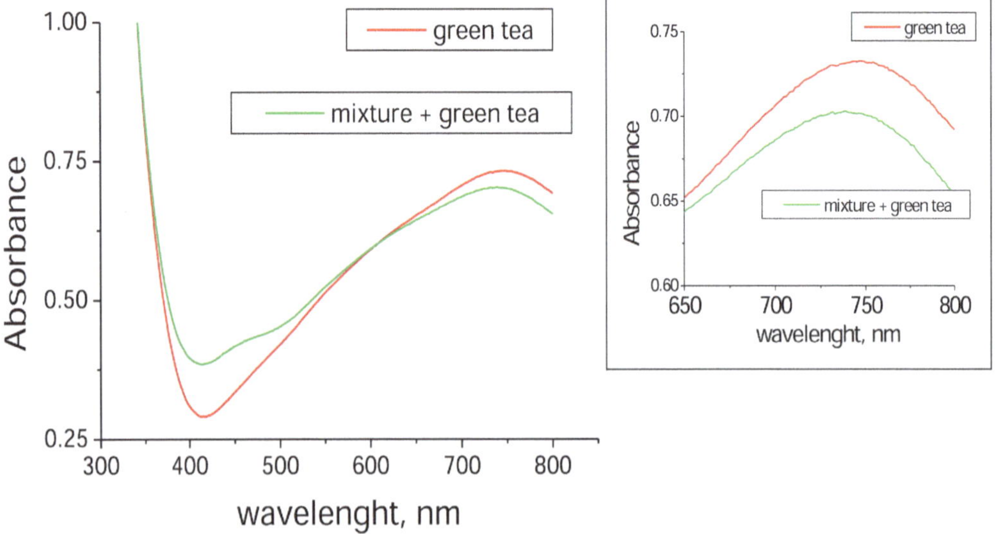

Fig. (33). Obtained spectra measuring total polyphenols in a green tea infusion, in the presence and absence of reaction mixture NaStz-nitrite. NaStz /nitrite molar ratio = 1/3. Medium: 0.01 M HCl. In the inset: detail between 650 and 800 nm.

NaStz-nitrite

In the case of green tea (GT), a new peak was observed at 417 nm, whose intensity increased correlatively to the dose of antimutagen

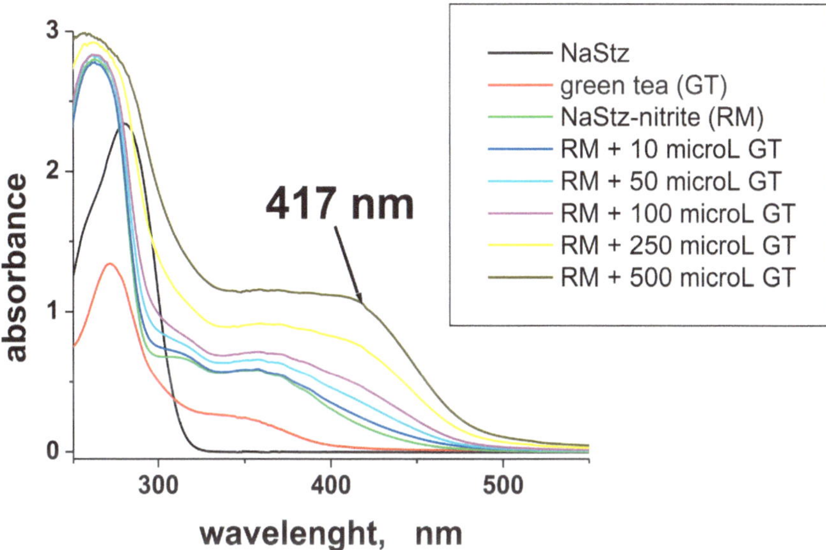

Fig. (34). Spectral pattern of sulfathiazole-nitrite mixture plus GT was the same both GT being added before or after nitrite.

Assuming overlapping of spectra, we work making the differences between them.

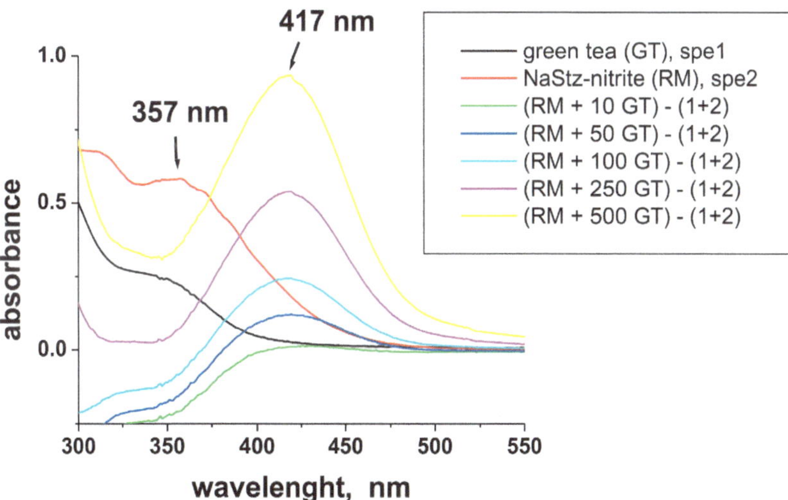

Fig. (35). Differential spectra of the reaction mixture with increasing amounts of green tea minus the sum of the spectra of the mixture and green tea alone showed increased of absorbance at 417 nm and decreased at 357 nm.

In summary, when increasing the concentration of GT, the absorbance at 417 nm increased and at 357 nm it decreased.

Glibenclamide

In the glibenclamide-nitrite system in 0.01 M HCl medium in 1: 1 DMSO-water no modification was observed in the glibenclamide peak, maintaining the absorbance maximum at 301 nm (Fig. **36**).

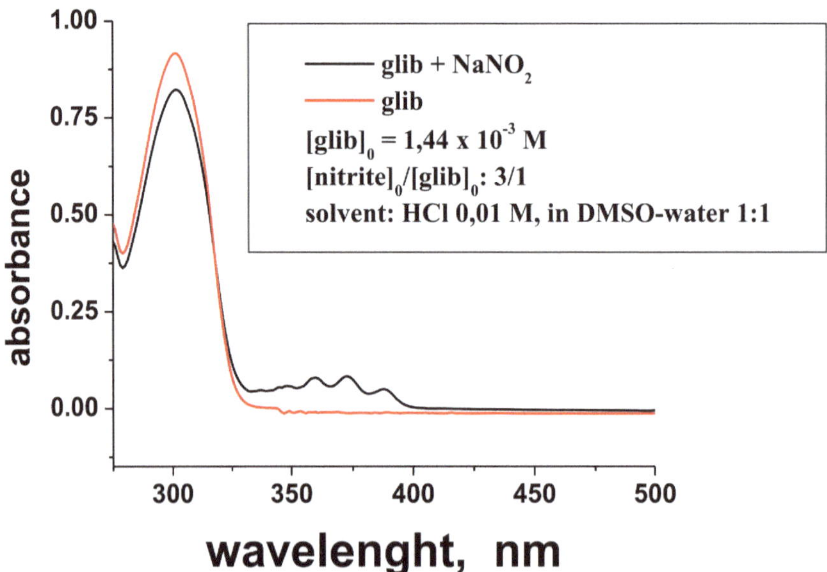

Fig. (36). Electronic spectra of glibenclamide in the presence and absence of NaNO$_2$. the transitions observed in the glib+ NaNO$_2$ spectrum between 350 and 400 nm are due to the nitrite spectrum alone.

This evidence of non-reactivity between glibenclamide and nitrite in acid medium is consistent with the lack of mutagenicity of said system in the Ames test with both strains tested (TA98 and TA100).

CONCLUDING REMARKS

Sulfonamides, which are widely used for their various properties (antimicrobial, antidiabetic, herbicides, analytical reagents, *etc*.) are potentially nitrosatable due to its amine and/or amide functions. Previously we found mutagenicity in reaction mixtures formed by selected sulfonamide and nitrite [11], so, we began to study the antimutagenic activity of L-ascorbic acid (AA) and green tea extracts on the acute toxicity and mutagenicity of these reaction mixtures by means of the *Allium* and Ames tests and by electronic spectroscopic analysis and we reach the following conclusions:

• AA and green tea infusion showed a high ability to inhibit the direct mutagenicity of reaction mixtures sulfonamide-nitrite (tested sulfonamides: sodium sulfathiazole, complex cobalt(III)-sulfathiazole [108], the latter not shown here), either added before or after the nitrite, at pH 1-2.

- No direct mutagenicity was observed in the glibenclamide-nitrite system in the Ames test. The UV-Vis spectra allow to check that there is no reaction between the said sulfonylurea and nitrite in the experimental conditions.

- For all the above, both AA and green tea infusions are presented as effective antimutagens to mitigate the mutagenicity of mixtures sulfonamide-nitrite in acidic media [142].

In brief, the possibility for dietary prevention and modification of mutagen formation is a subjet of current discussion and future avenues for further research [142].

CONSENT FOR PUBLICATION

Not applicable.

CONFLICT OF INTEREST

The author(s) confirm that this chapter content has no conflict of interest.

ACKNOWLEDGEMENT

We thanks the National University of Rosario for financial support. A.P. did her doctoral thesis with a CONICET grant.

REFERENCES

[1]   World Health Organization Environmental Health Criteria. **1985**. *apps.who.int/iris/bitstream/10665/38607/1/9241541911-corr-eng.pdf http://www.inchem.org/documents/ehc/ehc/ehc51.htm,*

[2]   Mundry, M. D.; Carballo, M. A. *Genética Toxicológica*; De los Cuatro Vientos: Buenos Aires, **2006**, pp. 45-46.

[3]   Bishop, J.M. The molecular genetics of cancer. *Science,* **1987**, *235*(4786), 305-311.
      [http://dx.doi.org/10.1126/science.3541204] [PMID: 3541204]

[4]   Cohen, S.M.; Arnold, L.L. Chem. carcinogenesis. *Toxicol. Sci.,* **2011**, *120*, 76-92.
      [http://dx.doi.org/10.1093/toxsci/kfq365]

[5]   Uhl, M.; Plewa, M.J.; Majer, B.J.; Knasmüller, S. Basic principles of genetic toxicology with an emphasis on plant bioassays.*Bioassays in Plant Cells for Improvement of Ecosystem and human Health: A course manual*; Maluszynska, J.; Plewa, M., Eds.; Katowice, Poland, **2003**, pp. 11-30.

[6]   Mundry, M.D.; Carballo, M.A. *Genética Toxicológica*; De los Cuatro Vientos: Buenos Aires, **2006**, p. 319.

[7]   Ben Rhouma, G.; Chebil, L.; Krifa, M.; Ghoul, M.; Chekir-Ghedira, L. Evaluation of mutagenic and antimutagenic activities of oligorutin and oligoesculin. *Food Chem.,* **2012**, *135*(3), 1700-1707.
      [http://dx.doi.org/10.1016/j.foodchem.2012.06.029] [PMID: 22953912]

[8]   Claxton, L.D.; Allen, J.; Auletta, A.; Mortelmans, K.; Nestmann, E.; Zeiger, E. Guide for the *Salmonella typhimurium*/mammalian microsome tests for bacterial mutagenicity. *Mutat. Res.,* **1987**, *189*(2), 83-91.
        [http://dx.doi.org/10.1016/0165-1218(87)90014-0] [PMID: 3309640]

[9]   Maron, D.M.; Ames, B.N. Revised methods for the *Salmonella* mutagenicity test. *Mutat. Res.,* **1983**, *113*(3-4), 173-215.
        [http://dx.doi.org/10.1016/0165-1161(83)90010-9] [PMID: 6341825]

[10]   DeMarini, D.M. Induction of mutation spectra by complex mixtures: approaches, problems, and possibilities. *Environ. Health Perspect.,* **1994**, *102* Suppl. 4, 127-130.
        [PMID: 7821286]

[11]   Trossero, C.; Pontoriero, A.; Hure, E.; Monti, L.; Gorr, C.; Mosconi, N.; Caffarena, G.; Rizzotto, M. Reaction mixtures formed by nitrite and selected sulfa-drugs showed mutagenicity in acidic medium. *Quim. Nova,* **2009**, *32*, 1151-1156.
        [http://dx.doi.org/10.1590/S0100-40422009000500013]

[12]   Fernandes, T.C.; Mazzeo, D.E.; Marin-Morales, M.A. Origin of nuclear and chromosomal alterations derived from the action of an aneugenic agent--Trifluralin herbicide. *Ecotoxicol. Environ. Saf.,* **2009**, *72*(6), 1680-1686.
        [http://dx.doi.org/10.1016/j.ecoenv.2009.03.014] [PMID: 19419762]

[13]   Leme, D.M.; Marin-Morales, M.A. Chromosome aberration and micronucleus frequencies in *Allium cepa* cells exposed to petroleum polluted water-a case study. *Mutat. Res.,* **2008**, *650*(1), 80-86.
        [http://dx.doi.org/10.1016/j.mrgentox.2007.10.006] [PMID: 18068420]

[14]   Vega, M.; Mosconi, N.; Toplikar, B.; Coca, V.; Rizzotto, M. The test of *Allium cepa* L .: an effective method for the detection of phyto, cyto and genotoxicity of the promutagen 2-aminofluorene. *BIOCELL,* **2016**, *40*(suppl. 4), 10.

[15]   Leme, D.M.; Marin-Morales, M.A. *Allium cepa* test in environmental monitoring: a review on its application. *Mutat. Res.,* **2009**, *682*(1), 71-81.
        [http://dx.doi.org/10.1016/j.mrrev.2009.06.002] [PMID: 19577002]

[16]   Venitt, S.; Parry, J.M. *Mutagenicity Testing: A Practical Approach*; IRL Press: USA, **1984**.

[17]   Bhattacharya, S. Natural Antimutagens: A Review. *Res. J. Med. Plant,* **2011**, *5*, 116-126.
        [http://dx.doi.org/10.3923/rjmp.2011.116.126]

[18]   Sreeranjini, S.; Siril, E.A. Evaluation of anti-genotoxicity of the leaf extracts of *Morinda citrifolia* Linn. *Plant Soil Environ.,* **2011**, *57*, 222-227.
        [http://dx.doi.org/10.17221/376/2010-PSE]

[19]   Oyeyemi, I.T.; Bakare, A.A. Genotoxic and anti-genotoxic effect of aqueous extracts of *Spondias mombin* L., *Nymphea lotus* L. and *Luffa cylindrica* L. on *Allium cepa* root tip cells. *Caryologia,* **2013**, *66*, 360-367.
        [http://dx.doi.org/10.1080/00087114.2013.857829]

[20]   Boone, C.W.; Kelloff, G.J.; Malone, W.E. Identification of cancer chemotherapy agents and their evaluation in animal models and human clinical trials: A review. *Cancer Res.,* **1990**, *50*, 2-9.
        [PMID: 2403415]

[21]   Srinivasan, K. Antimutagenic and cancer preventive potential of culinary spices and their bioactive compounds. *PharmaNutrition,* **2017**, *5*, 89-102.
        [http://dx.doi.org/10.1016/j.phanu.2017.06.001]

[22]   Shankel, D.M.; Pillai, S.P.; Telikepalli, H.; Menon, S.R.; Pillai, C.A.; Mitscher, L.A. Role of antimutagens/anticarcinogens in cancer prevention. *Biofactors,* **2000**, *12*(1-4), 113-121.
        [http://dx.doi.org/10.1002/biof.5520120118] [PMID: 11216471]

[23]   Edenharder, R.; Tang, X. Inhibition of the mutagenicity of 2-nitrofluorene, 3-nitrofluoranthene and 1-

nitropyrene by flavonoids, coumarins, quinones and other phenolic compounds. *Food Chem. Toxicol.,* **1997**, *35*(3-4), 357-372.
[http://dx.doi.org/10.1016/S0278-6915(97)00125-7] [PMID: 9207898]

[24]   Amoo, S.O.; Aremu, A.O.; Van Staden, J. Unraveling the medicinal potential of South African Aloe species. *J. Ethnopharmacol.,* **2014**, *153*(1), 19-41.
[http://dx.doi.org/10.1016/j.jep.2014.01.036] [PMID: 24509153]

[25]   Jia, Y.; Zhao, G.; Jia, J. Preliminary evaluation: the effects of *Aloe ferox* Miller and *Aloe arborescens* Miller on wound healing. *J. Ethnopharmacol.,* **2008**, *120*(2), 181-189.
[http://dx.doi.org/10.1016/j.jep.2008.08.008] [PMID: 18773950]

[26]   Bezanger-Beauquesne, L.; Pinkas, M.; Torck, M.; Trotin, F. *Plantes medicinales des regions temperees*; , **1980**.

[27]   Mueller, S.O.; Schmitt, M.; Dekant, W.; Stopper, H.; Schlatter, J.; Schreier, P.; Lutz, W.K. Occurrence of emodin, chrysophanol and physcion in vegetables, herbs and liquors. Genotoxicity and anti-genotoxicity of the anthraquinones and of the whole plants. *Food Chem. Toxicol.,* **1999**, *37*(5), 481-491.
[http://dx.doi.org/10.1016/S0278-6915(99)00027-7] [PMID: 10456676]

[28]   Ammar, R.B.; Sghaier, M.B.; Boubaker, J.; Bhouri, W.; Naffeti, A.; Skandrani, I.; Bouhlel, I.; Kilani, S.; Ghedira, K.; Chekir-Ghedira, L. Antioxidant activity and inhibition of aflatoxin B1-, nifuroxazide-, and sodium azide-induced mutagenicity by extracts from Rhamnus alaternus L. *Chem. Biol. Interact.,* **2008**, *174*(1), 1-10.
[http://dx.doi.org/10.1016/j.cbi.2008.04.006] [PMID: 18511029]

[29]   Gonzáez de Mejía, E.; Quintanar-Hernández, A.; Loarca-Piña, G. Antimutagenic activity of carotenoids in green peppers against some nitroarenes. *Mutat. Res.,* **1998**, *416*(1-2), 11-19.
[http://dx.doi.org/10.1016/S1383-5718(98)00070-9] [PMID: 9725989]

[30]   Salvadori, D.M.; Ribeiro, L.R.; Natarajan, A.T. Effect of beta-carotene on clastogenic effects of mitomycin C, methyl methanesulphonate and bleomycin in Chinese hamster ovary cells. *Mutagenesis,* **1994**, *9*(1), 53-57.
[http://dx.doi.org/10.1093/mutage/9.1.53] [PMID: 7516036]

[31]   Swami, S.B.; Thakor, N.J.; Haldankar, P.M.; Kalse, S.B. Jackfruit and its many functional components as related to human health: A review. *Compr. Rev. Food Sci. Food Saf.,* **2012**, *11*, 565-576.
[http://dx.doi.org/10.1111/j.1541-4337.2012.00210.x]

[32]   Ruiz-Montañez, G.; Burgos-Hernández, A.; Calderón-Santoyo, M.; López-Saiz, C.M.; Velázquez-Contreras, C.A.; Navarro-Ocaña, A.; Ragazzo-Sánchez, J.A. Screening antimutagenic and antiproliferative properties of extracts isolated from Jackfruit pulp (*Artocarpus heterophyllus* Lam). *Food Chem.,* **2015**, *175*, 409-416.
[http://dx.doi.org/10.1016/j.foodchem.2014.11.122] [PMID: 25577099]

[33]   Ramirez-Victoria, P.; Guzman-Rincon, J.; Espinosa-Aguirre, J.J.; Murillo-Romero, S. Antimutagenic effect of one variety of green pepper (Capsicum spp.) and its possible interference with the nitrosation process. *Mutat. Res.,* **2001**, *496*(1-2), 39-45.
[http://dx.doi.org/10.1016/S1383-5718(01)00217-0] [PMID: 11551479]

[34]   Joseph, B.; Raj, S.J. Phytopharmacological and phytochemical properties of three *ficus* species: An overview. *Int. J. Pharma Bio Sci.,* **2010**, *1*, 246-253.

[35]   Anwar, F.; Latif, S.; Ashraf, M.; Gilani, A.H. *Moringa oleifera*: a food plant with multiple medicinal uses. *Phytother. Res.,* **2007**, *21*(1), 17-25.
[http://dx.doi.org/10.1002/ptr.2023] [PMID: 17089328]

[36]   Satish, A.; Punith Kumar, R.; Rakshith, D.; Satish, S.; Ahmed, F. Antimutagenic and antioxidant activity of *Ficus benghalensis* stem bark and *Moringa oleifera* root extract. *Int. J. Chem. Anal. Sci.,* **2013**, *4*, 45-48.
[http://dx.doi.org/10.1016/j.ijcas.2013.03.008]

[37]   Shankel, D.M.; Pillai, S.P.; Telikepalli, H.; Menon, S.R.; Pillai, C.A.; Mitscher, L.A. Role of antimutagens/anticarcinogens in cancer prevention. *Biofactors,* **2000**, *12*(1-4), 113-121.
[http://dx.doi.org/10.1002/biof.5520120118] [PMID: 11216471]

[38]   Wall, M.E.; Wani, M.C.; Manikumar, G.; Hughes, T.J.; Taylor, H.; McGivney, R.; Warner, J. Plant antimutagenic agents, 3. Coumarins. *J. Nat. Prod.,* **1988**, *51*(6), 1148-1152.
[http://dx.doi.org/10.1021/np50060a016] [PMID: 3069958]

[39]   Vázquez-García, J.A.; Jimeno-S, D.; Cuevas-G, R.; Cházaro-B, M.; Muñiz-Castro, M.A. *Echeveria yalmanantlanensis* (Crassulaceae): a new species from Cerro Grande, Sierra de Manantlán, Western Mexico. *Brittonia,* **2013**, *65*, 273-279.
[http://dx.doi.org/10.1007/s12228-012-9274-9]

[40]   Jimeno-Sevilla, H.D.; Hernández-Ramírez, A.M.; Ornelas, J.F.; Marten-Rodríguez, S. Morphological and nectar traits in *Echeveria rosea* Lindley (Crassulaceae) linked to hummingbird pollination in central Veracruz, Mexico. *Haseltonia,* **2014**, 17-25.
[http://dx.doi.org/10.2985/026.019.0104]

[41]   Martínez Ruiz, M.G.; Gómez-Velasco, A.; Juárez, Z.N.; Hernández, L.R.; Bach, H. Exploring the biological activities of *Echeveria leucotricha. Nat. Prod. Res.,* **2013**, *27*(12), 1123-1126.
[http://dx.doi.org/10.1080/14786419.2012.708662] [PMID: 22845689]

[42]   López-Angulo, G.; Montes-Avila, J.; Páz Díaz-Camacho, S.; Vega-Aviña, R.; Báez-Flores, M.E.; Delgado-Vargas, F. Bioactive components and antimutagenic and antioxidant activities of two *Echeveria* DC. species. *Ind. Crops Prod.,* **2016**, *85*, 38-48.
[http://dx.doi.org/10.1016/j.indcrop.2016.02.044]

[43]   Gerardi, C.; Frassinetti, S.; Caltavuturo, L.; Leone, A.; Lecci, R.; Calabriso, N.; Carluccio, M.A.; Blando, F.; Mita, G. Anti-proliferative, anti-inflammatory and anti-mutagenic activities of a *Prunus mahaleb* L. anthocyanin-rich fruit extract. *J. Funct. Foods,* **2016**, *27*, 537-548.
[http://dx.doi.org/10.1016/j.jff.2016.09.024]

[44]   Calomme, M.; Pieters, L.; Vlietinck, A.; Vanden Berghe, D. Inhibition of bacterial mutagenesis by Citrus flavonoids. *Planta Med.,* **1996**, *62*(3), 222-226.
[http://dx.doi.org/10.1055/s-2006-957864] [PMID: 8693033]

[45]   Rustaiyan, A.; Masoudi, S. Chemical composition and biological activities of Iranian *Artemisia* species. *Phytochem. Lett.,* **2011**, *4*, 440-447.
[http://dx.doi.org/10.1016/j.phytol.2011.07.003]

[46]   Canadanovic-Brunett, J.M.; Djilas, S.M.; Cetkovic, G.S.; Tumbas, V.T. Free-radical scavenging activity of wormwood (*Artemisia absinthium*) extracts. *J. Sci. Food Agric.,* **2005**, *85*, 265-272.
[http://dx.doi.org/10.1002/jsfa.1950]

[47]   Taherkhani, M.; Rustaiyan, A.; Taherkhani, T. Chemical composition, antimicrobial activity, antioxidant and total phenolic content within the leaves essential oil of *Artemisia absinthium* L. growing wild in Iran. *Afr. J. Pharm. Pharmacol.,* **2013**, *7*, 30-36.
[http://dx.doi.org/10.5897/AJPP12.945]

[48]   Aicha, N.; Skandrani, I.; Ben Sghaier, M.; Bouhlel, I.; Kilani, S.; Ghedira, K.; Neffati, M.; Chraief, I.; Hammami, M.; Chekir-Ghedira, L. Chemical composition, mutagenic and antimutagenic activities of essential oils from (Tunisian) *Artemisia campestris* and *Artemisia herba-alba. J. Essent. Oil Res.,* **2008**, *20*, 471-477.
[http://dx.doi.org/10.1080/10412905.2008.9700061]

[49]   Taherkhani, M. Mutagenic and antimutagenic activities of *Artemisia absinthium* volatile oil by the bacterial reverse mutation assay in *Salmonella typhimurium* strains TA98 and TA100. *Asian Pac. J. Trop. Dis.,* **2014**, *4* Suppl. 2, S840-S844.
[http://dx.doi.org/10.1016/S2222-1808(14)60739-8]

[50]   Erickson, L. Rooibos tea: research into antioxidant and antimutagenic properties. *HerbalGram.,* **2003**,

59, 34-45.

[51]   van der Merwe, J.D.; Joubert, E.; Richards, E.S.; Manley, M.; Snijman, P.W.; Marnewick, J.L.; Gelderblom, W.C.A. A comparative study on the antimutagenic properties of aqueous extracts of *Aspalathus linearis* (rooibos), different *Cyclopia* spp. (honeybush) and *Camellia sinensis* teas. *Mutat. Res.,* **2006**, *611*(1-2), 42-53.
       [http://dx.doi.org/10.1016/j.mrgentox.2006.06.030] [PMID: 16949333]

[52]   Snijman, P.W.; Swanevelder, S.; Joubert, E.; Green, I.R.; Gelderblom, W.C.A. The antimutagenic activity of the major flavonoids of rooibos (*Aspalathus linearis*): some dose-response effects on mutagen activation-flavonoid interactions. *Mutat. Res.,* **2007**, *631*(2), 111-123.
       [http://dx.doi.org/10.1016/j.mrgentox.2007.03.009] [PMID: 17537670]

[53]   Woźniak, D.; Oszmiański, J.; Matkowski, A. Antimutagenic and antioxidant activity of the extract from Belamcanda chinensis (L.) DC. *Acta Pol. Pharm.,* **2006**, *63*(3), 213-218.
       [PMID: 20085227]

[54]   Thelen, P.; Scharf, J.G.; Burfeind, P.; Hemmerlein, B.; Wuttke, W.; Spengler, B.; Christoffel, V.; Ringert, R.H.; Seidlová-Wuttke, D. Tectorigenin and other phytochemicals extracted from leopard lily *Belamcanda chinensis* affect new and established targets for therapies in prostate cancer. *Carcinogenesis,* **2005**, *26*(8), 1360-1367.
       [http://dx.doi.org/10.1093/carcin/bgi092] [PMID: 15845653]

[55]   Wozniak, D.; Janda, B.; Kapusta, I.; Oleszek, W.; Matkowski, A. Antimutagenic and anti-oxidant activities of isoflavonoids from *Belamcanda chinensis* (L.) DC. *Mutat. Res.,* **2010**, *696*(2), 148-153.
       [http://dx.doi.org/10.1016/j.mrgentox.2010.01.004] [PMID: 20096370]

[56]   Seo, W.G.; Pae, H-O.; Oh, G-S.; Chai, K.Y.; Kwon, T.O.; Yun, Y-G.; Kim, N-Y.; Chung, H-T. Inhibitory effects of methanol extract of Cyperus rotundus rhizomes on nitric oxide and superoxide productions by murine macrophage cell line, RAW 264.7 cells. *J. Ethnopharmacol.,* **2001**, *76*(1), 59-64.
       [http://dx.doi.org/10.1016/S0378-8741(01)00221-5] [PMID: 11378282]

[57]   Kilani, S.; Ben Ammar, R.; Bouhlel, I.; Abdelwahed, A.; Hayder, N.; Mahmoud, A.; Ghedira, K.; Chekir-Ghedira, L. Investigation of extracts from (Tunisian) *Cyperus rotundus* as antimutagens and radical scavengers. *Environ. Toxicol. Pharmacol.,* **2005**, *20*(3), 478-484.
       [http://dx.doi.org/10.1016/j.etap.2005.05.012] [PMID: 21783629]

[58]   Gupta, S.; Saha, B.; Giri, A.K. Comparative antimutagenic and anticlastogenic effects of green tea and black tea: a review. *Mutat. Res.,* **2002**, *512*(1), 37-65.
       [http://dx.doi.org/10.1016/S1383-5742(02)00024-8] [PMID: 12220589]

[59]   Lee, I.P.; Kim, Y.H.; Kang, M.H.; Roberts, C.; Shim, J.S.; Roh, J.K. Chemopreventive effect of green tea (*Camellia sinensis*) against cigarette smoke-induced mutations (SCE) in humans. *J. Cell. Biochem. Suppl.,* **1997**, *27*, 68-75.
       [http://dx.doi.org/10.1002/(SICI)1097-4644(1997)27+<68::AID-JCB12>3.0.CO;2-H]   [PMID: 9591195]

[60]   Parvathy, K.; Negi, P.S.; Srinivas, P. Curcumin–amino acid conjugates: Synthesis, antioxidant and antimutagenic attributes. *Food Chem.,* **2010**, *120*, 523-530.
       [http://dx.doi.org/10.1016/j.foodchem.2009.10.047]

[61]   Silva, I.C.; Polaquini, C.R.; Regasini, L.O.; Ferreira, H.; Pavan, F.R. Evaluation of cytotoxic, apoptotic, mutagenic, and chemopreventive activities of semi-synthetic esters of gallic acid. *Food Chem. Toxicol.,* **2017**, *105*, 300-307.
       [http://dx.doi.org/10.1016/j.fct.2017.04.033] [PMID: 28454784]

[62]   Khajeh, M.; Yamini, Y.; Sefidkon, F.; Bahramifar, N. Comparison of essential oil composition of *Carum copticum* obtained by supercritical carbon dioxide extraction and hydrodistillation methods. *Food Chem.,* **2004**, *86*, 587-591.
       [http://dx.doi.org/10.1016/j.foodchem.2003.09.041]

[63]   Zahin, M.; Ahmad, I.; Aqil, F. Antioxidant and antimutagenic activity of *Carum copticum* fruit extracts. *Toxicol. In Vitro,* **2010**, *24*(4), 1243-1249.
[http://dx.doi.org/10.1016/j.tiv.2010.02.004] [PMID: 20149861]

[64]   Sharma, R.A.; Gescher, A.J.; Steward, W.P. Curcumin: the story so far. *Eur. J. Cancer,* **2005**, *41*(13), 1955-1968.
[http://dx.doi.org/10.1016/j.ejca.2005.05.009] [PMID: 16081279]

[65]   Shishu, I.P.K. Antimutagenicity of curcumin and related compounds against genotoxic heterocyclic amines from cooked food: The structural requirement. *Food Chem.,* **2008**, *111*, 573-579.
[http://dx.doi.org/10.1016/j.foodchem.2008.04.022]

[66]   Goli, A.H.; Barzegar, M.; Sahari, M.A.; Sahari, M.A. Antioxidant activity and total phenolic compounds of pistachio (*Pistachia vera*) hull extracts. *Food Chem.,* **2005**, *92*, 521-525.
[http://dx.doi.org/10.1016/j.foodchem.2004.08.020]

[67]   Rajaei, A.; Barzegar, M.; Mobarez, A.M.; Sahari, M.A.; Esfahani, Z.H. Antioxidant, anti-microbial and antimutagenicity activities of pistachio (*Pistachia vera*) green hull extract. *Food Chem. Toxicol.,* **2010**, *48*(1), 107-112.
[http://dx.doi.org/10.1016/j.fct.2009.09.023] [PMID: 19781589]

[68]   Bahadori, M.B.; Valizadeh, H.; Farimani, M.M. Chemical composition and antimicrobial activity of the volatile oil of *Salvia santolinifolia* Boiss. from Southeast of Iran. *Pharm. Sci.,* **2016**, *22*, 42-48.
[http://dx.doi.org/10.15171/PS.2016.08]

[69]   Bahadori, M.B.; Asghari, B.; Dinparast, L.; Zengin, G.; Sarikurkcu, C.; Abbas-Mohammadi, M.; Bahadori, S. *Salvia nemorosa* L.: A novel source of bioactive agents with functional connections. *Lebensm. Wiss. Technol.,* **2017**, *75*, 42-50.
[http://dx.doi.org/10.1016/j.lwt.2016.08.048]

[70]   Albach, D.C.; Jensen, S.R.; Özgökce, F.; Grayer, R.J. *Veronica*: Chemical characters for the support of phylogenetic relationships based on nuclear ribosomal and plastid DNA sequence data. *Biochem. Syst. Ecol.,* **2005**, *33*, 1087-1106.
[http://dx.doi.org/10.1016/j.bse.2005.06.002]

[71]   Barreira, J.C.M.; Dias, M.I.; Zivković, J.; Stojković, D.; Soković, M.; Santos-Buelga, C.; Ferreira, I.C.F.R. Phenolic profiling of Veronica spp. grown in mountain, urban and sandy soil environments. *Food Chem.,* **2014**, *163*, 275-283.
[http://dx.doi.org/10.1016/j.foodchem.2014.04.117] [PMID: 24912726]

[72]   Živkovic, J.; Barreira, J.C.M.; Stojkovic, D.; Cebovic, T.; Santos-Buelga, C.; Maksimovic, Z.; Ferreira, I.C.F.R. Phenolic profile, antibacterial, antimutagenic and antitumour evaluation of *Veronica urticifolia* Jacq. *J. Funct. Foods,* **2014**, *9*, 192-201.
[http://dx.doi.org/10.1016/j.jff.2014.04.024]

[73]   Elias, R.; De Méo, M.; Vidal-Ollivier, E.; Laget, M.; Balansard, G.; Dumenil, G. Antimutagenic activity of some saponins isolated from Calendula officinalis L., C. arvensis L. and Hedera helix L. *Mutagenesis,* **1990**, *5*(4), 327-331.
[http://dx.doi.org/10.1093/mutage/5.4.327] [PMID: 2204784]

[74]   Srivastav, S.; Singh, P.; Mishra, G.; Jha, K.; Khosa, R. *Achyranthes aspera*-an important medicinal plant: A review. *Journal of Natural Product and Plant Resources,* **2011**, *1*, 1-14.

[75]   Kirtikar, K.R.; Basu, B.D. *Indian Medicinal Plants,* 2nd ed.; Oriental Enterprises: New Connaught Place, Dehradun, Uttranchal, India, **2001**.

[76]   Stintzing, F.C.; Carle, R. Functional properties of anthocyanins and betalains in plants, food and in human nutrition. *Trends Food Sci. Technol.,* **2004**, *15*, 19-38.
[http://dx.doi.org/10.1016/j.tifs.2003.07.004]

[77]   Octaviani, C.D.; Lusiana, M.; Zuhrotun, A.; Diantini, A.; Subarnas, A.; Abdulah, R. Anticancer properties of daily-consumed vegetables *Amaranthus spinosus, Ipomoea aquatica, Apium graveolens*

and *Manihot utilisima* to LNCaP prostate cancer cell lines. *J. Natural Pharmaceuticals,* **2013**, *4*, 67-70.
[http://dx.doi.org/10.4103/2229-5119.110366]

[78]   Kumar, B.S.A.; Lakshman, K.; Jayaveera, K.N.; Shekar, D.S.; Nandeesh, R.; Velmurugan, C. Chemoprotective and antioxidant activities of methanolic extract of *Amaranthus spinosus* leaves on paracetamol induced-liver damage in rats. *Acta Medica Saliniana,* **2010**, *39*, 68-74.

[79]   Prajitha, V.; Thoppil, J.E. Genotoxic and antigenotoxic potential of the aqueous leaf extracts of *Amaranthus spinosus* Linn. using *Allium cepa* assay. *S. Afr. J. Bot.,* **2016**, *102*, 18-25.
[http://dx.doi.org/10.1016/j.sajb.2015.06.018]

[80]   Chung, K.T.; Wong, T.Y.; Wei, C.I.; Huang, Y.W.; Lin, Y. Tannins and human health: a review. *Crit. Rev. Food Sci. Nutr.,* **1998**, *38*(6), 421-464.
[http://dx.doi.org/10.1080/10408699891274273] [PMID: 9759559]

[81]   Sasaki, Y.F.; Matsumoto, K.; Imanishi, H.; Watanabe, M.; Ohta, T.; Shirasu, Y.; Tutikawa, K. *In vivo* anticlastogenic and antimutagenic effects of tannic acid in mice. *Mutat. Res.,* **1990**, *244*(1), 43-47.
[http://dx.doi.org/10.1016/0165-7992(90)90106-T] [PMID: 2110623]

[82]   Ishtikhar, M.; Ahmad, E.; Siddiqui, Z.; Ahmad, S.; Khan, M.V.; Zaman, M.; Siddiqi, M.K.; Nusrat, S.; Chandel, T.I.; Ajmal, M.R.; Khan, R.H. Biophysical insight into the interaction mechanism of plant derived polyphenolic compound tannic acid with homologous mammalian serum albumins. *Int. J. Biol. Macromol.,* **2018**, *107*(Pt B), 2450-2464.
[http://dx.doi.org/10.1016/j.ijbiomac.2017.10.136] [PMID: 29102789]

[83]   Chopra, R.N.; Nayar, S.L. *Chopra, I.C. Glossary of Indian Medicinal Plants*; CSIR: New Delhi, **1956**.

[84]   Somanabandhu, A.; Nitayangkura, S.; Mahidol, C.; Ruchirawat, S.; Likhitwitayawuid, K.; Shieh, H.L.; Chai, H.; Pezzuto, J.M.; Cordell, G.A. 1H- and 13C-nmr assignments of phyllanthin and hypophyllanthin: lignans that enhance cytotoxic responses with cultured multidrug-resistant cells. *J. Nat. Prod.,* **1993**, *56*(2), 233-239.
[http://dx.doi.org/10.1021/np50092a008] [PMID: 8385184]

[85]   Sripanidkulchai, B.; Tattawasart, U.; Laupatarakasem, P.; Vinitketkumneun, U.; Sripanidkulchai, K.; Furihata, C.; Matsushima, T. Antimutagenic and anticarcinogenic effects of *Phyllanthus amarus.* *Phytomedicine,* **2002**, *9*(1), 26-32.
[http://dx.doi.org/10.1078/0944-7113-00092] [PMID: 11924760]

[86]   Lansky, E.P.; Newman, R.A. *Punica granatum* (pomegranate) and its potential for prevention and treatment of inflammation and cancer. *J. Ethnopharmacol.,* **2007**, *109*(2), 177-206.
[http://dx.doi.org/10.1016/j.jep.2006.09.006] [PMID: 17157465]

[87]   Balasundram, N.; Sundram, K.; Samman, S. Phenolic compounds in plants and agri-industrial by-products: antioxidant activity, occurrence, and potential uses. *Food Chem.,* **2006**, *99*, 191-203.
[http://dx.doi.org/10.1016/j.foodchem.2005.07.042]

[88]   Negi, P.; Jayaprakasha, G.K.; Jena, B.S. Antioxidant and antimutagenic activities of pomegranate peel extracts. *Food Chem.,* **2003**, *80*, 393-397.
[http://dx.doi.org/10.1016/S0308-8146(02)00279-0]

[89]   Zahin, M.; Aqil, F.; Ahmad, I. Broad spectrum antimutagenic activity of antioxidant active fraction of *punica granatum* L. peel extracts. *Mutat. Res.,* **2010**, *703*(2), 99-107.
[http://dx.doi.org/10.1016/j.mrgentox.2010.08.001] [PMID: 20708098]

[90]   Connolly, J.D.; Kitahara, Y.; Overton, K.H.; Yoshikoshi, A. A direct correlation of dolabradiene and erythroxydiol Y. *Chem. Pharm. Bull. (Tokyo),* **1965**, *13*(5), 603-605.
[http://dx.doi.org/10.1248/cpb.13.603] [PMID: 5867719]

[91]   Di Giacomo, S.; Abete, L.; Cocchiola, R.; Mazzanti, G.; Eufemi, M.; Di Sotto, A. Caryophyllane sesquiterpenes inhibit DNA-damage by tobacco smoke in bacterial and mammalian cells. *Food Chem. Toxicol.,* **2018**, *111*, 393-404.

[http://dx.doi.org/10.1016/j.fct.2017.11.018] [PMID: 29154797]

[92] Kumar, A.; Varshney, V. Chemical constituents of *Morina* genus: A comprehensive review. *American Journal of Essential Oils and Natural Products,* **2013**, *1*, 1-15.

[93] Mocan, A.; Zengin, G.; Uysal, A.; Gunes, E.; Mollica, A.; Sena Degirmenci, N.; Alpsoy, L.; Aktumsek, A. Biological and chemical insights of *Morina persica* L.: A source of bioactive compounds with multifunctional properties. *J. Funct. Foods,* **2016**, *25*, 94-109.
[http://dx.doi.org/10.1016/j.jff.2016.05.010]

[94] Sreelatha, S.; Jeyachitra, A.; Padma, P.R. Antiproliferation and induction of apoptosis by *Moringa oleifera* leaf extract on human cancer cells. *Food Chem. Toxicol.,* **2011**, *49*(6), 1270-1275.
[http://dx.doi.org/10.1016/j.fct.2011.03.006] [PMID: 21385597]

[95] Abdul, A.B.; Adel, S.A.; Nirmala, D.T.; Siddig, I.A.; Zetty, N.Z.; Sharin, M.; Ruslay, S.; Syam, M.M. Anticancer activity of natural compound (zerumbone) extracted from *Zingiber zerumbet* in human HeLa cervical cancer cells. *Int. J. Pharmacol.,* **2008**, *4*, 160-186.
[http://dx.doi.org/10.3923/ijp.2008.160.168]

[96] Eltayeb, E.E.M.; Abdul, A.B.; Suliman, F.E.O.; Sukari, M.A.; Rasedee, A.; Fatah, S.S. Characterization of the inclusion complex of zerumbone with hydroxypropyl-β cyclodextrin. *Carbohydr. Polym.,* **2011**, *83*, 1707-1714.
[http://dx.doi.org/10.1016/j.carbpol.2010.10.033]

[97] Huang, G.C.; Chien, T.Y.; Chen, L.G.; Wang, C.C. Antitumor effects of zerumbone from *Zingiber zerumbet* in P-388D1 cells *in vitro* and *in vivo. Planta Med.,* **2005**, *71*(3), 219-224.
[http://dx.doi.org/10.1055/s-2005-837820] [PMID: 15770541]

[98] Prasannan, R.; Kalesh, K.A.; Shanmugam, M.K.; Nachiyappan, A.; Ramachandran, L.; Nguyen, A.H.; Kumar, A.P.; Lakshmanan, M.; Ahn, K.S.; Sethi, G. Key cell signaling pathways modulated by zerumbone: role in the prevention and treatment of cancer. *Biochem. Pharmacol.,* **2012**, *84*(10), 1268-1276.
[http://dx.doi.org/10.1016/j.bcp.2012.07.015] [PMID: 22842489]

[99] Santosh Kumar, S.C.; Srinivas, P.; Negi, P.S.; Bettadaiah, B.K. Antibacterial and antimutagenic activities of novel zerumbone analogues. *Food Chem.,* **2013**, *141*(2), 1097-1103.
[http://dx.doi.org/10.1016/j.foodchem.2013.04.021] [PMID: 23790891]

[100] Antunes, L.M.; Takahashi, C.S. Effects of high doses of vitamins C and E against doxorubicin-induced chromosomal damage in Wistar rat bone marrow cells. *Mutat. Res.,* **1998**, *419*(1-3), 137-143.
[http://dx.doi.org/10.1016/S1383-5718(98)00134-X] [PMID: 9804927]

[101] Tavan, E.; Maziere, S.; Narbonne, J.F.; Cassand, P. Effects of vitamins A and E on methylazoxymethanol-induced mutagenesis in Salmonella typhimurium strain TA100. *Mutat. Res.,* **1997**, *377*(2), 231-237.
[http://dx.doi.org/10.1016/S0027-5107(97)00079-1] [PMID: 9247619]

[102] Kuroda, Y. Antimutagenic activity of vitamins in cultured mammalian cells. *Basic Life Sci.,* **1990**, *52*, 233-256.
[PMID: 2327939]

[103] Sánchez-Navarrete, J.; Arriaga-Alba, M.; Ruiz-Pérez, N.J.; Toscano-Garibay, J.D. Antimutagenic activity of vitamin B1 against damages induced by chemical and physical mutagens in *Salmonella typhimurium* and *Escherichia coli. Toxicol. In Vitro,* **2017**, *45*(Pt 1), 202-206.
[http://dx.doi.org/10.1016/j.tiv.2017.09.015] [PMID: 28927723]

[104] Ferguson, A.R.; Huang, H. Genetic resources of kiwifruit: domestication and breeding. *Hortic. Rev. (Am. Soc. Hortic. Sci.),* **2007**, *33*, 1-121.

[105] Li, J-Q.; Li, X-W.; Soejarto, D.D. Actinidiaceae in flora of china hippocastanaceae through the aceae., **2007**.

[106] Hunter, D.C.; Skinne, M.A.; Ross Ferguson, A. *Fruits, Vegetables, and Herbs. CHAPTER 12 Kiwifruit*

and health; Elsevier Inc., **2016**, pp. 239-268.
[http://dx.doi.org/10.1016/B978-0-12-802972-5.00012-3]

[107] Vissers, M.C.M.; Carr, A.C.; Pullar, J.M.; Bozonet, S.M. The bioavailability of vitamin C from kiwifruit. *Adv. Food Nutr. Res.,* **2013**, *68*, 125-147.
[http://dx.doi.org/10.1016/B978-0-12-394294-4.00007-9] [PMID: 23394985]

[108] Pontoriero, A.C. *"Acción quimiopreventiva del ácido L-ascórbico y de extractos de té verde sobre la mutagenicidad y toxicidad aguda de mezclas de reacción sulfonamida-nitrito para las siguientes sulfonamidas o sus derivados: *sulfatiazol, *complejo sulfatiazol-cobalto(III), *glibenclamida"* National University of Rosario, Argentina,* **2013**.

[109] De Flora, S.; Izzoth, A.; Benniceili, C. Mechanisms of Antimutagenesis and Anticarcinogenesis, Role in Primary Protection.*Antimutagenesis and Anticarcinogenesis Mechanisms*; Bronezetti, G.; Waters, M.D.; Shanket, D.M., Eds.; Plenum Press: New York, **1992**, pp. 162-178.

[110] d'Ischia, M.; Napolitano, A.; Manini, P.; Panzella, L. Secondary targets of nitrite-derived reactive nitrogen species: nitrosation/nitration pathways, antioxidant defense mechanisms and toxicological implications. *Chem. Res. Toxicol.,* **2011**, *24*(12), 2071-2092.
[http://dx.doi.org/10.1021/tx2003118] [PMID: 21923154]

[111] Hebels, D.G.; Brauers, K.J.; van Herwijnen, M.H.; Georgiadis, P.A.; Kyrtopoulos, S.A.; Kleinjans, J.C.; de Kok, T.M. Time-series analysis of gene expression profiles induced by nitrosamides and nitrosamines elucidates modes of action underlying their genotoxicity in human colon cells. *Toxicol. Lett.,* **2011**, *207*(3), 232-241.
[http://dx.doi.org/10.1016/j.toxlet.2011.09.012] [PMID: 21946166]

[112] Stuff, J.E.; Goh, E.T.; Barrera, S.L.; Bondy, M.L.; Forman, M.R. Construction of an N-nitroso database for assessing dietary intake. *J. Food Compos. Anal.,* **2009**, *22* Suppl. 1, S42-S47.
[http://dx.doi.org/10.1016/j.jfca.2009.01.008] [PMID: 20161416]

[113] Loh, Y.H.; Jakszyn, P.; Luben, R.N.; Mulligan, A.A.; Mitrou, P.N.; Khaw, K-T. N-nitroso compounds and cancer incidence: the European Prospective Investigation into Cancer and Nutrition. *Am. J. Clin. Nutr.,* **2011**, *93*(5), 1053-1061.
[http://dx.doi.org/10.3945/ajcn.111.012377] [PMID: 21430112]

[114] Milkowski, A.; Garg, H.K.; Coughlin, J.R.; Bryan, N.S. Nutritional epidemiology in the context of nitric oxide biology: a risk-benefit evaluation for dietary nitrite and nitrate. *Nitric Oxide,* **2010**, *22*(2), 110-119.
[http://dx.doi.org/10.1016/j.niox.2009.08.004] [PMID: 19748594]

[115] Mirvish, S.S. Role of N-nitroso compounds (NOC) and N-nitrosation in etiology of gastric, esophageal, nasopharyngeal and bladder cancer and contribution to cancer of known exposures to NOC. *Cancer Lett.,* **1995**, *93*(1), 17-48.
[http://dx.doi.org/10.1016/0304-3835(95)03786-V] [PMID: 7600541]

[116] Cockburn, A.; Brambilla, G.; Fernández, M.L.; Arcella, D.; Bordajandi, L.R.; Cottrill, B.; van Peteghem, C.; Dorne, J.L. Nitrite in feed: from animal health to human health. *Toxicol. Appl. Pharmacol.,* **2013**, *270*(3), 209-217.
[http://dx.doi.org/10.1016/j.taap.2010.11.008] [PMID: 21095201]

[117] Kyrtopoulos, S.A. Ascorbic acid and the formation of N-nitroso compounds: possible role of ascorbic acid in cancer prevention. *Am. J. Clin. Nutr.,* **1987**, *45*(5) Suppl., 1344-1350.
[http://dx.doi.org/10.1093/ajcn/45.5.1344] [PMID: 3578122]

[118] Brambilla, G.; Martelli, A. Genotoxic and carcinogenic risk to humans of drug-nitrite interaction products. *Mutat. Res.,* **2007**, *635*(1), 17-52.
[http://dx.doi.org/10.1016/j.mrrev.2006.09.003] [PMID: 17157055]

[119] Lijinsky, W. Reaction of drugs with nitrous acid as a source of carcinogenic nitrosamines. *Cancer Res.,* **1974**, *34*(1), 255-258.
[PMID: 4148978]

[120]   Ajibade, P.A.; Kolawole, G.A.; O'Brien, P.; Helliwell, M.; Rafter, J. Cobalt(II) complexes of the antibiotic sulfadiazine, the X-ray single crystal structure of [Co(C$_{10}$H$_9$N$_4$O$_2$S)$_2$(CH$_3$OH)$_2$. *Inorg. Chim. Acta,* **2006**, *359*, 3111-3116.
[http://dx.doi.org/10.1016/j.ica.2006.03.030]

[121]   García-Raso, A.; Fiol, J.; Rigo, S.; López-López, A.; Molins, E.; Espinosa, E.; Borrás, E.; Alzuet, G.; Borrás, J.; Castiñeiras, A. Coordination behaviour of sulfanilamide derivatives.: Crystal structures of [Hg(sulfamethoxypyridazinato)$_2$], [Cd(sulfadimidinato)$_2$(H$_2$O)]·2H$_2$O and [Zn(sulfamethoxazolato)$_2$-(pyridine)$_2$(H$_2$O)$_2$]. *Polyhedron,* **2000**, *19*, 991-1004.
[http://dx.doi.org/10.1016/S0277-5387(00)00355-7]

[122]   Tricker, A.R.; Preussmann, R. Carcinogenic N-nitrosamines in the diet: occurrence, formation, mechanisms and carcinogenic potential. *Mutat. Res.,* **1991**, *259*(3-4), 277-289.
[http://dx.doi.org/10.1016/0165-1218(91)90123-4] [PMID: 2017213]

[123]   Wattenberg, L.W. Chemoprevention of cancer. *Cancer Res.,* **1985**, *45*(1), 1-8.
[PMID: 3880665]

[124]   Ikken, Y.; Cambero, I.; Marín, M.L.; Martínez, A.; Haza, A.I.; Morales, P.J. Antimutagenic Effect of Fruit and Vegetable Aqueous Extracts against N-Nitrosamines Evaluated by the Ames Test. *J. Agric. Food Chem.,* **1998**, *46*, 5194-5200.
[http://dx.doi.org/10.1021/jf980657s]

[125]   De Lucia, M.; Panzella, L.; Crescenzi, O.; Napolitano, A.; Barone, V.; d'Ischia, M. The catecholic antioxidant piceatannol is an effective nitrosation inhibitor *via* an unusual double bond nitration. *Bioorg. Med. Chem. Lett.,* **2006**, *16*(8), 2238-2242.
[http://dx.doi.org/10.1016/j.bmcl.2006.01.043] [PMID: 16455243]

[126]   Combet, E.; El Mesmari, A.; Preston, T.; Crozier, A.; McColl, K.E.L. Dietary phenolic acids and ascorbic acid: Influence on acid-catalyzed nitrosative chemistry in the presence and absence of lipids. *Free Radic. Biol. Med.,* **2010**, *48*(6), 763-771.
[http://dx.doi.org/10.1016/j.freeradbiomed.2009.12.011] [PMID: 20026204]

[127]   Ohsawa, K.; Nakagawa, S.Y.; Kimura, M.; Shimada, C.; Tsuda, S.; Kabasawa, K.; Kawaguchi, S.; Sasaki, Y.F. Detection of *in vivo* genotoxicity of endogenously formed N-nitroso compounds and suppression by ascorbic acid, teas and fruit juices. *Mutat. Res.,* **2003**, *539*(1-2), 65-76.
[http://dx.doi.org/10.1016/S1383-5718(03)00156-6] [PMID: 12948815]

[128]   Vermeer, I.T.; Moonen, E.J.; Dallinga, J.W.; Kleinjans, J.C.; van Maanen, J.M. Effect of ascorbic acid and green tea on endogenous formation of N-nitrosodimethylamine and N-nitrosopiperidine in humans. *Mutat. Res.,* **1999**, *428*(1-2), 353-361.
[http://dx.doi.org/10.1016/S1383-5742(99)00061-7] [PMID: 10518007]

[129]   Rao, G.S.; Osborn, J.C.; Adatia, M.R. Drug-nitrite interactions in human saliva: effects of food constituents on carcinogenic N-nitrosamine formation. *J. Dent. Res.,* **1982**, *61*(6), 768-771.
[http://dx.doi.org/10.1177/00220345820610062301] [PMID: 6953112]

[130]   Sram, R.J.; Binkova, B.; Rossner, P., Jr Vitamin C for DNA damage prevention. *Mutat. Res.,* **2012**, *733*(1-2), 39-49.
[http://dx.doi.org/10.1016/j.mrfmmm.2011.12.001] [PMID: 22178550]

[131]   Anesini, C.; Ferraro, G.E.; Filip, R. Total polyphenol content and antioxidant capacity of commercially available tea (Camellia sinensis) in Argentina. *J. Agric. Food Chem.,* **2008**, *56*(19), 9225-9229.
[http://dx.doi.org/10.1021/jf8022782] [PMID: 18778031]

[132]   Feng, W.Y. Metabolism of green tea catechins: an overview. *Curr. Drug Metab.,* **2006**, *7*(7), 755-809.
[http://dx.doi.org/10.2174/138920006778520552] [PMID: 17073579]

[133]   Singh, B.N.; Shankar, S.; Srivastava, R.K. Green tea catechin, epigallocatechin-3-gallate (EGCG): mechanisms, perspectives and clinical applications. *Biochem. Pharmacol.,* **2011**, *82*(12), 1807-1821.

[http://dx.doi.org/10.1016/j.bcp.2011.07.093] [PMID: 21827739]

[134]   Lee, S.Y.; Munerol, B.; Pollard, S.; Youdim, K.A.; Pannala, A.S.; Kuhnle, G.G.; Debnam, E.S.; Rice-Evans, C.; Spencer, J.P. The reaction of flavanols with nitrous acid protects against N-nitrosamine formation and leads to the formation of nitroso derivatives which inhibit cancer cell growth. *Free Radic. Biol. Med.,* **2006**, *40*(2), 323-334.
[http://dx.doi.org/10.1016/j.freeradbiomed.2005.08.031] [PMID: 16413414]

[135]   Mortelmans, K.; Zeiger, E. The Ames Salmonella/microsome mutagenicity assay. *Mutat. Res.,* **2000**, *455*(1-2), 29-60.
[http://dx.doi.org/10.1016/S0027-5107(00)00064-6] [PMID: 11113466]

[136]   Ammar, R.B.; Sghaier, M.B.; Boubaker, J.; Bhouri, W.; Naffeti, A.; Skandrani, I.; Bouhlel, I.; Kilani, S.; Ghedira, K.; Chekir-Ghedira, L. Antioxidant activity and inhibition of aflatoxin B1-, nifuroxazide-, and sodium azide-induced mutagenicity by extracts from *Rhamnus alaternus* L. *Chem. Biol. Interact.,* **2008**, *174*(1), 1-10.
[http://dx.doi.org/10.1016/j.cbi.2008.04.006] [PMID: 18511029]

[137]   Trossero, C. PhD Thesis, 'Estudios biológicos de drogas sulfa y sus derivados: * Propiedades antifúngicas del complejo Co(II)-sulfatiazol * Detección de mutagenicidad en mezclas Co(II)-sulfatiazol y ftalil sulfatiazol con nitrito de sodio en medio ácido mediante el test de Ames'. Universidad Nacional de Rosario (UNR), Argentina, **2005**.

[138]   Endo, H.; Noda, H.; Kinoshita, N.; Inui, N.; Nishi, Y. Formation of a transplacental mutagen, 1,3-Di(4-sulfamoylphenyl)triazene, from sodium nitrite and sulfanilamide in human gastric juice and in the stomachs of hamsters. *J. Natl. Cancer Inst.,* **1980**, *65*(3), 547-551.
[PMID: 6931934]

[139]   Mirvish, S.S. Experimental evidence for inhibition of N-nitroso compound formation as a factor in the negative correlation between vitamin C consumption and the incidence of certain cancers. *Cancer Res.,* **1994**, *54*(7) Suppl., 1948s-1951s.
[PMID: 8137317]

[140]   Arya, S.; Mahajan, M. Photometric methods for the determination of vitamin C. *Anal. Sci.,* **1998**, *14*, 889-894.
[http://dx.doi.org/10.2116/analsci.14.889]

[141]   Selimović, A.; Salkić, M.; Selimović, M. Direct Spectrophotometric Determination of L-Ascorbic acid in Pharmaceutical Preparations using Sodium Oxalate as a Stabilizer. Int. J. Basic & Appl. Sci. *IJBAS-IJENS,* **2011**, *11*, 106-109.

[142]   Rizzotto, M.; Pontoriero, A. Chemopreventive action of L-ascorbic acid and green tea infusions on the acute toxicity and mutagenicity of reaction mixtures nitrite-sulfonamide. *J. Forensic Toxicol. Pharmacol.,* **2015**, *4*(3), 66.

CHAPTER 3

Encapsulated Plant-Derived Polyphenols as Potential Cancer Treatment Agents

Merve Deniz Kose and **Oguz Bayraktar**[*]

Ege University, Department of Chemical Engineering, Faculty of Engineering, Bornova, İzmir, Turkey

Abstract: Cancer is one of the leading causes of death worldwide. There are many problems in cancer therapy due to the side-effects which limit its usage. Products derived from natural substances, particularly polyphenolic compounds which have very little toxic effects on normal cells, have gained a crucial interest as therapeutic weapon in clinical oncology due to their chemopreventive, antitumoral, radiosensibilizing and chemosensibilizing activities against different types of aggressive, recurrent and drug-resistant cancers.

Especially now, polyphenols and their applications are one of the most studied topics in the literature due to their promising results against cancer cells. In many studies, it has been reported that, polyphenols inhibited the development of tumors through variety of mechanisms and reduce the tumor cell mass. However, with all the advantages of polyphenols, in the literature it is stated that, issues like poor solubility, high degradation rate and high dose requirement restrict the applications of polyphenols. Still, these obstacles can be overcome by using encapsulation and nano-drug delivery systems for plant-derived polyphenols. With the encapsulation techniques it is possible to increase their bioavailability, stability of the polyphenols and their uptake in the targeted cells. Encapsulated polyphenols have been used against cancer in various scientific studies. And the obtained results were promising. With the encapsulation methods, greater accumulation of polyphenols has been observed on the cell membrane and cytoplasm due to smaller size.

In this chapter, plant-derived polyphenols, their stabilities and encapsulation of polyphenols in order to increase their stability and their potential as cancer treatment agents will be explained.

Keywords: Anticancerogenic, Cancer Treatments, Drug Delivery, Drug Delivery Systems, Encapsulation, Flavonoids, Nanoparticles, Phenolic Acids, Polyphenols.

---

[*] **Corresponding Author Oguz Bayraktar:** Ege University, Department of Chemical Engineering, Faculty of Engineering, Bornova, İzmir, Turkey; E-mails: oguz.bayraktar@ege.edu.tr, merve.deniz.kose@ege.edu.tr

Ferid Murad, Atta-ur-Rahman and Ka Bian (Eds.)

INTRODUCTION

Polyphenols are natural compounds, and they all consist of one or more than one benzenic cycles having one or several hydroxy functions. They can be obtained from the metabolism of shikimic acid and/or polyacetate which are secondary metabolites found in all vascular plants, and represent a big group of common and different substances, from simple molecules to complex structures [1]. Natural polyphenols are found mostly in the fresh fruits, vegetables, cereals and beverages. Fruits such as grapes, apple, pear, cherries and berries contain up to 200–300 mg polyphenols per 100 grams fresh weight. The obtained products from these fruits, as well contain polyphenols in great amounts. For instance, products like, a glass of red wine or a cup of tea or coffee contains about 100 mg polyphenols. Also, products like chocolate contributes to the daily polyphenol intake [2, 3]. Polyphenols are secondary metabolites of plants which are produced in order to protect against environmental conditions like temperature, ultraviolet radiation or aggression by pathogens [4]. However, in foods, polyphenols also can cause the bitterness, astringency, color, flavor, odor and oxidative stability.

The studies and associated analyses showed that development of cancers, cardiovascular diseases, diabetes, osteoporosis and neurodegenerative diseases can be prevented with long term consumption of plants rich with polyphenols [5]. Due to their positive effects on human health, polyphenols and other phenolic foods are subjected to the increasing scientific interest [6].

Over the years more than 8,000 polyphenolic compounds in various plant species have been classified. Primarily, they were obtained in conjugated forms, with one or more sugar residues linked to hydroxyl groups, even though there are linkages of the sugar (polysaccharide or monosaccharide) to an aromatic carbon. In addition to the sugar linkage, phenol can be linked with other compounds, like carboxylic and organic acids, amines, lipids and other phenolic groups [7].

Polyphenols can be categorized into different groups based on the number of phenol rings that they consist and the molecular structure diversity that hold these rings one to another. The main groups can be categorized as the flavonoids, phenolic acids, and stilbenoids. And again, it can be sub-group, as hydroxybenzoic acids, hydroxycinnamic acids, anthocyanins, proanthocyanidins, flavonols, flavones, flavanols, flavanones, isoflavones, stilbenes, and lignans.

Phenolic Acids

Phenolic acids can be divided into two subclasses: derivatives of benzoic acid and derivatives of cinnamic acid which are mostly found in foods. Other than certain red fruits, black radish and onions, the hydroxybenzoic acid content of edible plants is generally low [8]. The hydroxycinnamic acids are found more than hydroxybenzoic acids and consist chiefly of p-coumaric, caffeic, ferulic and sinapic acids. The antioxidant capacity of phenolic acids and their esters changed with the number of hydroxyl groups in the molecule that would be strengthened by steric interference.

Molecular structure of gallic acid is given in the Fig. (**1**).

Fig. (1). Molecular Structure of Gallic Acid (Hydroxybenzoic acid).

Flavonoids

In the literature, amongst the all polyphenols flavonoids are the most studied group. Flavonoids have consisted with two aromatic rings hold together by three carbon atoms that form an oxygenated heterocycle. There is more than 4,000 have been identified types of flavonoids. Most of them are the reason behind the attractive colors of the flowers, fruits and leaves [9]. Flavonoids can be categorized as six sub-groups: flavonols, flavones, flavanones, flavanols, anthocyanins and isoflavones based on the which type of heterocycle present. The differences of each group are the amount and placement of the hydroxyl groups and their extent of alkylation and/or glycosylation [3]. Quercetin, myricetin, catechins can be examples for some most known flavonoids. Molecular structure of flavonol is given in the Fig. (**2**).

Fig. (2). Molecular Structure of Flavonol.

Stilbenes

Stilbenes have two phenyl moieties held by a two-carbon methylene bridge. Most stilbenes in plants are produced in order to prevent an infection or injury or act as antifungal phytoalexins. However, the daily intake ratio of stilbenes is quite low. One of the best-known, naturally produced stilbene is resveratrol (3,4',5-trihydroxystilbene), which found largely in grapes and their skin. Red wine which is a product made from grapes also contains significant amount of resveratrol [10].

Fig. (3). Molecular Structure of Trans Stilbene.

Lignans

Lignans are diphenolic compounds that hold a 2,3-dibenzylbutane structure which is obtained by the dimerization of two cinnamic acid residues. Several lignans, like secoisolariciresinol, are phytoestrogens. Linseed is the richest dietary source for lignans, which contains almost 3.7 g/kg dry weight secoisolariciresinol and low quantities of matairesinol [10].

Fig. (4). Molecular structure of α-tocopherol/vitamin E.

PLANTS RICH IN POLYPHENOLS

Content of the Polyphenols

The phenolics compounds can be distributed in many parts of the plants. They can be found in the tissue, cellular and subcellular levels. While, insoluble phenolics are found in cell walls, the soluble phenolics are found inside of the plant cell vacuoles. However, some specific compounds like quercetin are presented in all plant products; such as fruits, vegetables, on the other hand for flavanones and isoflavones are more rare and specific to some food groups. Most of the time polyphenols found in foods as complex mixture. Higher level of phenolics present in the outer layers of plants rather than those found in their inner parts [8].

Polyphenol content of plants can be changed with numerous factors, such as ripeness of the fruit or vegetable when it was harvested, environmental factors like temperature, processing and storage. Total phenolic content of the foods is greatly changed by environmental conditions. In addition to the environmental factors specific factors like soil type, sun exposure, rainfall *etc* change the polyphenolic content [11]. It is stated that in most cases phenolic acid content decreases during ripening, whereas anthocyanin concentrations increase. For this reason, in the literature for the extraction of polyphenols from fruits unripe produce were selected for the higher phenolic acid content.

Many polyphenols, especially phenolic acids, are produced as plants response to different types of stress. They help to healing of injured areas. They show antimicrobial properties, and their concentrations higher after infection [10]. Storage is another important parameter that directly changes the phenolic content of the foods. Studies have showed that phenolic content of the foods can be changed during storage due to the oxidation of polyphenols [11]. These oxidation reactions resulted as formation of polymerized substances and degradation of the phenolic content which changes the quality of foods, especially in color and organoleptic characteristics which can be harmful as in browning of fruit. However sometimes these changes could be beneficial, as is the case with black tea. Disadvantages of storage can be avoided by using cold storage, in contrast to room temperature, it has slightly better effect on the phenolic content of apples, pears or onions [12]. In addition to the light, heat is another parameter that can change the phenolic content. For example, heat has a crucial effect on decreasing the amount of phenolic content. Onions and tomatoes lose between 75% and 80% of their initial phenolic content after boiling for 15 min, 65% after cooking in a microwave oven, and 30% after frying [13].

Polyphenols can be defined as a big group of highly effective antioxidants, since they exhibit potent free radical scavenging capability and protection against oxidation of transition metals and lipid peroxidation [14]. They have been used for a long time as healthier dietary options. However, indigestion and absorption processes, low bioavailability and instability of polyphenols mostly limits their health benefits. In fact, only a very small amount are absorbed when it is taken orally, due to the insufficient gastric residence time, low permeability, and water-solubility [15]. Because of these restrictions, conventional usage of polyphenols has been decreased over the years.

A different type of technologies has been developed to encapsulate polyphenols to overcome the shortcomings of stability of polyphenols, including spray drying, coacervation, emulsions, liposomes, micellar, nanoparticles, freeze-drying, co-crystallization and yeast encapsulation. This chapter will be focus on novel usage of polyphenols; specifically, novel usage of polyphenols on cancer studies.

Polyphenols are plant originated antioxidants present in number of foods and their products. They show more than 500 different molecules and structures. This variety should be considered when bioavailability, biological properties and health effects compared due to the fact all these parameters change with their specific chemical structures [16]. Another challenge is to determine the total phenolic content of foods due to the diversity of polyphenols which is crucial, for food and nutrition researchers and the food industry. Studies have been ranking the foods and beverages for the highest polyphenol content. In these studies, colorimetric redox assays have been performed which based on the generic reducing property of phenolic groups [17]. One of the most known and used test is the Folin assay [18]. In addition to the phenolic groups these assays can be interference with non-phenolic food components. However this interference could be eliminated with pretreatment solid phase extraction of polyphenols, which can be applied to a large variety of foods [19]. Data collected from the United States Department of Agriculture (USDA) database show the 15 foods with the highest ranking for the phenolic contents are given in Table **1**. The object of this table is to provide an information about food composition tables for flavonoids and to estimate their intake in several groups [20]. The food group with the highest number of polyphenolic content in the Table **1** is the seasoning group, followed by fruits, and seeds). Total phenolic contents changed between 15 000 mg per 100 g in cloves to 7.8 mg per 100 ml in rose´ wine [21].

Table 1. Polyphenol and antioxidant content in the 15 richest foods (mg per 100 g or mg per 100 ml) [21].

Food	Food Group	Polyphenols		Polyphenols AE*		Antioxidants		Common Properties
		Content	Rank	Content	Rank	Content	Rank	
Cloves	Seasonings	15188	1	15188	1	16047	1	Antibacterial, anticancer and antifungal [22]
Peppermint, dried	Seasonings	11960	2	7920	2	980	26	Antibacteria, anticancer [23]
Star Anise	Seasonings	5460	3	5460	3	1810	16	Antifungal antimycotoxigenic, anticancer [24]
Cocoa Powder	Cocoa Products	3448	4	3294	4	1104	24	Anti-cariogenic, antibacterial [25]
Mexican Oregano, Dried	Seasonings	2319	5	2137	5	-	-	Antifungal, antibacterial, anticancer [22]

(Table 1) cont.....

Food	Food Group	Polyphenols		Polyphenols AE*		Antioxidants		Common Properties
		Content	Rank	Content	Rank	Content	Rank	
Celery Seed	Seasonings	2094	6	1007	10	-	-	Antiproliferative, anticancer [26]
Black Chokeberry	Fruits	1756	7	1432	7	1752	17	Antibacterial antiviral [27]
Dark Chocolate	Cocoa Products	1664	8	1618	6	1860	13	Antiatherogenic, Anti-cariogenic [25, 28]
Flaxseed Meal	Seeds	1528	9	1220	8	-	-	Anticancer [29]
Black Elderberry	Fruits	1359	10	804	13	1950	12	Anti-inflammatory, anticancer [30 - 32]
Chestnut	Seeds	1215	11	1215	9	2757	9	Antiproliferative Antiangiogenic [33]
Common Sage Dried	Seasonings	1207	12	893	12	2920	8	Antimicrobial, Anticancer [22]
Rosemary Dried	Seasonings	1018	13	522	14	2519	10	Antibacterial, antifungal [22]
Spearmint, Dried	Seasonings	956	14	491	18	6575	3	Antibacterial, anticancer [23]
Common Thyme, Dried	Seasonings	878	15	464	19	1815	15	Antiviral, antifungal [22]

*Abbreviation: AE, (polyphenols as) aglycone equivalents.

EXTRACTION METHODS OF POLYPHENOLS

Due to their phenolic nature polyphenols are mostly more hydrophilic than lipophilic. Because of the hydrophilic properties, free polyphenols along with aglycones, glycosides and oligomers can be easily obtained by using solvents such as methanol, ethanol, acetonitrile and acetone, or by their mixtures with water [34]. However, extraction processes involve the use of organic solvents which might cause unwanted environmental and biological impact.

New studies are focused on new sustainable more environmental methods for the extraction of the polyphenols. For instance, with the supercritical fluids (SCFs) extraction of polyphenols can be higher due to the fact they can be affected from extraction conditions. And also, it is safer to the environment; therefore, using supercritical fluids create a better solution to other extraction methods which involve unsafe organic solvents and a high-energy demand. SCFs might be a good alternative to the conventional solvents and/or a pretreatment method in order to improve the separation [35]. The biggest health and safety benefits of SCFs (SC

CO_2 and SC H_2O) that they are non-cancerogenic, non-toxic, non-mutagenic, non-flammable and thermodynamically stable. Dense CO_2 is one of the "green" extraction solvent, especially when organic solvents and high process temperatures harmful to the natural compound and to the environment. A number of studies on the isolation, purification and fractionation of phenolic compounds have published over the decades. With every research, the traditional methods for extraction, sample preparation, separation, detection, and identification steps are regularly changed by new and better techniques.

For the first step of extraction, the suitable procedure for the sample must be decided. The decision process for the extraction method is shaped by the chemical structure of the substance, particle size of sample, also by the presence of interfering components. The important parameters, which are changing the extraction yield, are extraction time, temperature, solid-to-liquid ratio, the number of repeated extractions of the sample, and lastly chosen extraction solvents. Both extraction time and temperature can be changed the solubility. For instance a simultaneous increment in the temperature, increases solubility and mass transfer velocities while decreases viscosity and surface tension of solvents leading to a higher extraction rate [35]. In addition to the extraction steps for the removal of the undesirable components like waxes, fats, terpenes, and chlorophylls, additional steps such as pretreatments might be needed [36].

Extraction of phenolic compounds can be done from fresh, frozen or dried plant samples. Firstly, the feed can be pre-treated by milling, grinding, drying or homogenization. The type of the drying procedure will change the total phenolic content. With freeze-drying method higher phenolic content can be reached in plant samples when it is compared to air-drying [37]. Phenolic extracts containing high anthocyanin can also be produced by using an acidified organic solvent such as methanol or ethanol.

Conventional Methods

Even though there are many disadvantages, liquid-liquid and solid-liquid extraction are still the most preferred extraction procedures. Over the years, these conventional techniques have been extensively used, mostly they are easy to use, efficient, and wide-ranging applicable [38]. These processes include the use of conventional solvents like alcohols (methanol, ethanol), acetone, diethyl ether and ethyl acetate, often solutions of water with various concentrations.

The most common and extensively used conventional extraction methods are maceration and Soxhlet extraction. However, there are several disadvantages of these methods such as their low efficiency and potential environmental hazards due to the high amount of organic solvents used in the process. Other than environmental hazards, because of the residue of organic solvents remain in the final product can cause a possible hazardous effect on the human health. In order to avoid that in the final products additional purification steps are required. And that would have resulted in an increase of the time consumption and total process cost.

To sum up, polar phenolic acids like benzoic and cinnamic acids cannot be `extracted completely by using only pure organic solvents. In those cases, alcohol-water or acetone-water solutions are suggested to dissolve both hydrophilic and hydrophobic parts of the natural compounds. Highly nonpolar compounds like waxes, oils, sterols, chlorophyll can be obtained from the material by using less polar solvents like dichloromethane, chloroform, hexane and benzene [39]. The extraction yield and rate of polyphenolic compounds depend on the characteristics of the solvent. From literature, it was seen that methanol is more effective in the extraction of lower molecular weight polyphenols while for the extraction of the higher molecular weight flavanols, aqueous acetone is a suitable solvent [40]. However, in the process of extraction many phenolic compounds are go through degradation or undesirable oxidation. Therefore, extraction yield of the phenolic compounds is significantly decreased. To improve this problem high processing temperature in the extraction should be eliminated. Conventional extraction is typically done at temperatures between 20 °C to 50 °C. Temperatures over 70 °C are unwanted and cause decrease in the phenolic content. Long extraction duration is another problem due to the feasibility of the extraction procedures.

Modern Extraction Techniques

Problems with the conventional extraction procedures are high process temperatures and long processing times. These processes are especially problematic for the extraction of the phenolic compounds. There is an urge to finding a better alternative to the conventional extraction techniques.

Possible problems can be overcome by using systems like, ultrasound-assisted and microwave-assisted extraction or ultrasound-microwave-assisted extraction, supercritical fluid extraction and subcritical water extraction. Due to their simple process applications, shorter extraction times and less organic solvent consumption than conventional techniques supercritical fluid extraction and subcritical water extraction that have been popular [41].

Supercritical fluid technologies have been investigated for selective isolation of antioxidants from natural compounds. Since with the mild extraction conditions like shorter processing time and lower temperatures oxidation and/or degradation of natural compounds during extraction can be avoided. Also, new legal limitations and restrictions in the food and pharmaceutical industries, about using organic solvents and number of solvent residues have become even more critical than before.

Due to the direct impacts on the environment, isolation and fractionation of natural bioactive compounds using conventional production technologies is commonly renewed by alternative production technologies with low toxic wastes. With the alternative technologies, it is possible for the side-products to be used more efficiently during the process. And the most important features are higher quality and healthier nutrient products.

Several parameters affect the extraction yield by changing solubility, extraction of desired compounds in the supercritical fluid [42]. Quality of extraction highly depends on extraction parameters like the selected pressure and temperature which can significantly change the final phenolic content of the extracts. These modern extraction techniques have been accepted as eco-friendly and green due to the less organic solvent consumption and process parameters and they can be a good alternative to the conventional organic solvent-based extraction of polyphenols.

STABILITY OF POLYPHENOLS

The most important problems faced working with polyphenols are low bioavailability and stability problems during the process and storage. These problems limit their potential against cancer, aging, inflammation, cardiovascular and neurodegenerative diseases. Benefits of the encapsulation and the delivery systems that they can improve the stability and bioavailability of the polyphenols. Unfortunately, without the encapsulation bioavailability of these valuable natural bioactive compounds is crucially low [43].

It is stated that the polyphenol concentrations needed to obtain *in vitro* efficiency are generally superior to *in vivo* moderate levels. Bioavailability and integrity of the natural compounds change with the route of administration, and directly related with efficiency of these compounds [15]. Such as, only a small ratio of molecules is absorbed when it is administered orally due to the inadequate gastric residence time, low permeability and/or low solubility. The limiting factor for the applications of polyphenols for the industries, their instability during food processing, distribution or storage, or in the gastrointestinal tract (pH, enzymes, presence of other nutrients) [44]. In addition to the oral use, the topical use of natural polyphenols is also tricky due to their sensitivity to environmental factors, including physical, chemical, and biological conditions. Unfortunately, their quick oxidization, resulting in a brown color and/or unpleasant odors with most importantly, a considerable loss in the activity [45]. Furthermore, many polyphenols have an unpleasant taste which must be treated before their applications in the food supplements or oral medicines [19].

Hence, the administration of phenolic compounds need a finished formulation for the protecting natural bioactive compounds and be able to maintain the structural integrity of the polyphenol until the consumption or the administration. Among all the existing stabilization methods, encapsulation is an interesting and popular technique in order to improve their bioavailability and water solubility.

Bioavailability of Polyphenols

Each polyphenol has different bioavailability. In addition to that, there is no relation between the quantity of polyphenols in food and their bioavailability in human body.

Most plant-derived polyphenols like esters, glycosides or polymers cannot be absorbed from small intestine in their initial form. Only aglycones can be absorbed from the small intestine [1]. These compounds must be hydrolyzed by intestinal enzymes or by colonic microflora before absorption. During the absorption process, polyphenols go through an extensive changes; even they are conjugated in the intestinal cells and later in the liver by methylation, sulfation and/or glucuronidation [46]. Consequently, the final product come to the blood and tissues are very different from those taken from the food in the beginning due to the hydrolyzation. Because of that it is very hard to identify all the metabolites and to evaluate their biological activity. Fortunately, absorption rate and state of the metabolites going through in the plasma determined from the chemical structure of polyphenols not its concentration [20].

Even though most of the polyphenols were absorbed from small intestine after the hydrolyzed by intestinal enzymes, there are some indirect evidences for the absorption of polyphenols through the gut barrier. And it is known from the increase in the antioxidant capacity of the plasma after the consumption of polyphenol-rich foods [47].

In humans the absorption site of polyphenols changes. For example, some of the polyphenols are started to absorbed in the gastrointestinal tract while others absorbed in intestine or other part of the digestive tract. Most flavonoids except flavanols exist in glycosylated forms in foods. However, glycosides mechanism in the stomach is not clear yet. Most of the glycosides probably resist acidic medium during hydrolysis in the stomach and hence arrive intact in the intestine [48] where only aglycones and few glucosides can be absorbed. The most important part of polyphenol metabolism is the accumulation of polyphenols in the tissues. The accumulated polyphenols in the tissues are the concentration of biologically active molecules for exerting the beneficial effects of polyphenols.

In the literature many studies have shown that the especially metabolized polyphenols can go through tissues. Hence, it has been a strong indication for the beneficial health effects of the polyphenols depends on both the intake and bioavailability [1].

It is known that polyphenol-rich foods and its products may increase the antioxidant capacity of the plasma. After the consumption of the polyphenol rich products, hydrolyzed polyphenols and their metabolites will be present in the plasma which will increase the antioxidative capacity of plasma and their effects to other reducing agents (sparing effects of polyphenols on other endogenous antioxidants), or by their effect on the absorption of pro-oxidative food components, such as iron [2].

Reduced levels of oxidative damage have been associated with consumed antioxidant molecules present in the plasma. Supporting results have been obtained from the studies done with polyphenol rich food showing the protective effects of polyphenols against diseases. With these studies protective role of polyphenols on cell parts against oxidative damage can be shown.

Anti-Cancer Effect of Polyphenols

Effect of polyphenols on human cancer cell lines, mostly seen as protective and reduce the number of tumors or their growth. These beneficial effects have been seen working at various parts of the body, including mouth, stomach, colon, liver, lung or skin. In the literature most of the polyphenols, like quercetin, catechins, isoflavones, lignans, flavanones, ellagic acid, red wine polyphenols, resveratrol and curcumin have been studied and all of them showed protective effects against various cancer cells, even though they have a different action mechanisms [49].

Development of cancer is a multistage and step by step process. There are three major stages of cancer: initiation, promotion and progression. Initiation is a heritable aberration of a cell. Initiated cells can start a transformation to malignancy if promotion and progression continues. On the other hand, promotion can be altered by factors that do not change DNA sequences and include the selection and clonal expansion of initiated cells. Many action mechanisms have been known for chemoprotective effect of polyphenols. These are estrogenic/antiestrogenic activity, anti-proliferation, initiation of cell cycle arrest or apoptosis, prevention of oxidation, induction of detoxification enzymes, regulation of the host immune system, anti-inflammatory activity and changes in cellular signaling [50]. In the body, hydrolyzed polyphenols can produce potentially toxic quinones which are substrates of these enzymes. The daily intake of polyphenols might activate these enzymes for their own detoxication and, create a general boost in our defenses against toxic xenobiotics [51]. For the drug resistant tumor cells *in vitro* and *in vivo* studies were done in the literature, support using dietary polyphenols for human cancer as chemoprotection with combination either chemotherapeutic drugs or cytotoxic factors for more efficient treatment.

Protective Role of Polyphenols on Cancer Studies

As there are many types of polyphenols available in the nature, also there are various types of cancer. Even though, polyphenols show protective properties against oxidative damage due to the different action mechanisms, different polyphenols have been studied against different cancer types.

Prostate cancer (PCa) is the most common cancer for men. Risk factors for PCa include parameters like age, genetics, ethnicity, hormonal status, diet and lifestyle. In the literature many bioactive compounds have been studied against PCa. Green tea derived polyphenols, which can be given as green tea polyphenols (GTP) have gained a big interest for their protective properties, especially their important part in prostate cancer for chemoprevention and chemotherapy.

Many studies have showed protective effects of GTP using *in vitro* and *in vivo* methods and in human clinical trials. GTP shows greater advantages like inhibiting various stages of cancer development by changing key cellular proteins which are involved in diverse signal transduction pathways. Hence changing the expression of genes responsible for cell proliferation, angiogenesis and apoptosis. Among green tea catechins, epigallocatechin-3-gallate (EGCG) is best studied for its cancer preventive properties [52].

In the study done by Henning *et al.* phytoestrogens and tea polyphenols in human prostate tissue were measured. And it showed that tea polyphenols are bioavailable in human prostate. The obtained data showed that, at the end of the daily consumption of 1.42 L of green tea or black tea for 5 days, epigallocatechin, epicatechin, epigallocatechin gallate, epicatechin gallate reached concentrations ranging from 21 to 107 pmol/g tissue in prostate tissue samples [53].

More than 650,000 patients per year are diagnosed with head and neck cancer which become globally critical health problem. Unfortunately, this cancer shows a high recurrence rate, and causing second primary cancers in other locations, most of the time causing a poor prognosis. Another problem faced within this cancer is that, with the current medical and surgical treatments a considerable damage has done to speaking and swallowing functions. In addition to that, side effects such as nausea, vomiting, bone marrow suppression, and renal damage, significantly effecting the patients' quality of life. In order to improve the quality of the treatments polyphenols have been studied. For head and neck cancer cells the most studied phytochemicals are the carotenoids and phenolics. The chemopreventive activities of phytochemicals have been shown to be associated with their antioxidant properties [54]. Studies showed that phenolics can regulate the cancer cell signaling pathways, protect the healthy cell during the treatment which reduce the damage caused by invasive treatments of chemotherapy and radiotherapy.

By being the second most common cancer in worldwide cervical cancer is the major threat to the health of women age between 15 to 44. The most important and unanimously accepted factor causing the cervical cancer is the infection of human papillomavirus which is known as HPV. Working on specific steps of viral transformation processes, polyphenols have been shown inhibition of tumor cell growth selectively without significantly disturbing normal cells which could be a promising therapeutic tool for treatment of cervical cancer [55]. Due to these reasons polyphenols have been found to be promising agents toward cervical cancer. For the cervical cancer cells. epigallocatechin-3-gallate, curcumin, ferulic acid, resveratrol, are one of the few studied polyphenols.

Even though it is a multi-factorial chronic disease, resulting from the combination of multiple genetic and environmental factors, the most crucial and important factor is mostly a poor diet regimen for the colon or colorectal cancer. With the nutritional well-balanced diet and the plant-derived polyphenols it is possible to inhibit cancer development and propagation. In addition, polyphenols can be used as chemopreventive agents. Some of the studies reported that, polyphenols have a protective effect against colon cancer, for example; curcumin, gallic acid, ellagic acid, and epigallocatechin-3-gallate [56].

In study done by Hung *et al.* inhibitory effects of apple polyphenol (AP) *in vitro* and *in vivo* were investigated. As a result of study, it was seen that AP majorly suppressed migration, invasion, colony formation and adhesion of DLD-1 cells. In the study they also showed antitumoral and anti-metastatic effects of AP were also demonstrated *in vivo*. Collectively, AP significantly inhibited motility of DLD-1 cells *via* disruption of interaction between Snail and the FAK promoter and consequently diminished tumorigenesis and metastasis of DLD-1 cells [57]. The importance of their findings was indicate that AP diminished the metastatic capability of DLD-1 cells *via* Snail-mediated down-regulation of FAK expression and the subsequent inhibition of FAK signaling cascades such as paxillin, Src, Akt, Rho A, Rac-1 and Cdc42.

In other study done by Lin *et al.* showed that apple polyphenol phloretin inhibits colorectal cancer cell growth *via* inhibition of the type 2 glucose transporter. For this study, p53-mediated signals were crucial. With the inhibition of wild type p53 by dominant negative p53 will reduce the phloretin-induced colon cancer migration and its related signals. In the studies it was shown that with the activation of nuclear factor-kB(NF-kB) occurs *via* lipopolysaccharide (LPS) binding to the Toll-like receptor 4 (TLR4) in colon cancer. By changing the polysaccharide components in apple modified this pathway; which led to, supplementation of apple polysaccharide significantly inhibited the migratory ability *in vitro* on the LPS/TLR4/NF-kB pathway in colorectal cancer cells (HT-29 and SW620 cells. With this study beneficial properties of phloretin were observed. In addition to inducing growth arrest of cells in the G0/G1 phase, induce apoptotic cell death and inhibit tumor cells migration and metastasis. All these effects can be assigned to the phloretin-induced intracellular glucose deprivation [58].

Liver cancer or hepatocellular carcinoma (HCC) is one of the most common malignancy worldwide with a high mortality. Current treatments are not so efficient against HCC. In order to improve that new treatments are needed. Same with other types of cancers chemoprotective effects of polyphenols are effective against liver cancer which is an important way for making HCC to reverse, suppress or prevent carcinogenesis. In order to achieve that natural or synthetic chemical agents have been used. Among the studied polyphenols, quercetin along with 4-hydroxyflavone and luteolin were the most effective to inhibit liver cancer cell growth [59].

In a study done on liver cancer cells, the effect of apple polyphenol extract on the proliferation and invasion of rat ascites hepatoma cell line (AH109A) was examined *in vitro*. The apple polyphenol extract attenuated both proliferation and invasion of the hepatoma cell line in a dose-dependent approach up to 200 mg/mL. In an *in vivo* study, apple polyphenol also reduced the growth and metastasis of solid hepatomas and importantly inhibited the serum lipid peroxide level in rats transplanted with AH109A [60].

ENCAPSULATION OF POLYPHENOLS

New applications of polyphenols, have raised a new potential in the functional foods, nutraceutical and pharmaceutical industries, due to their beneficial effects to human health. Due to the increasing interest in polyphenols, improving their stability become the priority in the scientific studies. Protecting the natural compounds from the harsh environmental and process conditions that can change the stability, bioactivity and bioavailability. In addition to that, the unpleasant taste of polyphenols also limit their application in various industries. Just by using the encapsulation techniques these deficiencies can be effectively decreased.

Many structures can be obtained with encapsulation, but there are two main groups: one is mononuclear capsules, which have obtained from encapsulation of a single core by a shell matrix and the other one is aggregates which have more than a single core in a matrix [61]. Their properties like shape, size change with the type of encapsulation technique and the materials used for the encapsulation. The used technologies for encapsulation of polyphenols, include spray drying, coacervation, liposome entrapment, inclusion complexation, co-crystallization, nanoencapsulation, freeze drying, yeast encapsulation and emulsion.

Even though different techniques are used for encapsulation, three main steps are same for each encapsulation technique:

- The obtaining wall around the desired material
- Ensuring that unwanted leakage does not occur from the encapsulate
- Ensuring that unwanted materials are left out [62]

The aim of the encapsulation is to protect the core material from harsh environmental conditions, such as undesirable effects of light, temperature, moisture, and oxygen. By improving these conditions, the shelf life of the product is increased, and obtain a controlled delivery from the encapsulate [63]. The main reasons for the encapsulation have been summarized by Desai and Park as follows:

- Protection of the core material from degradation to improve its stability by protecting from harsh environmental conditions
- Changing the evaporation or release rate of the core material to the outer media
- Altering of the physical characteristics of the core material to create better handling such as easier tableting or stabile formulations for the pharmaceutical industries
- Modifying the release profile of the core material for the specific time
- To hide an unpleasant flavor, smell or taste of the core material
- Changing the concentration of the core material when only small amounts are required, while achieving uniform dispersion in the host material
- The separation of the reacted components with one another in the mixture [64]

With all these advantages encapsulation of polyphenols for the better and stabile formulations, protection of the natural bioactive compounds has been become a great potential for the industries such as pharmaceuticals, food and nutraceutical.

One of the biggest challenge working with the bioactive compounds are a very small portion of the compound is available when it is orally administrated. As previously mentioned, reasons for that are low permeability and solubility, inadequate gastric residence time, stability problems due to harsh process conditions in the gastrointestinal tract pH, presence of enzymes and other compounds [16]. The effectiveness of encapsulated bioactive natural compounds against diseases depends on preserving the bioavailability and the stability of the active ingredients. In order to deliver these compounds, encapsulates that can protect the stability of the bioactive compound until the time of consumption are needed. Also, with the encapsulation it is possible to deliver to physiological target within the organism. In addition to that with encapsulation it is possible to overcome limited stability and low solubility problems that come working with polyphenols [17]. Another challenge of polyphenols is their potential unpleasant taste or smell, which has to be hidden before added into food products or used as food supplements.

With the encapsulation of polyphenols rather than using their free forms can overcome these challenges of their instability, ease unpleasant tastes or flavors, as well as improve the bioavailability and half-life of the compound *in vivo* and *in vitro*.

Spray Drying

Due to the fact it is easy to use, flexible and continuous operation, spray drying encapsulation mostly has been preferred in the food industry in order to prepare dry, stable food additives and flavors [64]. Particles obtained with spray dryer have a good quality. For the encapsulation as shell material modified starch, maltodextrin, gum or other substances are used. To obtain homogenous mixture it is crucial to homogenize the core and shell mixture. After that the mixture is introduced to spray dryer and particles are obtained through a nozzle or spinning wheel. Water in the mixture is evaporated during the drying process by hot air in the system. The encapsulates are collected from bottom of the dryer [62]. For the spray dryer method only drawback is the solubility of the shell material in the water must be at an acceptable level. Therefore there are limited numbers of shell materials available [64]. By using spray drying method the stability of the products can be improved.

Coacervation

The object of encapsulation by using coacervation method is the phase separation of one or many hydrocolloids from the initial solution. The following position of the obtained coacervate phase around the active ingredient suspended or emulsified in the same reaction medium.

Coacervation encapsulation can be obtained simply with only one colloidal solute or through a complex coacervation. Even though for encapsulation of food ingredients complex coacervation is considered an expensive method due to high operational costs; however for compounds like valuable, unstable, such as polyphenols it is possible to use complex coacervation method for the encapsulation [65]. For the laboratory scale, coacervation technique can be very useful however for the industrial scale due to high operational costs will not be feasible.

Liposomes

Liposomes are colloidal encapsulates with combination membrane systems obtained from lipids in order to encapsulate aqueous mediums. By using both lipid and aqueous phases, liposomes can be used for encapsulation of water soluble and lipid soluble compounds. In addition to the encapsulation with the liposomes delivery and release of these compounds can be achieved. The formation of the liposomes is depending on the interaction hydrophilic-hydrophobic phospholipids and water molecules. The biggest benefit of liposome is the controlling the release rate of the desired compound and obtain a targeted delivery [66]. Liposome encapsulated bioactive compounds can be protected harsh conditions to sustain bioactivity and bioavailability and show significant levels of absorption in the gastrointestinal tract [67]. In the literature there are various techniques for obtaining liposomes. Different techniques can be used for different types of polyphenols.

Inclusion Encapsulation

Molecular inclusion is usually obtained by using cyclodextrins (CDs) as the shell material for the encapsulates. The external part of the cyclodextrin molecules is hydrophilic, whereas the internal part is hydrophobic. This characteristic structure of CDs makes a better alternative for the compounds for less polar such as essential oils due to the hydrophobic interaction between apolar internal cavity. The biggest benefit of working with CDs is the overcome the water solubility problems of less water-soluble phytochemicals [45]. In addition to that, with the encapsulation by using CDs increase the antioxidant activities of the polyphenols. Increment in the antioxidant activity might come from the prevention of the polyphenols from oxidation [68], and increasing their solubility in the biological medium [69]. The encapsulation efficiency of CDs inclusion is changed by the core materials. Generally, the higher the hydrophobicity and smaller the molecule is, the greater the affinity for the CDs.

Co-Crystallization

Encapsulation of bioactive compounds by using co-crystallization can be done where crystalline structure of sucrose is changed from a perfect to an irregular agglomerated crystal. With the obtained porous matrix active compound can be encapsulated [43]. The main advantages of encapsulation with co-crystallization method are increased solubility, wettability, homogeneity, dispersibility, hydration, anticaking, stability and flowability of the encapsulated materials. In addition to that especially for the pharmaceutical applications core materials in liquid form can be dried without any extra process step.

Co-crystallization can be a better encapsulation method for the products which have difficulties in tableting due to the agglomerated structure. Especially, in candy and pharmaceutical industries it can be a significant advantage due to the tableting processes [64].

Freeze Drying

Freeze-drying, also known as lyophilization, is a process used for the drying of almost all heat-sensitive materials and aromas. For the encapsulation process, core materials homogenized in the matrix solutions. After then, then co-lyophilize, usually resulting in different forms. Except for the long drying period required (generally 20 h) compounds. Other than that freeze-drying is a simple technique for encapsulating water-soluble essences and natural aromas, as well as drugs [64]. Freeze dried samples have shown good shelf life protection of phenolics during storage stability while the antioxidant activity remained the same or even improved slightly [70].

Yeast Encapsulation

Encapsulation of bioactive compounds by using yeast cells (*Saccharomyces cerevisiae*) as shell material has been one of the low cost high volume process. For yeast encapsulation, yeast cells are used to encapsulate the active compound. Cell wall and the membrane of the yeast cells allow the active compounds to pass through the cell and remain in there. Same as the other encapsulation techniques with the yeast encapsulation, protection of the active compounds from harsh process conditions can be achieved. Also release of the active compound through the cell is controlled the release profile of the encapsulate [71].

Emulsions

In the emulsion method, at least two immiscible liquids are needed. Emulsion can be done as oil in water or water in oil. In both way one of the liquid being dispersed as small droplets in each other [72]. One drawback of this method to prepare kinetically stable solutions. However, to overcome this problem stabilizers like emulsifiers or modifiers are generally added in the emulsions [73]. Encapsulation with emulsion method usually used when encapsulated bioactive compound is used as liquid state.

Nanoparticles in Cancer Therapy

In the recent years, nanoparticles have been widely studied to increase targeted delivery of drugs to the tumor site. Selectivity of nanoparticles can optimize dose requirement and reduce systemic toxicity which are one of the most common limits of anticancer drugs.

Nanoparticles accomplished this task due to their ability to accumulate in the solid tumor mass and their targeting mechanisms that can be either passive or active and to specifically trigger internalization inside tumor cells. These specifications have made nanoparticles an irreplaceable method for cancer therapy, imaging, and a combination of the two in the more recent theranostic approach [74].

The major challenges are faced with polyphenolic compounds, low solubility and poor permeability across the cells, which restrict the applications of the natural compounds in the therapeutic protocols [74]. Using of the encapsulation as effective delivery systems that can heal the side effects of these chemopreventive compounds is the crucial part in cancer treatments. With these systems improvements in absorption through membrane of cancer cells are possible [59].

However, dimensions of the carrier system and surface properties are most relevant factors for the interaction with the cell surfaces. With the nanoparticles the strict relationship polyphenols' solubility and absorption is changed. Nanoparticles become the beneficial pathway for cell penetration and possibly localization in the targeted site [75].

A study done by Minaei *et al.* investigated the role of nano-quercetin (phytosome) in doxorubicin-induced apoptosis. Quercetin, is one of the most known plant-derived phenolic compounds which plays a crucial part in controlling hemostasis, by having potent antioxidant and free-radical scavenging properties. When this flavonoid combined with chemotherapeutic drugs, the benefits of these agents in induction of apoptosis in cancer cells improves.

Their results suggest that, with the phytosome technology the benefits of chemotherapeutics can be elevated by increasing the permeability of tumor cells to chemical agents. Recently, in the literature the applications of phytosoms, which are advanced nanoparticles, for the drug delivery purposes have been started to study. The main advantages come with phytosoms including high bioavailability and improved molecular size which can increase the efficiency of chemotherapeutic agents passing through the biological membranes. In the study, nanoparticle complexes were prepared with quercetin and lecithin mixture. And the results showed that, high stability, high solubility and excellent size for absorption in tumor cells. With this study potential ability of nano quercetinas as supporting therapy to chemotherapy protocols was reported [76].

A study done by Kristl *et al.* were compared the effects of resveratrol (RSV)-loaded liposomes (LIP–RSVs) to free RSV on the performances of the cell metabolic activity and cell-redox system. And the results showed that liposomes distinctly qualify the uptake of RSV by the cancer cells and hence influence its intracellular fate. Encapsulation of RSV into liposomal bilayers prevents transformation of the active RSV from trans configuration into inactive cis form which is shown by HPLC analysis. The –OH groups, which are responsible for the antioxidant activity of the RSV, are likely positioned at the liposomal surface for scavenging of radicals. Encapsulation of RSV with liposomal bilayers provide an environment for storage and thus cell membranes are prevented against high RSV loading, which caused deteriorative effects on the cells [77]. Moreover, obtained results of this study shows that with the encapsulation of RSV with liposomes ensure the release of RSV into the cytosol is slow, which reduces its cytotoxicity. In summary, liposomal formulation provides a prolonged intracellular delivery of RSV with no cytotoxic results.

A study performed by Zaman *et al.*, encapsulation of curcumin was investigated. To improve its rapid degradation and poor bioavailability, they report a poly(lactic-co-glycolic acid) based curcumin nanoparticle formulation (Nano-CUR). This study shows that in comparison to free CUR, Nano-CUR in terms of cell growth inhibition, increase apoptosis, and arrests the cell cycle in cervical cancer cell lines. Internalization patterns of CUR and Nano-CUR were investigated with fluorescence microscopy and flow cytometry techniques. The results showed that an increase in the concentration of CUR and Nano-CUR in cervical cancer cells. Fluorescence microscopy analysis revealed that, free CUR incubated cells exhibited presence of CUR in the periphery and cytoplasm. Whereas, in the case of Nano-CUR, due to smaller size internalization was more efficient by endocytosis process. Therefore, greater accumulation of CUR was observed on the cell membrane and cytoplasm due to the greater interaction of Nano-CUR with the cell surface. Nano-CUR treatment decreased factors such as miRNAs, transcription factors, and proteins associated with carcinogenesis. Moreover, Nano-CUR effectively decreased the tumor burden in a pre-clinical orthotopic mouse model of cervical cancer by decreasing oncogenic miRNA-21, suppressing nuclear β-catenin, and abrogating expression of E6/E7 HPV oncoproteins including smoking compound benzo[a]pyrene (BaP) induced E6/E7 and IL-6 expression. These superior pre-clinical data suggest that Nano-CUR may be an effective therapeutic modality for cervical cancer [78].

Another study investigated nano-formulation of curcumin to extend its retention time in the body and enhance the bio-availability. High-pressure emulsification-solvent-evaporation was designed to obtain curcumin-loaded PLGA nanoparticles (C-NPs) were done by Tsai *et al*. In the study parameters for the curcumin-loaded PLGA nanoparticles has been optimized. And obtained results were favorable for characteristics, and storage stability of nano-particles. In addition, the pharmacokinetic parameters of the curcumin-loaded PLGA nanoparticles have been determined after intravenous and oral administration, as well as excretion matters with C-NPs in a freely-moving rat model. Curcumin exposure in the body was increased with both intravenous or oral administration given nanoparticles. These findings demonstrate that PLGA nano-formulation could potentially be applied to increase bioavailability of hydrophobic polyphenols [79].

Another study done by Hung *et al*. evaluate the emulsion-liposome blends for resveratrol delivery. The aim of this present study was to develop formulations with both lipid emulsions and liposomes for resveratrol delivery. The formulations were prepared with coconut oil as the oil phase, soybean lecithin and Brij surfactants as the emulsifiers, and glycerol formal as a solubilizer. Resveratrol, the main active polyphenol in red wine, was encapsulated into different combinations of emulsions and liposomes to investigate its physicochemical characteristics and cardiovascular protection. The mixtures of emulsion-liposome were prepared with coconut oil, soybean lecithin, glycerol formal, and non-ionic surfactants. Multiple systems were investigated by evaluating the droplet size, surface charge, drug encapsulation, release rate, and stability. The liposomal particles in the systems had smaller diameters by comparing with emulsions. With the encapsulation almost 70% of drug were encapsulated into the particles. Also, due to the encapsulation of resveratrol into these systems drug release rate was decreased in both the presence and absence of plasma *in vitro*. The emulsion-liposome blends which incorporated Brij 98 (F5) showed the slowest release at zero- order for resveratrol delivery. Treatment using resveratrol in the particle formulations dramatically suppressed vascular intimal thickening, which was tested in an experimental model in which endothelial injury was produced in normal rat carotid arteries. Intraperitoneal injection of the multiple systems was showed almost no toxicity in both liver and kidney. The results showed that encapsulation with the emulsion-liposome systems is a convincing way to enhance the preventative and therapeutic benefits of resveratrol [80].

In Table **2** studies done with encapsulation of polyphenols and their anticancer activities were given. As seen from the studies given at Table **2** with the encapsulation of polyphenols poor bioavailability, low solubility and stability problems were overcome and the treatment for the cancer cells were achieved.

Table 2. Encapsulated polyphenols with anticancer activity and their mechanisms of action.

Encapsulated Polyphenol	Materials	Targets	Anticancer activity	References
Quercetin	Polylactide	Brain	↑antitoxic effect ↓ cell proliferation	[74]
	PLGA	Brain, liver		[76]
	Glyceryl monoste	Stomach, intestine		[75]
Resveratrol	Poly-caprolactone-PEG	Neuronal cell line	↓ cell growth and ↓tumor growth	[77]
	mPEG–PCL	Glioma cells		[80]
Curcumin	PLGA	Leukemia, colon, breast, prostate cancer cells	↓cell growth ↓ tumor growth ↓cell viability	[15, 56]
	Alginate-chitosan	Cervical cancer cells		[78]
	Silk	Breast cancer cells		[79]
	Casein	Cervical cancer cells		[55]
	Poly(butyl) cyanoacrylate	Neuroblastoma cells		[81]
Epigallocatechin gallate	PLA-PEG	Pancreatic cancer	↓colony formation and ↓cell viability	[15]
β-Lapachone	PLA-PEG	Lung, prostate, breast cancer cells	↓cell viability	[81]
Daidzein	PEGylated phospholipid	Cardiovascular system		[81]
Tea polyphenol (TP)	Chitosan	Colon cancer	↑ Photothermal destruction	[82]
		Prostate cancer		[52]
Thymoquinone	PLGA	Leukemic cells		
Courmarin	PLGA nanoparticles	Skin cancer	↓Cell viability ↑Apoptosis	[81]
Baicalein	ligands of folate and hyaluronic acid	lung cancer	↓Tumor growth *in vivo*	[15, 81]
Ferulic acid	BSA	Liver		[59]
	Bovine serum albumin	Liver		[59]
Chrysin	Nanosuspension	hepatocellular carcinoma	↓Cell growth	[81]
Honokiol	MPEG micelles	lung cancer cell	↓Cell growth Induction of cell cycle arrest	[81]

(Table 2) cont.....

Encapsulated Polyphenol	Materials	Targets	Anticancer activity	References
Luteolin	Phytosome	Breast cancer cells	↓Cell viability ↑Sensitivity to doxorubicin	
	PLA-PEG-OMe nanoparticles	Lung cancer	↓Tumor growth ↓Colony formation ↓Tumor size in animals	[15, 81]

In Table (**2**) anticancer activity of encapsulated some polyphenols studied in the literature are given.

CONCLUDING REMARKS

It is known that polyphenols or polyphenol-rich foods offer a significant protection against the development and progression of many chronic pathological conditions including cancer, diabetes, cardiovascular problems and aging. Even though there are many studies in the literature showing the biological effects of polyphenols, still mechanism of some polyphenols in the human body is yet to be discovered. The utilization of polyphenols as potential cancer treatment agents is unfortunately limited due to their limited absorption, low tissue bioavailability and high chemical instability. For this reason, encapsulation technologies can be potential solutions to these limitations by enhancing bioavailability, stability along with targeted delivery of polyphenols with a controlled manner. By using encapsulation technologies polyphenols can effectively be used for treatment of various diseases. The sizes of the carriers encapsulating polyphenols can range from nano to micro scale. The number of studies performed in the past few years concerning with nanomedicine in cancer therapy has resulted in a greater knowledge of carrier properties which are more relevant to selective drug delivery and efficacy. Even with the unknown territory it is known that polyphenols offer great hope for the prevention of chronic human diseases. Same as most nanoparticle research, evidence of the improvement of interaction with cells is, currently obtained from preliminary *in vitro* studies on cell cultures. Although lack of clinical studies in humans, the data obtained from *in vitro* and in animal model studies were resulted with positive outcomes. There are still a lot to discover on the role of polyphenols in human health which makes it a fertile subject for the research. This knowledge, as provided in this chapter, resulted especially useful to exploit the great potential of polyphenols in cancer prevention and therapy. The results were promising in this field. Therefore, the researches in this area will be encouraging.

CONSENT FOR PUBLICATION

Not applicable.

CONFLICT OF INTEREST

The authors confirm that this chapter content has no conflict of interest.

ACKNOWLEDGEMENT

Declared none.

REFERENCES

[1]   D'Archivio, M.; Filesi, C.; Di Benedetto, R.; Gargiulo, R.; Giovannini, C.; Masella, R. Polyphenols, dietary sources and bioavailability. *Ann. Ist. Super. Sanita,* **2007,** *43*(4), 348-361.
[PMID: 18209268]

[2]   Scalbert, A.; Manach, C.; Morand, C.; Rémésy, C.; Jiménez, L. Dietary polyphenols and the prevention of diseases. *Crit. Rev. Food Sci. Nutr.,* **2005,** *45*(4), 287-306.
[http://dx.doi.org/10.1080/1040869059096] [PMID: 16047496]

[3]   Spencer, J.P.E.; Abd El Mohsen, M.M.; Minihane, A-M.; Mathers, J.C. Biomarkers of the intake of dietary polyphenols: strengths, limitations and application in nutrition research. *Br. J. Nutr.,* **2008,** *99*(1), 12-22.
[http://dx.doi.org/10.1017/S0007114507798938] [PMID: 17666146]

[4]   Beckman, C.H. Phenolic-Storing Cells: Keys to Programmed Cell Death and Periderm Formation in Wilt Disease Resistance and in General Defence Responses in Plants? *Physiol. Mol. Plant Pathol.,* **2000,** *57*(3), 101-110.
[http://dx.doi.org/10.1006/pmpp.2000.0287]

[5]   Graf, B.A.; Milbury, P.E.; Blumberg, J.B. Flavonols, flavones, flavanones, and human health: epidemiological evidence. *J. Med. Food,* **2005,** *8*(3), 281-290.
[http://dx.doi.org/10.1089/jmf.2005.8.281] [PMID: 16176136]

[6]   Arts, I.C.W.; Hollman, P.C.H. Polyphenols and disease risk in epidemiologic studies. *Am. J. Clin. Nutr.,* **2005,** *81*(1) Suppl., 317S-325S.
[http://dx.doi.org/10.1093/ajcn/81.1.317S] [PMID: 15640497]

[7]   Kondratyuk, T.P.; Pezzuto, J.M. Natural Product Polyphenols of Relevance to Human Health. *Pharm. Biol.,* **2004,** *42,* 46-63.
[http://dx.doi.org/10.3109/13880200490893519]

[8]   de Simón, B.F.; Pérez-Ilzarbe, J.; Hernández, T.; Gómez-Cordovés, C.; Estrella, I. Importance of Phenolic Compounds for the Characterization of Fruit Juices. *J. Agric. Food Chem.,* **1992,** *40*(9), 1531-1535.
[http://dx.doi.org/10.1021/jf00021a012]

[9]   de Groot, H.; Rauen, U. Tissue injury by reactive oxygen species and the protective effects of flavonoids. *Fundam. Clin. Pharmacol.,* **1998,** *12*(3), 249-255.
[http://dx.doi.org/10.1111/j.1472-8206.1998.tb00951.x] [PMID: 9646056]

[10]   Pandey, K.B.; Rizvi, S.I. Plant polyphenols as dietary antioxidants in human health and disease. *Oxid. Med. Cell. Longev.,* **2009,** *2*(5), 270-278.
[http://dx.doi.org/10.4161/oxim.2.5.9498] [PMID: 20716914]

[11]   Manach, C.; Williamson, G.; Morand, C.; Scalbert, A.; Rémésy, C. Bioavailability, Polyphenols: Food Sources and. *Am. J. Clin. Nutr.,* **2004,** *79,* 727-747.

[http://dx.doi.org/10.1093/ajcn/79.5.727] [PMID: 15113710]

[12]   Price, K.R.; Bacon, J.R.; Rhodes, M.J.C. Effect of Storage and Domestic Processing on the Content and Composition of Flavonol Glucosides in Onion (Allium Cepa). *J. Agric. Food Chem.,* **1997**, *45*(3), 938-942.
[http://dx.doi.org/10.1021/jf9605916]

[13]   Crozier, A.; Lean, M.E.J.; McDonald, M.S.; Black, C. Quantitative Analysis of the Flavonoid Content of Commercial Tomatoes, Onions, Lettuce, and Celery. *J. Agric. Food Chem.,* **1997**, *45*(3), 590-595.
[http://dx.doi.org/10.1021/jf960339y]

[14]   Zhou, L.; Elias, R.J. Antioxidant and pro-oxidant activity of (-)-epigallocatechin-3-gallate in food emulsions: Influence of pH and phenolic concentration. *Food Chem.,* **2013**, *138*(2-3), 1503-1509.
[http://dx.doi.org/10.1016/j.foodchem.2012.09.132] [PMID: 23411273]

[15]   Munin, A.; Edwards-Lévy, F. Encapsulation of natural polyphenolic compounds; a review. *Pharmaceutics,* **2011**, *3*(4), 793-829.
[http://dx.doi.org/10.3390/pharmaceutics3040793] [PMID: 24309309]

[16]   Manach, C.; Williamson, G.; Morand, C.; Scalbert, A.; Rémésy, C. Bioavailability and bioefficacy of polyphenols in humans. I. Review of 97 bioavailability studies. *Am. J. Clin. Nutr.,* **2005**, *81*(1) Suppl., 230S-242S.
[http://dx.doi.org/10.1093/ajcn/81.1.230S] [PMID: 15640486]

[17]   Vinson, J.A.; Su, X.; Zubik, L.; Bose, P. Phenol antioxidant quantity and quality in foods: fruits. *J. Agric. Food Chem.,* **2001**, *49*(11), 5315-5321.
[http://dx.doi.org/10.1021/jf0009293] [PMID: 11714322]

[18]   Singleton, V.L.; Rossi, J.A., Jr; Rossi, J.A., Jr Colorimetry of Total Phenolics with Phosphomolybdic-Phosphotungstic Acid Reagents. *Am. J. Enol. Vitic.,* **1965**, *16*(3), 144-158.

[19]   Brat, P.; Georgé, S.; Bellamy, A.; Du Chaffaut, L.; Scalbert, A.; Mennen, L.; Arnault, N.; Amiot, M.J. Daily polyphenol intake in France from fruit and vegetables. *J. Nutr.,* **2006**, *136*(9), 2368-2373.
[http://dx.doi.org/10.1093/jn/136.9.2368] [PMID: 16920856]

[20]   Ovaskainen, M-L.; Törrönen, R.; Koponen, J.M.; Sinkko, H.; Hellström, J.; Reinivuo, H.; Mattila, P. Dietary intake and major food sources of polyphenols in Finnish adults. *J. Nutr.,* **2008**, *138*(3), 562-566.
[http://dx.doi.org/10.1093/jn/138.3.562] [PMID: 18287367]

[21]   Pérez-Jiménez, J.; Neveu, V.; Vos, F.; Scalbert, A. Identification of the 100 richest dietary sources of polyphenols: an application of the Phenol-Explorer database. *Eur. J. Clin. Nutr.,* **2010**, *64* Suppl. 3, S112-S120.
[http://dx.doi.org/10.1038/ejcn.2010.221] [PMID: 21045839]

[22]   Upadhyay, R.K. Essential Oils : Anti - Microbial, Antihelminthic, Antiviral, Anticancer And Anti - Insect Properties. *J. Appl. Biosci.,* **2010**, *36*(1), 1-22.

[23]   Imai, H.; Osawa, K.; Yasuda, H.; Hamashima, H.; Arai, T.; Sasatsu, M. Inhibition by the essential oils of peppermint and spearmint of the growth of pathogenic bacteria. *Microbios,* **2001**, *106* Suppl. 1, 31-39.
[PMID: 11549238]

[24]   Aly, S.E.; Sabry, B.A.; Shaheen, M.S.; Hathout, A.S. Assessment of Antimycotoxigenic and Antioxidant Activity of Star Anise (Illicium Verum) *in vitro. J. Saudi Soc. Agric. Sci.,* **2016**, *15*(1), 20-27.
[http://dx.doi.org/10.1016/j.jssas.2014.05.003]

[25]   Ferrazzano, G.F.; Amato, I.; Ingenito, A.; De Natale, A.; Pollio, A. Anti-cariogenic effects of polyphenols from plant stimulant beverages (cocoa, coffee, tea). *Fitoterapia,* **2009**, *80*(5), 255-262.
[http://dx.doi.org/10.1016/j.fitote.2009.04.006] [PMID: 19397954]

[26]   Boivin, D.; Lamy, S.; Lord-Dufour, S.; Jackson, J.; Beaulieu, E.; Côté, M.; Moghrabi, A.; Barrette, S.;

Gingras, D.; Béliveau, R. Antiproliferative and Antioxidant Activities of Common Vegetables: A Comparative Study. *Food Chem.,* **2009,** *112*(2), 374-380.
[http://dx.doi.org/10.1016/j.foodchem.2008.05.084]

[27]   Kokotkiewicz, A.; Jaremicz, Z.; Luczkiewicz, M. Aronia plants: a review of traditional use, biological activities, and perspectives for modern medicine. *J. Med. Food,* **2010,** *13*(2), 255-269.
[http://dx.doi.org/10.1089/jmf.2009.0062] [PMID: 20170359]

[28]   Mulvihill, E.E.; Huff, M.W. Antiatherogenic properties of flavonoids: implications for cardiovascular health. *Can. J. Cardiol.,* **2010,** *26* Suppl. A, 17A-21A.
[http://dx.doi.org/10.1016/S0828-282X(10)71056-4] [PMID: 20386755]

[29]   Kaur, R.; Kaur, M.; Gill, B.S. Phenolic Acid Composition of Flaxseed Cultivars by Ultra-Performance Liquid Chromatography (UPLC) and Their Antioxidant Activities: Effect of Sand Roasting and Microwave Heating. *J. Food Process. Preserv.,* **2017,** *41*(5), e13181.
[http://dx.doi.org/10.1111/jfpp.13181]

[30]   David, L.; Moldovan, B.; Vulcu, A.; Olenic, L.; Perde-Schrepler, M.; Fischer-Fodor, E.; Florea, A.; Crisan, M.; Chiorean, I.; Clichici, S.; Filip, G.A. Green synthesis, characterization and anti-inflammatory activity of silver nanoparticles using European black elderberry fruits extract. *Colloids Surf. B Biointerfaces,* **2014,** *122*, 767-777.
[http://dx.doi.org/10.1016/j.colsurfb.2014.08.018] [PMID: 25174985]

[31]   Thole, J.M.; Kraft, T.F.; Sueiro, L.A.; Kang, Y-H.; Gills, J.J.; Cuendet, M.; Pezzuto, J.M.; Seigler, D.S.; Lila, M.A. A comparative evaluation of the anticancer properties of European and American elderberry fruits. *J. Med. Food,* **2006,** *9*(4), 498-504.
[http://dx.doi.org/10.1089/jmf.2006.9.498] [PMID: 17201636]

[32]   Dai, J.; Mumper, R.J. Plant phenolics: extraction, analysis and their antioxidant and anticancer properties. *Molecules,* **2010,** *15*(10), 7313-7352.
[http://dx.doi.org/10.3390/molecules15107313] [PMID: 20966876]

[33]   Mojžišová, G.; Mojžiš, J.; Pilátová, M.; Varinská, L.; Ivanová, L.; Strojný, L.; Richnavský, J. Antiproliferative and antiangiogenic properties of horse chestnut extract. *Phytother. Res.,* **2013,** *27*(2), 159-165.
[http://dx.doi.org/10.1002/ptr.4688] [PMID: 22451355]

[34]   Tsao, R. Chemistry and biochemistry of dietary polyphenols. *Nutrients,* **2010,** *2*(12), 1231-1246.
[http://dx.doi.org/10.3390/nu2121231] [PMID: 22254006]

[35]   Brunner, G. Supercritical Fluids: Technology and Application to Food Processing. *J. Food Eng.,* **2005,** *67*(1–2), 21-33.
[http://dx.doi.org/10.1016/j.jfoodeng.2004.05.060]

[36]   Díaz-Reinoso, B.; Moure, A.; Domínguez, H.; Parajó, J.C. Supercritical CO2 extraction and purification of compounds with antioxidant activity. *J. Agric. Food Chem.,* **2006,** *54*(7), 2441-2469.
[http://dx.doi.org/10.1021/jf052858j] [PMID: 16569029]

[37]   Abascal, K.; Ganora, L.; Yarnell, E. The Effect of Freeze-Drying and Its Implicationsfor Botanical Medicine: A Review. *Phytother. Res.,* **2004,** *2005*(19), 655-660.

[38]   Qiu, Y.; Liu, Q.; Beta, T. Antioxidant Properties of Commercial Wild Rice and Analysis of Soluble and Insoluble Phenolic Acids. *Food Chem.,* **2010,** *121*(1), 140-147.
[http://dx.doi.org/10.1016/j.foodchem.2009.12.021]

[39]   Stalikas, C.D. Extraction, separation, and detection methods for phenolic acids and flavonoids. *J. Sep. Sci.,* **2007,** *30*(18), 3268-3295.
[http://dx.doi.org/10.1002/jssc.200700261] [PMID: 18069740]

[40]   Metivier, R.P.; Francis, F.J.; Clydesdale, F.M. Solvent Extraction of Anthocyanins From Wine Pomace. *J. Food Sci.,* **1980,** *45*(4), 1099-1100.
[http://dx.doi.org/10.1111/j.1365-2621.1980.tb07534.x]

[41]   Solana, M.; Boschiero, I.; Dall'Acqua, S.; Bertucco, A. A Comparison between Supercritical Fluid and Pressurized Liquid Extraction Methods for Obtaining Phenolic Compounds from Asparagus Officinalis L. *J. Supercrit. Fluids,* **2015,** *100,* 201-208.
[http://dx.doi.org/10.1016/j.supflu.2015.02.014]

[42]   Kikic, I.; Lora, M.; Bertucco, A. A Thermodynamic Analysis of Three-Phase Equilibria in Binary and Ternary Systems for Applications in Rapid Expansion of a Supercritical Solution (RESS), Particles from Gas-Saturated Solutions (PGSS), and Supercritical Antisolvent (SAS). *Ind. Eng. Chem. Res.,* **1997,** *36*(12), 5507-5515.
[http://dx.doi.org/10.1021/ie970376u]

[43]   Fang, Z. Encapsulation of Polyphenols a Review. *Trends Food Sci. Technol.,* **2010,** *21*(10), 510-523.
[http://dx.doi.org/10.1016/j.tifs.2010.08.003]

[44]   Foegeding, A.E.; Plundrich, N.; Schneider, M.; Campbell, C.; Lila, M.A. Protein-Polyphenol Particles for Delivering Structural and Health Functionality. *Food Hydrocoll.,* **2017,** *72,* 163-173.
[http://dx.doi.org/10.1016/j.foodhyd.2017.05.024]

[45]   Puligundla, P.; Mok, C.; Ko, S.; Liang, J.; Recharla, N. Nanotechnological Approaches to Enhance the Bioavailability and Therapeutic Efficacy of Green Tea Polyphenols. *J. Funct. Foods,* **2017,** *34,* 139-151.
[http://dx.doi.org/10.1016/j.jff.2017.04.023]

[46]   Day, A.J.; Williamson, G. Biomarkers for exposure to dietary flavonoids: a review of the current evidence for identification of quercetin glycosides in plasma. *Br. J. Nutr.,* **2001,** *86*(86) Suppl. 1, S105-S110.
[http://dx.doi.org/10.1079/BJN2001342] [PMID: 11520427]

[47]   Duthie, G.G.; Pedersen, M.W.; Gardner, P.T.; Morrice, P.C.; Jenkinson, A.M.; McPhail, D.B.; Steele, G.M. The effect of whisky and wine consumption on total phenol content and antioxidant capacity of plasma from healthy volunteers. *Eur. J. Clin. Nutr.,* **1998,** *52*(10), 733-736.
[http://dx.doi.org/10.1038/sj.ejcn.1600635] [PMID: 9805220]

[48]   Gee, J.M.; DuPont, M.S.; Day, A.J.; Plumb, G.W.; Williamson, G.; Johnson, I.T. Intestinal transport of quercetin glycosides in rats involves both deglycosylation and interaction with the hexose transport pathway. *J. Nutr.,* **2000,** *130*(11), 2765-2771.
[http://dx.doi.org/10.1093/jn/130.11.2765] [PMID: 11053519]

[49]   Johnson, I.T.; Williamson, G.; Musk, S.R. Anticarcinogenic factors in plant foods: a new class of nutrients? *Nutr. Res. Rev.,* **1994,** *7*(1), 175-204.
[http://dx.doi.org/10.1079/NRR19940011] [PMID: 19094297]

[50]   García-Lafuente, A.; Guillamón, E.; Villares, A.; Rostagno, M.A.; Martínez, J.A. Flavonoids as anti-inflammatory agents: implications in cancer and cardiovascular disease. *Inflamm. Res.,* **2009,** *58*(9), 537-552.
[http://dx.doi.org/10.1007/s00011-009-0037-3] [PMID: 19381780]

[51]   Talalay, P.; De Long, M.J.; Prochaska, H.J. Identification of a common chemical signal regulating the induction of enzymes that protect against chemical carcinogenesis. *Proc. Natl. Acad. Sci. USA,* **1988,** *85*(21), 8261-8265.
[http://dx.doi.org/10.1073/pnas.85.21.8261] [PMID: 3141925]

[52]   Khan, N.; Mukhtar, H. Modulation of signaling pathways in prostate cancer by green tea polyphenols. *Biochem. Pharmacol.,* **2013,** *85*(5), 667-672.
[http://dx.doi.org/10.1016/j.bcp.2012.09.027] [PMID: 23041649]

[53]   Henning, S.M.; Aronson, W.; Niu, Y.; Conde, F.; Lee, N.H.; Seeram, N.P.; Lee, R-P.; Lu, J.; Harris, D.M.; Moro, A.; Hong, J.; Pak-Shan, L.; Barnard, R.J.; Ziaee, H.G.; Csathy, G.; Go, V.L.W.; Wang, H.; Heber, D. Tea polyphenols and theaflavins are present in prostate tissue of humans and mice after green and black tea consumption. *J. Nutr.,* **2006,** *136*(7), 1839-1843.
[http://dx.doi.org/10.1093/jn/136.7.1839] [PMID: 16772446]

[54]   Chang, H.P.; Sheen, L.Y.; Lei, Y.P. The protective role of carotenoids and polyphenols in patients with head and neck cancer. *J. Chin. Med. Assoc.,* **2015,** *78*(2), 89-95.
[http://dx.doi.org/10.1016/j.jcma.2014.08.010] [PMID: 25306067]

[55]   Di Domenico, F.; Foppoli, C.; Coccia, R.; Perluigi, M. Antioxidants in cervical cancer: chemopreventive and chemotherapeutic effects of polyphenols. *Biochim. Biophys. Acta,* **2012,** *1822*(5), 737-747.
[http://dx.doi.org/10.1016/j.bbadis.2011.10.005] [PMID: 22019724]

[56]   Santos, I.S.; Ponte, B.M.; Boonme, P.; Silva, A.M.; Souto, E.B. Nanoencapsulation of polyphenols for protective effect against colon-rectal cancer. *Biotechnol. Adv.,* **2013,** *31*(5), 514-523.
[http://dx.doi.org/10.1016/j.biotechadv.2012.08.005] [PMID: 22940401]

[57]   Hung, C-H.; Huang, C-C.; Hsu, L-S.; Kao, S-H.; Wang, C-J. Apple Polyphenol Inhibits Colon Carcinoma Metastasis *via* Disrupting Snail Binding to Focal Adhesion Kinase. *J. Funct. Foods,* **2015,** *12*, 80-91.
[http://dx.doi.org/10.1016/j.jff.2014.10.031]

[58]   Lin, S-T.; Tu, S-H.; Yang, P-S.; Hsu, S-P.; Lee, W-H.; Ho, C-T.; Wu, C-H.; Lai, Y-H.; Chen, M-Y.; Chen, L-C. Apple Polyphenol Phloretin Inhibits Colorectal Cancer Cell Growth *via* Inhibition of the Type 2 Glucose Transporter and Activation of p53-Mediated Signaling. *J. Agric. Food Chem.,* **2016,** *64*(36), 6826-6837.
[http://dx.doi.org/10.1021/acs.jafc.6b02861] [PMID: 27538679]

[59]   Stagos, D.; Amoutzias, G.D.; Matakos, A.; Spyrou, A.; Tsatsakis, A.M.; Kouretas, D. Chemoprevention of liver cancer by plant polyphenols. *Food Chem. Toxicol.,* **2012,** *50*(6), 2155-2170.
[http://dx.doi.org/10.1016/j.fct.2012.04.002] [PMID: 22521445]

[60]   Miura, D.; Miura, Y.; Yagasaki, K. Effect of apple polyphenol extract on hepatoma proliferation and invasion in culture and on tumor growth, metastasis, and abnormal lipoprotein profiles in hepatoma-bearing rats. *Biosci. Biotechnol. Biochem.,* **2007,** *71*(11), 2743-2750.
[http://dx.doi.org/10.1271/bbb.70359] [PMID: 17986774]

[61]   Schrooyen, P.M.M.; van der Meer, R.; De Kruif, C.G. Microencapsulation: its application in nutrition. *Proc. Nutr. Soc.,* **2001,** *60*(4), 475-479.
[http://dx.doi.org/10.1079/PNS2001112] [PMID: 12069400]

[62]   Gibbs, B.F.; Kermasha, S.; Alli, I.; Mulligan, C.N. Encapsulation in the food industry: a review. *Int. J. Food Sci. Nutr.,* **1999,** *50*(3), 213-224.
[http://dx.doi.org/10.1080/096374899101256] [PMID: 10627837]

[63]   Shahidi, F.; Han, X.Q. Encapsulation of food ingredients. *Crit. Rev. Food Sci. Nutr.,* **1993,** *33*(6), 501-547.
[http://dx.doi.org/10.1080/10408399309527645] [PMID: 8216812]

[64]   Desai, K.G.H.; Jin Park, H. Recent Developments in Microencapsulation of Food Ingredients. *Dry. Technol.,* **2005,** *23*, 1361-1394.
[http://dx.doi.org/10.1081/DRT-200063478]

[65]   Deladino, L.; Anbinder, P.S.; Navarro, A.S.; Martino, M.N. Encapsulation of Natural Antioxidants Extracted from Ilex Paraguariensis. *Carbohydr. Polym.,* **2008,** *71*(1), 126-134.
[http://dx.doi.org/10.1016/j.carbpol.2007.05.030]

[66]   Schäfer, V.; von Briesen, H.; Andreesen, R.; Steffan, A.M.; Royer, C.; Tröster, S.; Kreuter, J.; Rübsamen-Waigmann, H. Phagocytosis of nanoparticles by human immunodeficiency virus (HIV)-infected macrophages: a possibility for antiviral drug targeting. *Pharm. Res.,* **1992,** *9*(4), 541-546.
[http://dx.doi.org/10.1023/A:1015852732512] [PMID: 1495900]

[67]   Takahashi, M.; Inafuku, K.; Miyagi, T.; Oku, H.; Wada, K.; Imura, T.; Kitamoto, D. Efficient preparation of liposomes encapsulating food materials using lecithins by a mechanochemical method. *J. Oleo Sci.,* **2006,** *56*(1), 35-42.

[http://dx.doi.org/10.5650/jos.56.35] [PMID: 17693697]

[68]   Mercader-Ros, M.T.; Lucas-Abellán, C.; Fortea, M.I.; Gabaldón, J.A.; Núñez-Delicado, E. Effect of HP-B-Cyclodextrins Complexation on the Antioxidant Activity of Flavonols. *Food Chem.,* **2010,** *118*(3), 769-773.
[http://dx.doi.org/10.1016/j.foodchem.2009.05.061]

[69]   Haiyun, D.; Jianbin, C.; Guomei, Z.; Shaomin, S.; Jinhao, P. Preparation and spectral investigation on inclusion complex of beta-cyclodextrin with rutin. *Spectrochim. Acta A Mol. Biomol. Spectrosc.,* **2003,** *59*(14), 3421-3429.
[http://dx.doi.org/10.1016/S1386-1425(03)00176-8] [PMID: 14607238]

[70]   Delgado-Vargas, F.; Jiménez, A.R.; Paredes-López, O. Natural pigments: carotenoids, anthocyanins, and betalains--characteristics, biosynthesis, processing, and stability. *Crit. Rev. Food Sci. Nutr.,* **2000,** *40*(3), 173-289.
[http://dx.doi.org/10.1080/10408690091189257] [PMID: 10850526]

[71]   Bishop, J.R.P.; Nelson, G.; Lamb, J. Microencapsulation in yeast cells. *J. Microencapsul.,* **1998,** *15*(6), 761-773.
[http://dx.doi.org/10.3109/02652049809008259] [PMID: 9818954]

[72]   McClements, D.J.; Decker, E.A.; Park, Y.; Weiss, J. Structural design principles for delivery of bioactive components in nutraceuticals and functional foods. *Crit. Rev. Food Sci. Nutr.,* **2009,** *49*(6), 577-606.
[http://dx.doi.org/10.1080/10408390902841529] [PMID: 19484636]

[73]   Benichou, A.; Aserin, A.; Garti, N. Double emulsions stabilized with hybrids of natural polymers for entrapment and slow release of active matters. *Adv. Colloid Interface Sci.,* **2004,** *108-109*, 29-41.
[http://dx.doi.org/10.1016/j.cis.2003.10.013] [PMID: 15072926]

[74]   Bonferoni, M.C.; Rossi, S.; Sandri, G.; Ferrari, F. Nanoparticle formulations to enhance tumor targeting of poorly soluble polyphenols with potential anticancer properties. *Semin. Cancer Biol.,* **2017,** *46*, 205-214.
[http://dx.doi.org/10.1016/j.semcancer.2017.06.010] [PMID: 28673607]

[75]   Barzegar, A.; Moosavi-Movahedi, A.A. Intracellular ROS Protection Efficiency and Free Radical-Scavenging Activity of Curcumin. *Artif. Cells Nanomed. Biotechnol.,* **2016,** *44*, 128-134.
[http://dx.doi.org/10.3109/21691401.2014.926456] [PMID: 24959911]

[76]   Minaei, A.; Sabzichi, M.; Ramezani, F.; Hamishehkar, H.; Samadi, N. Co-delivery with nano-quercetin enhances doxorubicin-mediated cytotoxicity against MCF-7 cells. *Mol. Biol. Rep.,* **2016,** *43*(2), 99-105.
[http://dx.doi.org/10.1007/s11033-016-3942-x] [PMID: 26748999]

[77]   Kristl, J.; Teskač, K.; Caddeo, C.; Abramović, Z.; Šentjurc, M. Improvements of cellular stress response on resveratrol in liposomes. *Eur. J. Pharm. Biopharm.,* **2009,** *73*(2), 253-259.
[http://dx.doi.org/10.1016/j.ejpb.2009.06.006] [PMID: 19527785]

[78]   Zaman, M.S.; Chauhan, N.; Yallapu, M.M.; Gara, R.K.; Maher, D.M.; Kumari, S.; Sikander, M.; Khan, S.; Zafar, N.; Jaggi, M.; Chauhan, S.C. Curcumin Nanoformulation for Cervical Cancer Treatment. *Sci. Rep.,* **2016,** *6*(1), 20051.
[http://dx.doi.org/10.1038/srep20051] [PMID: 26837852]

[79]   Tsai, Y.M.; Jan, W.C.; Chien, C.F.; Lee, W.C.; Lin, L.C.; Tsai, T.H. Optimised nano-formulation on the bioavailability of hydrophobic polyphenol, curcumin, in freely-moving rats. *Food Chem.,* **2011,** *127*(3), 918-925.
[http://dx.doi.org/10.1016/j.foodchem.2011.01.059] [PMID: 25214079]

[80]   Hung, C.F.; Chen, J.K.; Liao, M.H.; Lo, H.M.; Fang, J.Y. Development and evaluation of emulsion-liposome blends for resveratrol delivery. *J. Nanosci. Nanotechnol.,* **2006,** *6*(9-10), 2950-2958.
[http://dx.doi.org/10.1166/jnn.2006.420] [PMID: 17048503]

[81]   Davatgaran-Taghipour, Y.; Masoomzadeh, S.; Farzaei, M.H.; Bahramsoltani, R.; Karimi-Soureh, Z.; Rahimi, R.; Abdollahi, M. Polyphenol nanoformulations for cancer therapy: experimental evidence and clinical perspective. *Int. J. Nanomedicine,* **2017**, *12*, 2689-2702.
        [http://dx.doi.org/10.2147/IJN.S131973] [PMID: 28435252]

[82]   Liang, J.; Yan, H.; Puligundla, P.; Gao, X.; Zhou, Y.; Wan, X. Applications of Chitosan Nanoparticles to Enhance Absorption and Bioavailability of Tea Polyphenols: A Review. *Food Hydrocoll.,* **2017**, *69*, 286-292.
        [http://dx.doi.org/10.1016/j.foodhyd.2017.01.041]

CHAPTER 4

The Role of Traditional Chinese Herbal Medicines in Management of Patients with Cancer-related Fatigue

Marcin Włodarczyk[1,*], Paweł Siwiński[1], Aleksandra Tarasiuk[2], Jakub Włodarczyk[2] and Aleksandra Sobolewska-Włodarczyk[2]

[1] *Department of General and Colorectal Surgery, Faculty of Military Medicine, Medical University of Lodz, Poland*

[2] *Department of Biochemistry, Faculty of Medicine, Medical University of Lodz, Poland*

Abstract: World Health Organization (WHO) estimates that in 2015 cancer was the primary cause of death of 8.8 million people, which transfers to every sixth death globally. The number of newly diagnosed cancer cases annually is expected to reach more than 23 million over the next 2 decades. Cancer describes a large group of diseases originating in uncontrolled growth of abnormal cells in the body, debilitating for the patient and usually requiring complex long-term treatment. Surgery, chemotherapy and radiotherapy are considered as the most common conventional cancer therapies. These treatment strategies, however, are associated with limitations and clinical results are often unsatisfactory. Therefore, combined and more effective therapies in cancer treatment must be implemented.

Traditional herbal medicines (THM) have been used in treatment of cancer for thousands of years in majority of Asian countries. It is also a common practice nowadays to combine THM with Western cancer management schemes, consolidating a variety of natural agents into one treatment strategy. The use of herbal products in cancer therapy, over the last years, has received much attention also in Western countries becoming more popular among patients, with a prevalence reaching up to 80%. Large number of these medications is also widely approved as a form of complementary and alternative medicine in cancer treatment in both Europe and United States.

Clinical challenge in management of cancer is cancer-related fatigue (CRF), which is a persistent sense of tiredness associated with the treatment or the disease itself that cannot be eliminated by rest. THM in the recent years presents with a wide range of opportunities among which management of adverse treatment effects and fatigue emerge as worth investigating. Herbal medicines may be considered as an effective and safe treatment of CRF.

---

* **Corresponding author Marcin Włodarczyk:** Department of General and Colorectal Surgery, Faculty of Military Medicine, Medical University of Lodz; Hallera 1 Sq, 90-647 Lodz, Poland; E-mail: marcin.wlodarczyk@umed.lodz.pl

Ferid Murad, Atta-ur-Rahman and Ka Bian (Eds.)
All rights reserved-© 2019 Bentham Science Publishers

In conclusion, herbal medicines possess a wide range of activities in relation to cancer treatment. Natural medical agents may reduce cancer-related fatigue as well as damage to gastrointestinal, respiratory and nervous systems. However, considering, little scientific knowledge about efficacy and safety of herbal products consecutive controlled clinical studies are needed to fully verify this matter.

Keywords: Cancer, Fatigue, Traditional Chinese Herbal Medicine.

INTRODUCTION

Cancer is considered one of the main causes of morbidity and mortality worldwide. World Health Organization (WHO) estimates that in 2018 cancer was the primary cause of death of 9.6 million people in the world, which transfers to every sixth death globally. The number of newly diagnosed cancer cases annually is expected to reach more than 23 million over the next two decades [1]. Cancer describes a large group of diseases originating in uncontrolled growth of abnormal cells in the body, debilitating for the patient and usually requiring complex long-term treatment. Surgery, chemotherapy and radiotherapy are considered as the most common conventional cancer therapies. These treatment strategies, however, are associated with limitations and clinical results are often unsatisfactory.

A significant number of patients, due to late diagnosis do not qualify for primary surgery and the applied systemic therapy is related to gradual resistance of cancer cells against treatment. In this group of patients, the chemotherapy and radiotherapy although effective, have serious side effects and complications from gastrointestinal, respiratory and nervous systems [2]. Therefore, combined and more effective therapies in cancer treatment must be implemented.

Cancer-related fatigue (CRF) can be defined as a chronic subjective feeling of physical, emotional or cognitive fatigue associated with cancer or its treatment, which is disproportionate to the physical activity and interferes with the normal functioning. This state is characterized by weakness, constant need for rest, "lack of energy", fast fatigue, aversion to physical or mental strain, impaired concentration and drowsiness [3, 4]. The syndrome can occur in 80-96% of those treated with cytostatics and often leads to a serious deterioration of the quality of life. Symptoms reach the highest intensity after 48-72 hours after drug administration and gradually reduce their severity until they disappear completely after treatment. It has been stated that 30% of patients experience weakness after 6 months from the end of treatment, and symptoms may persist even several years after that time [5, 6]. No criteria for recognizing this syndrome have been developed so far. Diagnosis is made on the basis of the interview, an auxiliary role is played by the severity of the ailments. The exact reason of CRF is hard to define, thus making the development of complex treatment particularly challenging.

Traditional chinese herbal medicines have been used in treatment of cancer for thousands of years and it is also a common practice nowadays to combine them with Western cancer management schemes, consolidating a variety of natural agents into one treatment strategy [7]. The use of herbal products in cancer therapy, over the last years, has received much attention in the Western countries and is becoming more popular among patients, with a prevalence reaching up to 80% [7]. Large number of these medications is widely approved as a form of complementary and alternative medicine in cancer treatment in both Europe and United States.

Traditional chinese herbal medicines in the recent years presents with a wide range of opportunities among which management of adverse treatment effects and fatigue emerge as worth investigating. Herbal medicines may be considered as an effective and safe treatment of CRF, however further studies are required to increase the strength of evidence.

Prevalence of Cancer-related Fatigue

CRF is a debilitating and highly prevalent symptom associated with cancer and its treatment. It can affect various aspects of patient's life including physical, mental and emotional functioning and usually has a negative impact on patients' quality of life [8]. The exact prevalence rate of CRF in cancer patients is difficult to ascertain and the estimates differ considerably between studies. The differences in various calculations likely reflect the subjective nature of the condition, difficulties in precise assessment as well as diverse diagnostic criteria that have been used. According to a systematic review of fourty studies on CRF, its prevalence rates fluctuate between 46 and 96% and the symptoms can be present long after treatment cessation in at least a quarter of patients [9]. The numbers also seem to correlate with the type of cancer treatment. Additional studies report that from 80 up to 96% of patients receiving chemotherapy and 60 to 93% of those on radiotherapy report significant fatigue [10].

CRF prevalence was also a subject of two US national surveys commissioned by the Fatigue Coalition, a multidisciplinary group of practitioners, researchers, and patient advocates [11, 12]. The results of the survey, apart from providing the symptom prevalence data, also emphasize the need for education on CRF both among patients and doctors. Out of 419 examined patients, 74 percent reported fatigue at some point during the course of their illness, but only 50% of patients had discussed fatigue with their clinician. What is more, only one-fourth of these cases received an adequate intervention proposal. According to the results, clinicians believed that pain affected patients to a greater degree than fatigue, whereas patients admitted that CRF had a more significant impact on their daily activities than pain. While the second large study presented with similar numbers of patients affected by the condition, it underlined the important economic aspect of CRF. Overall, 75% of employed patients were forced to change their employment status as a result of fatigue, and 65% reported that their caregivers had to take at least one day off from work in a typical month [12].

Pathogenesis of Cancer-Related Fatigue

Despite multiple studies on the CRF pathogenesis, the mechanisms underlying the development of the condition have not been fully explained. Owing to its multi-factorial nature the exact causes of CRF are difficult to define [13]. Although the underlying etiology of fatigue have not been yet fully understood, a variety of different etiologic factors contributing to fatigue have been proposed [14]. Potential factors to consider include the effect of tumor progression, side effects of therapy, comorbid medical conditions as well as genetic predisposition and environmental factors. To date, the mechanisms that have received most scientific attention and support are hypothalamic-pituitary-adrenal (HPA) axis dysregulation, influence of inflammatory processes, direct impact of cancer treatment and the anemia hypothesis [15 - 17].

First main hypothesis proposed for CRF is the HPA axis dysfunction resulting in endocrine changes that causes or contributes to fatigue. The HPA axis regulates the development of immune cells and cytokine production and is the central regulatory system controlling release of the stress hormone cortisol. In a multistage pathway, the paraventricular nucleus of the hypothalamus stimulated by physical or physiological stress secretes corticotropin-releasing hormone (CRH), which acts synergistically with vasopressin to release adrenocorticotropic hormone (ACTH) from the anterior pituitary. ACTH then stimulates the release of cortisol from the adrenal cortex. Studies evidenced that patients with chronic fatigue syndrome present with low levels of circulating cortisol [18]. Serum cortisol level shows a diurnal pattern with highest concentrations prior to awakening and a linear decline throughout the day [18]. A study performed by Bower *et al.* revealed that breast cancer survivors with persistent fatigue (in comparison with non-fatigued survivors) had a flatter cortisol slope and elevated levels of evening cortisol compared to individuals who did not experience fatigue [17]. These results suggest that alterations in HPA axis activity could influence fatigue.

Another potential etiology of fatigue is associated with activation of the proinflammatory cytokine network. This hypothesis suggests that the toxic downstream effects of dysregulated inflammatory pathways contribute to CRF and other concomitant conditions [19, 20]. The symptoms of fatigue and other behavioral changes appear as an effect of alterations in neural processes generated by the central nervous system (CNS) as a response to abnormal peripheral inflammatory cytokines release [21, 22]. Proinflammatory cytokines, such as tumor necrosis factor alpha (TNF-α) and IL-1β, are implicated in many of the mechanisms proposed for the etiology of CRF. IL-1, IL-6 and TNF-α have been shown to suppress erythropoiesis, resulting in anemia [23]. TNF-α has been associated with alterations in CNS neurotransmission, and among others also linked to development of cachexia resulting in severe fatigue [14, 16]. Additionally, in a quantitative review, CRF was associated with increased circulating levels of IL-6, IL-1 receptor antagonist, and neopterin [24].

Both cancer and its treatment by chemotherapy, surgery and radiotherapy elevate the levels of proinflammatory cytokines, including TNF-α, IL-1 and IL-6 [15]. In the pre-treatment period, the tumor itself may be a source for proinflammatory cytokines, while during treatment, cytokines may be produced in response to tissue damage from radiation or chemotherapy [25, 26]. Recent studies revealed that elevated serum levels of IL-1 receptor antagonist were associated with exacerbated fatigue in patients undergoing radiation therapy for early-stage breast or prostate cancer [27]. Alterations in IL-6 levels associated with fatigue during treatment were also found in breast cancer patients undergoing chemotherapy [28]. Consecutive studies proved that acute increase in markers of inflammation were correlated with increase in fatigue in patients with gastrointestinal cancer undergoing chemoradiation therapy [29, 30].

Another potential process leading to fatigue is the coexistence of anemia. Anemia is common in cancer patients and can be found at diagnosis, as a consequence of the neoplastic disease itself or due to cancer treatment. The exact mechanism by which anemia causes fatigue in patients with cancer is hard to define and a multifactorial mechanism is postulated. Bleeding, hemolysis, bone marrow infiltration, and nutritional deficiencies may all contribute to the development of anemia in patients with cancer. In addition, inflammatory cytokines, such as TNF-α, IL-1, IL-6, and interferon gamma (IFNγ), have been implicated in the suppression of erythrogenesis, resulting in anemia and fatigue [31]. Anemia is also a common complication of myelosuppressive chemotherapy, however it is less prevalent than fatigue [32]. On average, over one third of patients become anemic after three cycles of chemotherapy [33].

Primary research did not reveal a clear correlation between hemoglobin levels and the severity of CRF symptoms, however with the development of new evaluation instruments designed specifically for this purpose, a connection between anemia and fatigue has been established [34, 35]. Although the precise relationship between fatigue severity and patients' quality of life still remains to be fully elucidated, so far several studies reported an improvement in patients' life quality and relief of symptoms associated with CRF once correction of anemia has been achieved [36, 37]. Therefore, further investigation would presumably provide an important insight into the more general mechanisms of fatigue and related symptoms.

Clinical Manifestations of Cancer-related Fatigue

Fatigue seldom occurs as a single condition and commonly clusters with other significant symptoms including emotional distress, exhaustion and lack of energy, mood disorders, loss of drive, sleep disturbances and pain [38, 39]. Given the multifarious manifestations of CRF numerous attempts have been made to determine the condition [40, 41]. Regardless of the definition, CRF significantly impairs the quality of life and the physical performance ability of many of the affected patients [41].

Fatigue can often be manifested by sleep disturbances, ranging from hypersomnia to insomnia. The correlation between fatigue and sleep disturbances has been widely discussed in the symptom research literature [42 - 44]. Although common, sleep problems in individuals with cancer are likely under-reported [45]. Insomnia symptoms have been proven to exist in 30 to 50% of cancer patients, and 20 to 40% can be qualified as insomnia syndrome [46, 47]. Fatigue resulting from sleep problems often manifests as excessive daytime sleepiness. Poor sleep hygiene can result in tiredness during daytime, impaired physical activity and cognitive function deterioration.

Nutritional deficits significantly contribute to fatigue [48]. A nutritional problem may be manifested by poor appetite, gastrointestinal symptoms, weight loss, and low albumin may signal a nutritional problem. Oral intake can be adversely affected by anorexia, nausea, vomiting, mucositis, odynophagia, bowel obstruction, or constipation. Patients with neoplastic disease are also more likely to develop serious electrolyte imbalance, including sodium, potassium, calcium, and magnesium level fluctuations, which may amplify fatigue. Therapeutic actions directed at improving or maintaining nutritional status can decrease or prevent CRF. Refering the patient to a an experienced dietician may help to assess the severity of symptoms and provide essential dietary recommendations. Nutritional assessment should comprise of weight gain or loss evaluation, verifying and establishing adequate caloric intake, and controlling fluid and electrolyte imbalances.

Psychiatric spectrum of symptoms can also represent the presence of fatigue associated with cancer and its treatment. The exact relationship between CRF and emotional distress is not fully understood. There is a strong correlation between fatigue and depression, however in some cases it may be difficult to distinguish between the two as origin of emotional distress [49, 50]. Fatigue can present as symptom of depression, however excessive fatigue can also induce emotional distress when valued roles and activities are affected. Some studies state that despite the existing link between depression and fatigue, they follow a different time course in patients with cancer and respond variously to implemented treatment [51, 52]. As an example, placebo-controlled, randomized trials showed that patients randomly assigned to receive an antidepressant failed to demonstrate any improvement in CRF, despite notable benefits in relieving depression symptoms [53, 54].

Cancer patients often experience disruptions in their physical activity and deconditioning is one of the frequently observed symptoms in patients with CRF [55]. The underlying cause of deconditioning could be assigned to nutritional deficiencies, lack of physical activity, cardiopulmonary dysfunction or medication inducing sarcopenia. Deconditioning can significantly affect the functional status of an individual and have negative effect on the overall cause of disease and treatment. Exercise may be beneficial in improving CRF in certain patients, however safe and effective physical activity course needs to be developed individually in order to regain strength and build stamina. In order to implement appropriate therapeutic actions, the extent of debilitation caused by fatigue and establishing individual's functional status should be fully reviewed.

CRF has a multidimensional correlation with pain. Pain frequently coexists with fatigue and may present as a significant symptom, implementing possible correlations between those two [56]. Pain can significantly affect patients' sleep, decrease the physical strength and influence emotional distress, all of which may lead to fatigue development. Although current medical agents give a wide range of possibilities in pain management, fatigue may be in fact aggravated by the sedating side effects of some analgesics. Moreover opioids, commonly used in relieving pain in cancer patients, can disturb sleep patterns due to central apnea and alterations in sleep architecture, resulting in unrefreshing sleep and further fatigue progression [56].

Treatment of Cancer-related Fatigue

The treatment of CRF is multidirectional and pharmacotherapy needs to be optimized to an individual patient. It should always be assessed whether the fatigue syndrome is due to the progression of the neoplastic disease [57]. If possible, the CNS-inhibitory drugs dose is reduced or treatment is discontinued, including antiemetics, antihistamines, anxiolytics and sleeping pills. An important element of treatment is the implementation of effective analgesic therapy, but when the pain is well controlled, it may be necessary to reduce the dose of analgesics. An important element of treatment is the fight against anemia. It is also important to treat comorbidities and compensate for existing metabolic disorders (including disorders of calcium concentration, dehydration, hypoxia). It is advisable to modify the lifestyle by limiting the night vigil and increasing daily activity and physical exercises appropriate to the patient's abilities.

Due to the lack of clinical evidence on the effectiveness of pharmacological treatment, its standards have not been defined. Glucocorticoids (dexamethasone or prednisone) or antidepressants (selective serotonin reuptake inhibitors) are used in order to relieve the symptoms [58, 59].

Recent data indicate that only a part of CRF patients attempt to treat the syndrome on their own, although the methods used are often suboptimal or inappropriate. About 40% of patients with tumors with symptoms of chronic fatigue do not receive any treatment aimed at reducing the perception of CRF symptoms, about 40% of patients are recommended to relax, 10% of patients are proposed to modify their diet and take vitamins, and about 6% of patients are recommended different pharmaceuticals [12].

Chinese Herbal Medicines in Treatment of Cancer-related Fatigue

The usage of herbal remedies has grown excessively over the past few decades [60]. Despite the fact that treatments including herbal plants have indicated promising potential with the viability of a decent number of natural items clearly established, a lot of them stay untested and their use is either ineffectively observed or not checked at all. This results in lack of information about their method of activity, potential antagonistic responses, contraindications, and connections with existing standard pharmaceuticals and practical nourishments to advance safe as well as rational application of these components. Chinese herbal medicine formulas that follow the general principles of Chinese medicine to treat patients with CRF are: 'replenishing vital energy and nourishing blood, 'clearing heat and eliminating dampness', and 'coordinating Yin and Yang in the body' [61, 62].

Traditional Chniese Medicine (TCM) identifies CRF as deficiency pattern, which for the most part is caused by the disharmony of yin and yang, hypofunction of *zang-fu* organs, *qi* stagnation and blood stasis [63]. Chinese herbal medicine (CHM) is one of six branches of TCM and it pays particular attention to restorage and adjustment of energy, body and spirit to support mental as well as physical wellness [64, 65]. It has been stated that CHM has potential beneficial effects on supporting the treatment of cancer in multiple ways, such as, retarding cancer progression, boosting immune system, alleviating chemotherapy or radiotherapy-induced complications and side effects, such as pain, fatigue [66]. As described above, treatment of CRF should be multi-directional due to the multitude of factors that can cause it. Initially, thorough assessment and identification of the basis of fatigue should be stated [4]. There are some CHMs that are found to improve patient's life after cancer treatment as well as CRF and difficulties people may encounter due to its occurrence.

CHMs, used alone or in a combination with chemotherapy or as adjuvant, indicate that patients experience relief in CRF compared to placebo, chemotherapy or supportive care based on single trials [63]. The herbal medicine formula Yang Wei Kang Liu (YWKLF) is mostly used to inhibit the metastasis of human gastric cancer to prolong patient survival [67, 68]. It has been stated that combination of chemotherapy with oral administration of YWKLF significantly increased the survival of stage IV gastric cancer patients, which may be related to activation of major pro-apoptotic pathways in gastric cancer cells [67]. Moreover, due to its properties and the impact it has on apoptosis, it is used in the treatment of CRF.

List of CHMs is very long and not all of them are described in literature. Common formulas used in treatment of CRF involve modified *Guipi Decoction, Shiquan Dabu Decoction, modified Shenlingbaizhu Powder, Yougui Pill, Zuojin Pill, Wendan decoction, modified Chaihu Shugan Powder, modified Danggui Buxue Decoction, Xuefu Zhuyu Decoction.* Apart from CRF, these formulas aim to alleviate other symptoms, such as nausea, dizziness, pain or insomnia [69]. However, not only combinations of CHM have been studied. A plant that grows in the mountains of Eastern Asia – ginseng (*Panax ginseng*) as well as American ginseng (*Panax quinquefolius, Panacis quinquefolis*) which is native to eastern North America (though it is also cultivated in China) have been examined in several clinical trials likewise [70 - 72].

Other studies investigated several CHMs (medicinal formulae consisting of several Chinese herbs in combination) in relation to their efficacy in treating the side effects associated with orthodox cancer treatment, including CRF.

LCS101 Formula consists of: *Astragalus membranaceus, Poriae cocos, Atractylodes macrocephala, Lycium chinense, Ligustrum lucidum, Paeonia lactiflora, Paeonia obovate, Citrus reticulate, Ophiopogon japonicas, Milletia reticulate, Oldenlandia diffusa, Scutellaria barbata, Prunella vulgaris and Glehnia littoralis* [73]. Some data suggest that LCS101 used as an adjuvant to conventional chemotherapy indicate that at the end of treatment, 70% of 20 female breast cancer patients reported that they had either no or mildly severe levels of fatigue; 60% had none to mildly severe weakness; 85% had none to mildly severe pain; 70% had none to mildly severe nausea; and 80% reported none to mildly severe vomiting. Results showed that 20% reported severe impairment of overall function, and 40% severely impaired quality of life. Significantly, 85% reported that they believed the botanical compound helped reduce their symptoms. Results also indicated that no toxic side effects were attributed to the LCS101 treatment by the study participants [73, 74].

Chinese herbal injections have been proven beneficial to patients with gastric cancer by improving clinical efficacy and relieving adverse reactions of chemotherapy [75]. Shenqi Fuzheng injection which consists mainly of *Codonopsis lanceolata* and *Astragalus membranaceus* has been evaluated in recent studies [76]. Data suggested that treatment of CRF with Shenqi Fuzheng injection combined with chemotherapy compared to chemotherapy alone in patients with advanced lung cancer may play a beneficial role [73, 77]. The researchers stated that the efficacy rate in the treatment group (57.1%) was significantly greater than the control (31.2%). Moreover, in the treatment group, symptoms of fatigue, anorexia, and nausea as well as vomiting were significantly lower compared with the control group. Also, the occurrence of leukopenia and thrombocytopenia in the treatment group was lower than in the control group. The authors concluded that Shenqi Fuzheng injection combined with chemotherapy for advanced lung cancer can reduce drug toxicity, alleviate patient's fatigue, loss of appetite, gastrointestinal symptoms and improve quality of life [73, 76, 78].

Fatigue is not only a physical problem - emotional, psychological and social aspects are also bound to be taken into consideration. Also, not every CHM works exactly the same. Therefore it is difficult to describe specific mechanism of various CHMs in treatment of CRF [79]. To date, little information is known about the mechanism of anti-fatigue effects of CHMs.

In literatures, a few possible explanations for the anti-fatigue effects are proposed. Mechanism of *Panax Ginseng* involve normalization of lactic dehydrogenase, malondialdehyde and glutathione peroxidase levels through protection of the corpuscular membrane by preventing lipid oxidation via modifying several enzyme activities [80].

Another mechanism of alleviating fatigue by *Ginseng* involves promotion of the biosynthesis of protein and DNA-RNA and prevention of the decrease of the protein and nucleic acid synthesis [81]. *Radix codonopsis* enhances immunity through stimulating the formation of thymic T lymphocytes [82]. According to study, another CHM - Tanshinone cause the rapid oxidation of NADH in mitochondria and thus alleviate the accumulation of injury factors due to the deposition of NADH [83].

A research performed in mice showed that *Baoyuan Jiedu Decoction* (BYJD) improves the life quality of cancer cachexia mice and prevents muscle atrophy by downregulating expression of Atrogin-1 and MuRF-1 [84].

Key herbs of Kangai injection are: *Astragalus membranaceus*, ginseng, oxymatrine, and *Sophora flavescens*. A study by Wu *et al.* examined the efficacy of Kangai injection combined with chemotherapy versus control (chemotherapy alone) in 80 patients with advanced gastric cancer. They found that in the treatment group NK-cell activity and CD4/CD8 ratio was significantly higher after treatment, and CD3 and CD4 were increased. However, there was no significant difference in the efficacy rate between the treatment group (45%) and the control group (40%). There was also less leukopenia, nausea and/or vomiting, peripheral nerve toxicity in the treatment group compared with the control group, less fatigue and better appetite appeared in the treatment group. The authors also stated that treatment was more effective in relieving pain and assisting patients to gain weight compared with the control medication. The conclusion was that treatment of advanced gastric cancer with Kangai injection combined with chemotherapy may significantly reduce the negative impact of chemotherapy on the patient's immune function and reduce side effects such as CRF, thereby improving quality of life [75].

Astragalus membranaceus (*Astragalus propinquus*) which is the main constituent of LCS101 Formula, Shenqui Fuzheng Injection and Kongi Injection is one of the 50 fundamental herbs used in TCM [85]. This herb is a component in Lectranal, a food supplement used in treatment of seasonal allergic rhinitis though there is limited evidence of its effectiveness [85, 86]. Chemical constituents of *A. membranaceus* roots include polysaccharides and triterpenoids (such as astragalosides), as well as isoflavones (including kumatakenin, calycosin, and formononetin) and their glycosides and malonates [87, 88]. The extract of *A. membranaceus* (TA-65) is believed to be responsible for activation of telomerase, extending the lengths of the shortest telomeres which protect the terminal DNA at the ends of all chromosomes [89, 90].

The pilot study conducted by Zhao *et al.* suggests that spore powder of *Ganoderma lucidum* may have beneficial effects on CRF and quality of life in breast cancer patients undergoing endocrine therapy without any significant adverse effects [91]. *G. lucidum* is a potent immune system regulator, a promising anti-cancer agent, and stress reducer. This mushroom is frequently used in TCM in a form of spore powder. It is believed to have anti-oxidative effects when supplemented. It also has a therapeutic effect on insulin resistance, reduces the risk of prostate cancer, and can help treat a variety of conditions associated with metabolic syndrome [92 - 95]. Its bioactive ingredients such as fungal immunomodulatory proteins (FIPs) have immune building properties and can stimulate different cells and cellular components that enable immune response. Some of the molecules and cells that FIPs influence include T and B lymphocytes, natural killer cells, and macrophages [96]. Improved function of these cells is stated to promote cytokine expression such as IL-2, IL-4 and IFNγ which support lymphocyte proliferation, immune cell initiation, and tumor inhibiting factors. Immunostimulation from FIPs could possibly cause increased expression of costimulatory molecules and major histocompatibility complexes (MHC) which help to create a pathway for immune response [97].

Effectiveness and Safety of CHM in CRF

Although clinical studies of CHM for CRF have been conducted and reported with potential positive results, there is no systematic review on effectiveness and safety of CHM for CRF to justify their clinical use. Therefore, this subsection aims to assess the effectiveness and safety of CHM for the treatment of CRF. Even though there are some parameters that can be measured in order to establish the efficiency and safety of CHM treatment in CRF, *e.g.* abnormal cytokine activation, 5-hydroxy tryptophan (5-HT) neurotransmitter dysregulation, abnormal hypothalamic-pituitary-adrenal (HPA) axis function, and unusual metabolism of adenosine triphosphate (ATP) in muscle, the role of CHM used for CRF is questionable [14, 98 - 100]. For example, breast cancer survivors with persistent and gradually aggravating fatigue after treatment had increased levels of immune markers related with proinflammatory cytokines such as IL-6 and TNF-α. Nevertheless, no serious adverse effects during clinical trials have been recognized so far [101]. Consequently, Zhao *et al.* observed that patients who were administrated with spore powder of *Ganoderma lucidum* 1000 mg three times a day for four weeks experienced only mild discomforts such as dizziness and dry mouth, no serious adverse effects occurred during the trial [91]. Moreover, tests for safety and toxicity showed no significant change in different parameters of the renal function test (sodium, potassium, and urea creatinine) and liver function test (total protein, albumin, total bilirubin, alkaline phosphate, and alanine transaminase) during the study period.

In 2013, Debra L. Barton *et al.* stated in a randomized, double-blind trial that 200 mg daily (over an 8-week period) of *Panax ginseng* (Wisconsin Ginseng) may improve CRF [72]. It has been also reported that despite its activity against CRF the treatment may not be noticeable until two months after starting taking medication. Equally important, it has been shown that patients who currently experienced radiation and/or chemotherapy had factually essentially better general fatigue scores at four as well as eight weeks in the ginseng arm vs the placebo arm. Excelling results in those taking cancer treatment may suggest that ginseng may be a deterrent rather than treatment intervention, despite the fact that all patients had to have a certain level of fatigue to enter the trial. This depends on the way that in spite of the fact that it would be normal for fatigue to increment all through cancer treatment, fatigue scores diminished (enhanced) indeed in the process of treatment. Interestingly, in 2015 Yennurajalingman *et al.* conducted a clinical trial revealing that high-dose of *Panax ginseng* is free from harm [70]. *Panax ginseng* significantly improved QOL scores probably accordingly to its effectiveness on CRF and related symptoms such as pain, sleep disturbances, and anorexia – about 63% of the participants observed mild to immense improvement in perceiving these symptoms of CRF while experiencing *Panax ginseng* therapy. Another studies that used animal models shown that *Panax ginseng* modulates proinflammatory cytokines due to the properties of the active compounds such as ginsenosides and polysaccharides which are constituents of the ginseng extract [80, 102, 103]. Withal, further studies are needed to discern the mechanism of action of *Panax ginseng* on CRF. Some studies suggest the dysregulation of inflammatory cytokines can promote and enhance CRF and its related symptoms [104 - 107]. In 2017 Yennurajalingman *et al.* stated that oral administration of *Panax ginseng* at a dose of 400 mg twice a day and a matching placebo leaded to meaningful enhancement in CRF with minimum adverse or unwanted secondary effects [71]. Contrarily to above-mentioned studies, in this case the management of CRF and other contaminant symptoms was not relatively higher to placebo after four weeks of oral administration of *Panac ginseng*. These data indicate that in comparison to their previous clinical trial concerning *Panax ginseng* treatment is not advisable for managing fatigue in patients with advanced cancer. Wherefore, additionally clinical trials are still required. Table **1** summerize the chinese herbal medicines used in cancer-related fatigue.

Systematic review and meta-analysis by Jennifer Finnegan-John from 2013 as well as Vincent C.H. Chung *et al.* from 2016 underline how effective CHM can be in the treatment of CRF [62, 113]. As a result there emerges an insufficient character of complementary therapies, (including treatment with CHM) in decreasing CRF among cancer patients. Data obtained from clinical trials to date is not dominant to clearly ascertain the preponderance of CHM over the other ways of treatment of CRF. On that account, CHM may be delivered alongside other established useful interventions for CRF (such as exercise or psychosocial programs). It is really complex to determine whether combinations of interventions may perform together to attain a better results than interventions used alone. This hypothesis could be tested in future trials of interventions for CRF [113]. It has been also stated that CHM may be treated and used as the additive to conventional care in cancer patients for reducing pain or/and constipation. However, there is no proof that CHM may be applied in treating anorexia and fatigue in cancer patients [62].

Chinese Herbal Components	Type of Cancer	Pre-Clinical or Clinical Evidence of Activity
Bojungikki-tang [108]	Breast, gastric, colorectal and lung cancer	Bojunkgikki-tang extract granules vs no intervention Lack of relief in fatigue severity
G. Lucidum [109]	Breast cancer	Spore powder of G. Lucidum vs placebo Strong positive effect on decreasing fatigue
Kangai injection [110]	Colorectal cancer	Kangai injection plus FOLFOX4 vs FOLFOX4 Decreasing fatigue severity
Fufang Eijiao jiang [111]	Lung, breast, ovarian, intestinal, gastric and kidney cancer	Fufang Eijiao jiang plus chemotherapy vs chemotherapy Statistically greater number of patients with fatigue relief
Renshen yangrong decoction [111]	Non-small cell lung cancer and oesophageal cancer	Renshen Yangrong decoction plus rhEPO *vs* rhEPO Statistically greater number of patients with fatigue relief
ginseng [112]	Breast, colon and lung cancer	Wisconsin Ginseng vs placebo Decreasing fatigue more than a placebo did, as measured by various scales of fatigue, vitality, and well-being.

Future Perspectives and Implications for Research

Until today only a limited number of clinical studies reviewed the use of CHM for CRF. A vast majority of published research present with methodological shortcomings and the significance of their findings merits further analysis. Jeong *et al.*, in a pilot study, revealed that *Bojungikki-tang*, granules that contain a mixture of extracts of 10 medicinal plants, may have beneficial effects on CRF in cancer patients, without any significant adverse effects [101]. Although the results appear to be consistent with findings of Barton et al, reporting high doses of *American Ginseng* to be effective in relieving CRF, both studies retain an inherent risk of subjectivity [112]. The scientific strength of the results is limited by the heterogeneity of study groups, inadequate randomization procedure and short follow-up period.

An urgent demand for additional research on CHM in managing fatigue symptoms has also been strongly emphasized by the biggest meta-analysis up to date. Followed by a systematic search of several databases, Su *et al.* identified 10 randomized trials of CHM for CRF involving a total of 751 patients [85]. The results of the analysis underlined the high risk of bias and significant flaws in terms of methodology in majority of the studies, despite their promising results. Most of the papers were focused only on short term results, failed to fully demonstrate the randomization procedures and presented a great clinical heterogeneity in study groups as well as intervention procedures. Therefore, CHF use for CRF requires further research to fully elucidate the safety and beneficial effects in medical therapy.

Increasing evidence has shown that CHMs have promising therapeutic effects in different types of cancer. It has been shown that CHMs can be used to reduce side-effects of chemotherapy and also as a chemopreventive therapy in order to reduce the incidence of cancer in vulnerable populations. In literature there is evidence of positive effect of herbal compounds on cancer cells proliferation, apoptosis, adhesion and migration. In addition, it is supposed that CHMs may suppress angiogenesis and therefore reduce tumor growth [114]. To date, the precise mechanism of the therapeutic effects of CHMs remains poorly investigated and needs to be elucidated. A few examples of effects of CHMs on lung, liver and colon cancers are presented below.

According to the study by Liu *et al.* adjunctive therapy with CHMs could improve overall survival of lung cancer patients [115]. The combined Chinese–Western therapy significantly improves the survival and reduces symptoms of patients with advanced non-small cell lung cancer (NSCLC) compared with chemotherapy without CHM [116]. Study of Yang *et al.* showed that the progression free survival (PFS) was better in NSCLC patients treated with gefitinib plus CHM than with gefitinib only [117]. While improving the overall survival of patients, there is also evidence that administration of CHM can alleviate symptoms such as fatigue and cough [118].

CHMs such as *Jia Wei Xiao Yao San* and *Chai Hu Shu Gan Tang* are effective herbal agents that improve survival of liver cancer patients [118]. Saikosaponind is a major ingredient of *Chai Hu Shu Gan Tang* that effectively inhibits proliferation, suppresses invasion and induces apoptosis in cancer cells. Mechanism involve inhibiting the activated T lymphocytes via suppression of NF-κB, NF-AT and AP-1 signaling pathways [119].

In case of metastatic colorectal cancer it has been reported that patients treated with chemotherapy combined with CHM had a longer median survival time (40 months) than those treated without CHM (12 months) [120]. Also metaanalysis of CHM, as adjuvant therapy in CRC, has shown a modest increase in the 1-year and in the 3-year survival (OR 2.41; 2.4), reduction in cancer progression (OR 0.5) and improved quality of life (OR 3.43) [121]. Authors stated that chemotherapy coupled with CHM could reduce the risk of recurrence and metastasis as well as prolong the disease-free survival of patients with CRC. Moreover, CHM-base adjuvant therapy enhance the sensitivity to chemotherapy, reduce the chemotherapy-induced side effects and protect liver function, so as to alleviate radiotherapy or chemotherapy-induced fatigue [122].

Finally, future investigation of CHMs' efficacy in relieving CRF should include establishing a reliable and valid assessment of the syndrome itself. Currently available practice guidelines used to assess CRF include a variety of either unidimensional or multidimensional tools. Therefore, precise validation of particular agents' influence on symptoms relief lacks credibility. The instruments used in this evaluation should be tested in clinical environment to ensure that the results of various interventions can be thoroughly compared. Particular attention should be devoted to experimental design, because CRF symptoms are highly affected by subjectivity, unified definitions have not been established and therapy endpoints are particularly difficult to determine in a quantative indicator.

All the currently available data on the clinical use of herbal medicines leads to believe that CHM may present as an effective and safe method of CRF treatment. However, more carefully designed, large, multicenter trials are desirable to establish the true extent of beneficial effects of natural products administration. Future research should focus on standardization of instruments to define and measure fatigue. Establishing internationally recognized and validated scales will enable outcomes comparison between different clinical approaches. Additional attention should also be directed in the future to careful evaluation of any adverse effects of the therapy, determining the precise intervention scheme for specific types of cancer and establishing the cost-utility of the therapy.

CONCLUSIONS

CHMs possess a wide range of activities in relation to cancer treatment. Natural medical agents may significantly reduce CRF as well as damage to gastrointestinal, respiratory and nervous systems. Some reports promote the hypothesis that CHM may be useful, safe as well as effective in the treatment of CRF. However, considering insufficient and differing methodological quality of these experiments and variety of CHM therapies, data should be elucidated and interpreted with reasonable carefulness. Undoubtfully, further studies are required to extend the current knowledge and provide undeniable proof that CHMs may be not only effective in the treatment of CRF but also safe.

CONSENT FOR PUBLICATION

Not applicable.

CONFLICT OF INTEREST

The authors confirm that this chapter content has no conflict of interest.

ACKNOWLEDGEMENT

Declared none.

REFERENCES

[1]   WHO Cancer. *WHO.*, **2018**.

[2]   Raji, M.A. Management of chemotherapy-induced side-effects. *Lancet Oncol.*, **2005**, *6*(6), 357.
        [http://dx.doi.org/10.1016/S1470-2045(05)70182-0] [PMID: 15925813]

[3]   Jean-Pierre, P; Figueroa-Moseley, CD; Kohli, S; Fiscella, K; Palesh, OG; Morrow, GR Assessment of
        Cancer-Related Fatigue: Implications for Clinical Diagnosis and Treatment. *Oncologist.*, **2007**,
        12(suppl_1), 11-21.

[4]   Yeh, E-T.; Lau, S-C.; Su, W-J.; Tsai, D-J.; Tu, Y-Y.; Lai, Y-L. An examination of cancer-related
        fatigue through proposed diagnostic criteria in a sample of cancer patients in Taiwan. *BMC Cancer,*
        2011, *11*(1), 387.
        [http://dx.doi.org/10.1186/1471-2407-11-387] [PMID: 21896191]

[5]   Lawrence, D.P.; Kupelnick, B.; Miller, K.; Devine, D.; Lau, J. Evidence report on the occurrence,
        assessment, and treatment of fatigue in cancer patients. *J. Natl. Cancer Inst. Monogr.*, **2004**, *2004*(32),
        40-50.
        [http://dx.doi.org/10.1093/jncimonographs/lgh027] [PMID: 15263040]

[6]   Bower, J.E. Prevalence and causes of fatigue after cancer treatment: the next generation of research. *J.
        Clin. Oncol.*, **2005**, *23*(33), 8280-8282.
        [http://dx.doi.org/10.1200/JCO.2005.08.008] [PMID: 16219929]

[7]   de Araújo Júnior, R.F.; de Souza, T.P.; Pires, J.G.L.; Soares, L.A.; de Araújo, A.A.; Petrovick, P.R.;
        Mâcedo, H.D.; de Sá Leitão Oliveira, A.L.; Guerra, G.C. A dry extract of *Phyllanthus niruri* protects
        normal cells and induces apoptosis in human liver carcinoma cells. *Exp. Biol. Med. (Maywood),* **2012**,
        237(11), 1281-1288.
        [http://dx.doi.org/10.1258/ebm.2012.012130] [PMID: 23239439]

[8]   Sood, A.; Barton, D.L.; Bauer, B.A.; Loprinzi, C.L. A critical review of complementary therapies for
        cancer-related fatigue. *Integr. Cancer Ther.*, **2007**, *6*(1), 8-13.
        [http://dx.doi.org/10.1177/1534735406298143] [PMID: 17351022]

[9]   Prue, G.; Rankin, J.; Allen, J.; Gracey, J.; Cramp, F. Cancer-related fatigue: A critical appraisal. *Eur.
        J. Cancer,* **2006**, *42*(7), 846-863.
        [http://dx.doi.org/10.1016/j.ejca.2005.11.026] [PMID: 16460928]

[10]   Flechtner, H.; Bottomley, A. Fatigue and quality of life: lessons from the real world. *Oncologist,* **2003**,
        8(90001) Suppl. 1, 5-9.
        [http://dx.doi.org/10.1634/theoncologist.8-suppl_1-5] [PMID: 12626781]

[11]   Vogelzang, N.J.; Breitbart, W.; Cella, D.; Curt, G.A.; Groopman, J.E.; Horning, S.J.; Itri, L.M.;

Johnson, D.H.; Scherr, S.L.; Portenoy, R.K. Patient, caregiver, and oncologist perceptions of cancer-related fatigue: results of a tripart assessment survey. The Fatigue Coalition. *Semin. Hematol.,* **1997**, *34*(3) Suppl. 2, 4-12.
[PMID: 9253778]

[12] Curt, G.A.; Breitbart, W.; Cella, D.; Groopman, J.E.; Horning, S.J.; Itri, L.M.; Johnson, D.H.; Miaskowski, C.; Scherr, S.L.; Portenoy, R.K.; Vogelzang, N.J. Impact of cancer-related fatigue on the lives of patients: new findings from the Fatigue Coalition. *Oncologist,* **2000**, *5*(5), 353-360.
[http://dx.doi.org/10.1634/theoncologist.5-5-353] [PMID: 11040270]

[13] *NCCN Guidelines Cancer-Related Fatigue NCCN.org.,*

[14] Barsevick, A.; Frost, M.; Zwinderman, A.; Hall, P.; Halyard, M. I'm so tired: biological and genetic mechanisms of cancer-related fatigue. *Qual. Life Res.,* **2010**, *19*(10), 1419-1427.
[http://dx.doi.org/10.1007/s11136-010-9757-7] [PMID: 20953908]

[15] Morrow, G.R.; Andrews, P.L.; Hickok, J.T.; Roscoe, J.A.; Matteson, S. Fatigue associated with cancer and its treatment. *Support. Care Cancer,* **2002**, *10*(5), 389-398.
[http://dx.doi.org/10.1007/s005200100293] [PMID: 12136222]

[16] Ryan, JL; Carroll, JK; Ryan, EP; Mustian, KM; Fiscella, K; Morrow, GR Mechanisms of Cancer-Related Fatigue. *Oncologist.,* **2007**, *12*(suppl_1), 22-34.
[http://dx.doi.org/10.1634/theoncologist.12-S1-22]

[17] Bower, J.E. Cancer-related fatigue--mechanisms, risk factors, and treatments. *Nat. Rev. Clin. Oncol.,* **2014**, *11*(10), 597-609.
[http://dx.doi.org/10.1038/nrclinonc.2014.127] [PMID: 25113839]

[18] Cleare, A.J. The neuroendocrinology of chronic fatigue syndrome. *Endocr. Rev.,* **2003**, *24*(2), 236-252.
[http://dx.doi.org/10.1210/er.2002-0014] [PMID: 12700181]

[19] Wang, X.S. Pathophysiology of cancer-related fatigue. *Clin. J. Oncol. Nurs.,* **2008**, *12*(5) Suppl., 11-20.
[http://dx.doi.org/10.1188/08.CJON.S2.11-20] [PMID: 18842520]

[20] Cleeland, C.S.; Bennett, G.J.; Dantzer, R.; Dougherty, P.M.; Dunn, A.J.; Meyers, C.A.; Miller, A.H.; Payne, R.; Reuben, J.M.; Wang, X.S.; Lee, B.N. Are the symptoms of cancer and cancer treatment due to a shared biologic mechanism? A cytokine-immunologic model of cancer symptoms. *Cancer,* **2003**, *97*(11), 2919-2925.
[http://dx.doi.org/10.1002/cncr.11382] [PMID: 12767108]

[21] Haroon, E.; Raison, C.L.; Miller, A.H. Psychoneuroimmunology meets neuropsychopharmacology: translational implications of the impact of inflammation on behavior. *Neuropsychopharmacology,* **2012**, *37*(1), 137-162.
[http://dx.doi.org/10.1038/npp.2011.205] [PMID: 21918508]

[22] Dantzer, R.; O'Connor, J.C.; Freund, G.G.; Johnson, R.W.; Kelley, K.W. From inflammation to sickness and depression: when the immune system subjugates the brain. *Nat. Rev. Neurosci.,* **2008**, *9*(1), 46-56.
[http://dx.doi.org/10.1038/nrn2297] [PMID: 18073775]

[23] Konsman, J.P.; Parnet, P.; Dantzer, R. Cytokine-induced sickness behaviour: mechanisms and implications. *Trends Neurosci.,* **2002**, *25*(3), 154-159.
[http://dx.doi.org/10.1016/S0166-2236(00)02088-9] [PMID: 11852148]

[24] Schubert, C.; Hong, S.; Natarajan, L.; Mills, P.J.; Dimsdale, J.E. The association between fatigue and inflammatory marker levels in cancer patients: a quantitative review. *Brain Behav. Immun.,* **2007**, *21*(4), 413-427.
[http://dx.doi.org/10.1016/j.bbi.2006.11.004] [PMID: 17178209]

[25] Stone, H.B.; Coleman, C.N.; Anscher, M.S.; McBride, W.H. Effects of radiation on normal tissue:

consequences and mechanisms. *Lancet Oncol.,* **2003**, *4*(9), 529-536.
[http://dx.doi.org/10.1016/S1470-2045(03)01191-4] [PMID: 12965273]

[26]   Aggarwal, B.B.; Vijayalekshmi, R.V.; Sung, B. Targeting inflammatory pathways for prevention and therapy of cancer: short-term friend, long-term foe. *Clin. Cancer Res.,* **2009**, *15*(2), 425-430.
[http://dx.doi.org/10.1158/1078-0432.CCR-08-0149] [PMID: 19147746]

[27]   Bower, J.E.; Ganz, P.A.; Tao, M.L.; Hu, W.; Belin, T.R.; Sepah, S.; Cole, S.; Aziz, N. Inflammatory biomarkers and fatigue during radiation therapy for breast and prostate cancer. *Clin. Cancer Res.,* **2009**, *15*(17), 5534-5540.
[http://dx.doi.org/10.1158/1078-0432.CCR-08-2584] [PMID: 19706826]

[28]   Liu, L.; Mills, P.J.; Rissling, M.; Fiorentino, L.; Natarajan, L.; Dimsdale, J.E.; Sadler, G.R.; Parker, B.A.; Ancoli-Israel, S. Fatigue and sleep quality are associated with changes in inflammatory markers in breast cancer patients undergoing chemotherapy. *Brain Behav. Immun.,* **2012**, *26*(5), 706-713.
[http://dx.doi.org/10.1016/j.bbi.2012.02.001] [PMID: 22406004]

[29]   Wang, X.S.; Williams, L.A.; Krishnan, S.; Liao, Z.; Liu, P.; Mao, L.; Shi, Q.; Mobley, G.M.; Woodruff, J.F.; Cleeland, C.S. Serum sTNF-R1, IL-6, and the development of fatigue in patients with gastrointestinal cancer undergoing chemoradiation therapy. *Brain Behav. Immun.,* **2012**, *26*(5), 699-705.
[http://dx.doi.org/10.1016/j.bbi.2011.12.007] [PMID: 22251605]

[30]   Rotstein, S.; Blomgren, H.; Petrini, B.; Wasserman, J.; Baral, E. Long term effects on the immune system following local radiation therapy for breast cancer. I. Cellular composition of the peripheral blood lymphocyte population. *Int. J. Radiat. Oncol. Biol. Phys.,* **1985**, *11*(5), 921-925.
[http://dx.doi.org/10.1016/0360-3016(85)90114-2] [PMID: 3157666]

[31]   Dicato, M. Anemia in cancer: some pathophysiological aspects. *Oncologist,* **2003**, *8* Suppl. 1, 19-21.
[http://dx.doi.org/10.1634/theoncologist.8-suppl_1-19] [PMID: 12626784]

[32]   Groopman, J.E.; Itri, L.M. Chemotherapy-induced anemia in adults: incidence and treatment. *J. Natl. Cancer Inst.,* **1999**, *91*(19), 1616-1634.
[http://dx.doi.org/10.1093/jnci/91.19.1616] [PMID: 10511589]

[33]   Glaspy, J.; Degos, L.; Dicato, M.; Demetri, G.D. Comparable efficacy of epoetin alfa for anemic cancer patients receiving platinum- and nonplatinum-based chemotherapy: a retrospective subanalysis of two large, community-based trials. *Oncologist,* **2002**, *7*(2), 126-135.
[http://dx.doi.org/10.1634/theoncologist.7-2-126] [PMID: 11961196]

[34]   Yellen, S.B.; Cella, D.F.; Webster, K.; Blendowski, C.; Kaplan, E. Measuring fatigue and other anemia-related symptoms with the Functional Assessment of Cancer Therapy (FACT) measurement system. *J. Pain Symptom Manage.,* **1997**, *13*(2), 63-74.
[http://dx.doi.org/10.1016/S0885-3924(96)00274-6] [PMID: 9095563]

[35]   Gabrilove, J.L.; Cleeland, C.S.; Livingston, R.B.; Sarokhan, B.; Winer, E.; Einhorn, L.H. Clinical evaluation of once-weekly dosing of epoetin alfa in chemotherapy patients: improvements in hemoglobin and quality of life are similar to three-times-weekly dosing. *J. Clin. Oncol.,* **2001**, *19*(11), 2875-2882.
[http://dx.doi.org/10.1200/JCO.2001.19.11.2875] [PMID: 11387360]

[36]   Demetri, G.D.; Kris, M.; Wade, J.; Degos, L.; Cella, D. Quality-of-life benefit in chemotherapy patients treated with epoetin alfa is independent of disease response or tumor type: results from a prospective community oncology study. *J. Clin. Oncol.,* **1998**, *16*(10), 3412-3425.
[http://dx.doi.org/10.1200/JCO.1998.16.10.3412] [PMID: 9779721]

[37]   Littlewood, T.J.; Kallich, J.D.; San Miguel, J.; Hendricks, L.; Hedenus, M. Efficacy of darbepoetin alfa in alleviating fatigue and the effect of fatigue on quality of life in anemic patients with lymphoproliferative malignancies. *J. Pain Symptom Manage.,* **2006**, *31*(4), 317-325.
[http://dx.doi.org/10.1016/j.jpainsymman.2005.08.013] [PMID: 16632079]

[38]   Goldstein, D.; Bennett, B.; Friedlander, M.; Davenport, T.; Hickie, I.; Lloyd, A. Fatigue states after

cancer treatment occur both in association with, and independent of, mood disorder: a longitudinal study. *BMC Cancer,* **2006**, *6*(1), 240.
[http://dx.doi.org/10.1186/1471-2407-6-240] [PMID: 17026776]

[39]   Jacobsen, P.B.; Hann, D.M.; Azzarello, L.M.; Horton, J.; Balducci, L.; Lyman, G.H. Fatigue in women receiving adjuvant chemotherapy for breast cancer: characteristics, course, and correlates. *J. Pain Symptom Manage.,* **1999**, *18*(4), 233-242.
[http://dx.doi.org/10.1016/S0885-3924(99)00082-2] [PMID: 10534963]

[40]   Mock, V.; Atkinson, A.; Barsevick, A.M.; Berger, A.M.; Cimprich, B.; Eisenberger, M.A.; Hinds, P.; Kaldor, P.; Otis-Green, S.A.; Piper, B.F. Cancer-related fatigue. *J. Natl. Compr. Canc. Netw.,* **2007**, *5*(10), 1054-1078.
[http://dx.doi.org/10.6004/jnccn.2007.0088] [PMID: 18053429]

[41]   Barsevick, A.M.; Cleeland, C.S.; Manning, D.C.; O'Mara, A.M.; Reeve, B.B.; Scott, J.A.; Sloan, J.A. ASCPRO recommendations for the assessment of fatigue as an outcome in clinical trials. *J. Pain Symptom Manage.,* **2010**, *39*(6), 1086-1099.
[http://dx.doi.org/10.1016/j.jpainsymman.2010.02.006] [PMID: 20538190]

[42]   Berger, A.M.; Farr, L.A.; Kuhn, B.R.; Fischer, P.; Agrawal, S. Values of sleep/wake, activity/rest, circadian rhythms, and fatigue prior to adjuvant breast cancer chemotherapy. *J. Pain Symptom Manage.,* **2007**, *33*(4), 398-409.
[http://dx.doi.org/10.1016/j.jpainsymman.2006.09.022] [PMID: 17397701]

[43]   Berger, A.M.; Farr, L. The influence of daytime inactivity and nighttime restlessness on cancer-related fatigue. *Oncol. Nurs. Forum,* **1999**, *26*(10), 1663-1671.
[PMID: 10573683]

[44]   Lee, K.A. Sleep and fatigue. *Annu. Rev. Nurs. Res.,* **2001**, *19*, 249-273.
[http://dx.doi.org/10.1891/0739-6686.19.1.249] [PMID: 11439783]

[45]   Dahiya, S.; Ahluwalia, M.S.; Walia, H.K. Sleep disturbances in cancer patients: underrecognized and undertreated. *Cleve. Clin. J. Med.,* **2013**, *80*(11), 722-732.
[http://dx.doi.org/10.3949/ccjm.80a.12170] [PMID: 24186891]

[46]   Savard, J.; Morin, C.M. Insomnia in the context of cancer: a review of a neglected problem. *J. Clin. Oncol.,* **2001**, *19*(3), 895-908.
[http://dx.doi.org/10.1200/JCO.2001.19.3.895] [PMID: 11157043]

[47]   Savard, J.; Simard, S.; Blanchet, J.; Ivers, H.; Morin, C.M. Prevalence, clinical characteristics, and risk factors for insomnia in the context of breast cancer. *Sleep,* **2001**, *24*(5), 583-590.
[http://dx.doi.org/10.1093/sleep/24.5.583] [PMID: 11480655]

[48]   Berger, A.M.; Mitchell, S.A.; Jacobsen, P.B.; Pirl, W.F. Screening, evaluation, and management of cancer-related fatigue: Ready for implementation to practice? *CA Cancer J. Clin.,* **2015**, *65*(3), 190-211.
[http://dx.doi.org/10.3322/caac.21268] [PMID: 25760293]

[49]   Jacobsen, P.B.; Donovan, K.A.; Weitzner, M.A. Distinguishing fatigue and depression in patients with cancer. *Semin. Clin. Neuropsychiatry,* **2003**, *8*(4), 229-240.
[PMID: 14613050]

[50]   Roscoe, J.A.; Morrow, G.R.; Hickok, J.T.; Bushunow, P.; Matteson, S.; Rakita, D.; Andrews, P.L. Temporal interrelationships among fatigue, circadian rhythm and depression in breast cancer patients undergoing chemotherapy treatment. *Support. Care Cancer,* **2002**, *10*(4), 329-336.
[http://dx.doi.org/10.1007/s00520-001-0317-0] [PMID: 12029433]

[51]   Visser, M.R.M.; Smets, E.M.A. Fatigue, depression and quality of life in cancer patients: how are they related? *Support. Care Cancer,* **1998**, *6*(2), 101-108.
[http://dx.doi.org/10.1007/s005200050142] [PMID: 9540167]

[52]   Jean-Pierre, P.; Morrow, G.R.; Roscoe, J.A.; Heckler, C.; Mohile, S.; Janelsins, M.; Peppone, L.;

Hemstad, A.; Esparaz, B.T.; Hopkins, J.O. A phase 3 randomized, placebo-controlled, double-blind, clinical trial of the effect of modafinil on cancer-related fatigue among 631 patients receiving chemotherapy: a University of Rochester Cancer Center Community Clinical Oncology Program Research base study. *Cancer,* **2010**, *116*(14), 3513-3520.
[http://dx.doi.org/10.1002/cncr.25083] [PMID: 20564068]

[53]   Stockler, M.R.; O'Connell, R.; Nowak, A.K.; Goldstein, D.; Turner, J.; Wilcken, N.R.; Wyld, D.; Abdi, E.A.; Glasgow, A.; Beale, P.J.; Jefford, M.; Dhillon, H.; Heritier, S.; Carter, C.; Hickie, I.B.; Simes, R.J. Effect of sertraline on symptoms and survival in patients with advanced cancer, but without major depression: a placebo-controlled double-blind randomised trial. *Lancet Oncol.,* **2007**, *8*(7), 603-612.
[http://dx.doi.org/10.1016/S1470-2045(07)70148-1] [PMID: 17548243]

[54]   Morrow, G.R.; Hickok, J.T.; Roscoe, J.A.; Raubertas, R.F.; Andrews, P.L.; Flynn, P.J.; Hynes, H.E.; Banerjee, T.K.; Kirshner, J.J.; King, D.K. Differential effects of paroxetine on fatigue and depression: a randomized, double-blind trial from the University of Rochester Cancer Center Community Clinical Oncology Program. *J. Clin. Oncol.,* **2003**, *21*(24), 4635-4641.
[http://dx.doi.org/10.1200/JCO.2003.04.070] [PMID: 14673053]

[55]   Skapinakis, P.; Lewis, G.; Mavreas, V. Temporal relations between unexplained fatigue and depression: longitudinal data from an international study in primary care. *Psychosom. Med.,* **2004**, *66*(3), 330-335.
[http://dx.doi.org/10.1097/01.psy.0000124757.10167.b1] [PMID: 15184691]

[56]   Neil, S.E.; Klika, R.J.; Garland, S.J.; McKenzie, D.C.; Campbell, K.L. Cardiorespiratory and neuromuscular deconditioning in fatigued and non-fatigued breast cancer survivors. *Support. Care Cancer,* **2013**, *21*(3), 873-881.
[http://dx.doi.org/10.1007/s00520-012-1600-y] [PMID: 23052910]

[57]   Franc, M.; Michalski, B.; Kuczerawy, I.; Szuta, J.; Skrzypulec-Plinta, V. Cancer related fatigue syndrome in neoplastic diseases. *Przegl. Menopauz.,* **2014**, *13*(6), 352-355.
[http://dx.doi.org/10.5114/pm.2014.47989] [PMID: 26327879]

[58]   Eguchi, K.; Honda, M.; Kataoka, T.; Mukouyama, T.; Tsuneto, S.; Sakamoto, J.; Oba, K.; Saji, S. Efficacy of corticosteroids for cancer-related fatigue: A pilot randomized placebo-controlled trial of advanced cancer patients. *Palliat. Support. Care,* **2015**, *13*(5), 1301-1308.
[http://dx.doi.org/10.1017/S1478951514001254] [PMID: 25370595]

[59]   Chan, R. Cochrane review summary for cancer nursing: drug therapy for the management of cancer-related fatigue. *Cancer Nurs.,* **2011**, *34*(3), 250-251.
[http://dx.doi.org/10.1097/NCC.0b013e31820aeb72] [PMID: 21512346]

[60]   WHO guidelines on safety monitoring of herbal medicines in pharmacovigilance systems. *World Heal Organ Geneva.,* **2004**, *82* http://www.regione.emiliaromagna.it/agenziasan/mnc/pdf/documenti/oms/who_guid_pharmacovig.pdf

[61]   Smith, ME; Bauer-Wu, S *Traditional Chinese Medicine For Cancer-Related Symptoms.,* **2012**.
[http://dx.doi.org/10.1016/j.soncn.2011.11.007]

[62]   Chung, V.C.H.; Wu, X.; Lu, P.; Hui, E.P.; Zhang, Y.; Zhang, A.L.; Lau, A.Y.; Zhao, J.; Fan, M.; Ziea, E.T.; Ng, B.F.; Wong, S.Y.; Wu, J.C. Chinese Herbal Medicine for Symptom Management in Cancer Palliative Care: Systematic Review And Meta-analysis. *Medicine (Baltimore),* **2016**, *95*(7)e2793
[http://dx.doi.org/10.1097/MD.0000000000002793] [PMID: 26886628]

[63]   Yang, L.; Li, T.T.; Chu, Y.T.; Chen, K.; Tian, S.D.; Chen, X.Y.; Yang, G.W. Traditional Chinese medical comprehensive therapy for cancer-related fatigue. *Chin. J. Integr. Med.,* **2016**, *22*(1), 67-72.
[http://dx.doi.org/10.1007/s11655-015-2105-6] [PMID: 26108523]

[64]   Li, X.; Yang, G.; Li, X.; Zhang, Y.; Yang, J.; Chang, J.; Sun, X.; Zhou, X.; Guo, Y.; Xu, Y.; Liu, J.; Bensoussan, A. Traditional Chinese medicine in cancer care: a review of controlled clinical studies published in chinese. *PLoS One,* **2013**, *8*(4)e60338

[http://dx.doi.org/10.1371/journal.pone.0060338] [PMID: 23560092]

[65]   Liu, J.; Wang, S.; Zhang, Y.; Fan, H.T.; Lin, H.S. Traditional Chinese medicine and cancer: History, present situation, and development. *Thorac. Cancer,* **2015**, *6*(5), 561-569.
[http://dx.doi.org/10.1111/1759-7714.12270] [PMID: 26445604]

[66]   Qi, F.; Li, A.; Inagaki, Y.; Gao, J.; Li, J.; Kokudo, N.; Li, X.K.; Tang, W. Chinese herbal medicines as adjuvant treatment during chemo- or radio-therapy for cancer. *Biosci. Trends,* **2010**, *4*(6), 297-307.
[PMID: 21248427]

[67]   Li, J.; Sun, G-Z.; Lin, H-S.; Pei, Y.X.; Qi, X.; An, C.; Yu, J.; Hua, B.J. The herb medicine formula "Yang Wei Kang Liu" improves the survival of late stage gastric cancer patients and induces the apoptosis of human gastric cancer cell line through Fas/Fas ligand and Bax/Bcl-2 pathways. *Int. Immunopharmacol.,* **2008**, *8*(9), 1196-1206.
[http://dx.doi.org/10.1016/j.intimp.2008.04.007] [PMID: 18602065]

[68]   Sun, G.; Wu, Z.; Lu, J.; Lu, W.; Wang, X. The molecular mechanisms of Yang Wei Kang Liu powder on anticancer and reducing chemotherapy side-effect in combination with chemotherapy. *Chinese-German J. Clin. Oncol.,* **2010**, *9*(5), 287-291.
[http://dx.doi.org/10.1007/s10330-010-0021-y]

[69]   Ling, Y. Traditional Chinese medicine in the treatment of symptoms in patients with advanced cancer. *Ann. Palliat. Med.,* **2013**, *2*(3), 141-152.
[http://dx.doi.org/10.3978/j.issn.2224-5820.2013.04.05] [PMID: 25842096]

[70]   Yennurajalingam, S.; Reddy, A.; Tannir, N.M.; Chisholm, G.B.; Lee, R.T.; Lopez, G.; Escalante, C.P.; Manzullo, E.F.; Frisbee Hume, S.; Williams, J.L.; Cohen, L.; Bruera, E. High-Dose Asian Ginseng (Panax Ginseng) for Cancer-Related Fatigue: A Preliminary Report. *Integr. Cancer Ther.,* **2015**, *14*(5), 419-427.
[http://dx.doi.org/10.1177/1534735415580676] [PMID: 25873296]

[71]   Yennurajalingam, S.; Tannir, N.M.; Williams, J.L.; Lu, Z.; Hess, K.R.; Frisbee-Hume, S.; House, H.L.; Lim, Z.D.; Lim, K.H.; Lopez, G.; Reddy, A.; Azhar, A.; Wong, A.; Patel, S.M.; Kuban, D.A.; Kaseb, A.O.; Cohen, L.; Bruera, E. A Double-Blind, Randomized, Placebo-Controlled Trial of *Panax Ginseng* for Cancer-Related Fatigue in Patients With Advanced Cancer. *J. Natl. Compr. Canc. Netw.,* **2017**, *15*(9), 1111-1120.
[http://dx.doi.org/10.6004/jnccn.2017.0149] [PMID: 28874596]

[72]   Barton, D.L.; Liu, H.; Dakhil, S.R.; Linquist, B.; Sloan, J.A.; Nichols, C.R.; McGinn, T.W.; Stella, P.J.; Seeger, G.R.; Sood, A.; Loprinzi, C.L. Wisconsin Ginseng (Panax quinquefolius) to improve cancer-related fatigue: a randomized, double-blind trial, N07C2. *J. Natl. Cancer Inst.,* **2013**, *105*(16), 1230-1238.
[http://dx.doi.org/10.1093/jnci/djt181] [PMID: 23853057]

[73]   Weber, D.; O'Brien, K. Cancer and Cancer-Related Fatigue and the Interrelationships With Depression, Stress, and Inflammation. *J. Evid. Based Complementary Altern. Med.,* **2017**, *22*(3), 502-512.
[http://dx.doi.org/10.1177/2156587216676122] [PMID: 30208733]

[74]   Samuels, N.; Maimon, Y.; Zisk-Rony, R.Y. Effect of the Botanical Compound LCS101 on Chemotherapy-Induced Symptoms in Patients with Breast Cancer: A Case Series Report. *Integr. Med. Insights,* **2013**, *8*, 1-8.
[http://dx.doi.org/10.4137/IMI.S10841] [PMID: 23400272]

[75]   Zhang, D.; Zheng, J.; Ni, M.; Wu, J.; Wang, K.; Duan, X.; Zhang, X.; Zhang, B. Comparative efficacy and safety of Chinese herbal injections combined with the FOLFOX regimen for treating gastric cancer in China: a network meta-analysis. *Oncotarget,* **2017**, *8*(40), 68873-68889.
[http://dx.doi.org/10.18632/oncotarget.20320] [PMID: 28978164]

[76]   Du, J.; Cheng, B.C.Y.; Fu, X-Q.; Su, T.; Li, T.; Guo, H.; Li, S.M.; Wu, J.F.; Yu, H.; Huang, W.H.; Cao, H.; Yu, Z.L. *In vitro* assays suggest Shenqi Fuzheng Injection has the potential to alter melanoma

immune microenvironment. *J. Ethnopharmacol.,* **2016**, *194*, 15-19.
[http://dx.doi.org/10.1016/j.jep.2016.08.038] [PMID: 27566207]

[77]   Zhao, J; Wu, A; Shi, L. [Clinical observation on treatment of advanced gastric cancer by combined use of Shenqi Fuzheng injection, docetaxel, flurouracil and calcium folinate]. *Zhongguo Zhong xi yi jie he za zhi Zhongguo Zhongxiyi jiehe zazhi = Chinese J Integr Tradit West Med.,* **2007**, *27*(8), 736-738.

[78]   Qi, F.; Zhao, L.; Zhou, A.; Zhang, B.; Li, A.; Wang, Z.; Han, J. The advantages of using traditional Chinese medicine as an adjunctive therapy in the whole course of cancer treatment instead of only terminal stage of cancer. *Biosci. Trends,* **2015**, *9*(1), 16-34.
[http://dx.doi.org/10.5582/bst.2015.01019] [PMID: 25787906]

[79]   Yang, Y.; Ting, W.; Xiao, L.; Shufei, F.; Wangxiao, T.; Xiaoying, W.; Xiumei, G.; Boli, Z. Immunoregulation of Shenqi Fuzheng Injection Combined with Chemotherapy in Cancer Patients: A Systematic Review and Meta-Analysis. *Evid. Based Complement. Alternat. Med.,* **2017**, *2017*5121538
[http://dx.doi.org/10.1155/2017/5121538] [PMID: 28154607]

[80]   Wang, J.; Li, S.; Fan, Y.; Chen, Y.; Liu, D.; Cheng, H.; Gao, X.; Zhou, Y. Anti-fatigue activity of the water-soluble polysaccharides isolated from Panax ginseng C. A. Meyer. *J. Ethnopharmacol.,* **2010**, *130*(2), 421-423.
[http://dx.doi.org/10.1016/j.jep.2010.05.027] [PMID: 20580802]

[81]   Guan, F; Li, Z; Liao, Y Clinical investigation of acanthopanax root injection for improving the postoperative fatigue syndrome of the patients with gastrointestinal tumors. *Guo Ji Yi Yao Wei Sheng Dao Bao,* **2008**, (14), 78-81.

[82]   Gu, Y; Xu, H; Jiang, Y. Clinical effect of Shenqi Fuzheng Injection (SQFZI) on cancer-related fatigue. *Zhong Guo Zhong Xi Yi Jie He Za Zhi.,* **2009**, (29), 363-364.

[83]   Ge, J; Zhang, Y; He, H. Clinical observation on TanshinoneIIA Sulfonic Sodium injection combined with thymosin in the treatment of cancer-related fatigue. *Lin Chuan Yi Yao.,* **2009**, (18), 56.

[84]   Zhang, Y.; Han, X.; Ouyang, B.; Wu, Z.; Yu, H.; Wang, Y.; Liu, G.; Ji, X. Chinese Herbal Medicine Baoyuan Jiedu Decoction Inhibited Muscle Atrophy of Cancer Cachexia through Atrogin-1 and MuRF-1. *Evid. Based Complement. Alternat. Med.,* **2017**, *2017*6268378
[http://dx.doi.org/10.1155/2017/6268378] [PMID: 28286533]

[85]   Su, C-X.; Wang, L-Q.; Grant, S.J.; Liu, J-P. Chinese herbal medicine for cancer-related fatigue: a systematic review of randomized clinical trials. *Complement. Ther. Med.,* **2014**, *22*(3), 567-579.
[http://dx.doi.org/10.1016/j.ctim.2014.04.007] [PMID: 24906595]

[86]   Matkovic, Z; Zivkovic, V; Korica, M; Plavec, D; Pecanic, S; Tudoric, N Efficacy and safety of Astragalus membranaceus in the treatment of patients with seasonal allergic rhinitis. *Phyther Res.,* **2009**, *24*(2) doi:10.1002/ptr.2877.

[87]   Guo, R.; Pittler, M.H.; Ernst, E. Herbal medicines for the treatment of allergic rhinitis: a systematic review. *Ann. Allergy Asthma Immunol.,* **2007**, *99*(6), 483-495.
[http://dx.doi.org/10.1016/S1081-1206(10)60375-4] [PMID: 18219828]

[88]   Xu, Q.; Ma, X.; Liang, X. Determination of astragalosides in the roots of Astragalus spp. using liquid chromatography tandem atmospheric pressure chemical ionization mass spectrometry. *Phytochem. Anal.,* **2007**, *18*(5), 419-427.
[http://dx.doi.org/10.1002/pca.997] [PMID: 17624885]

[89]   Lin, L.Z.; He, X.G.; Lindenmaier, M.; Nolan, G.; Yang, J.; Cleary, M.; Qiu, S.X.; Cordell, G.A. Liquid chromatography-electrospray ionization mass spectrometry study of the flavonoids of the roots of Astragalus mongholicus and A. membranaceus. *J. Chromatogr. A,* **2000**, *876*(1-2), 87-95.
[http://dx.doi.org/10.1016/S0021-9673(00)00149-7] [PMID: 10823504]

[90]   Harley, C.B.; Liu, W.; Blasco, M.; Vera, E.; Andrews, W.H.; Briggs, L.A.; Raffaele, J.M. A natural product telomerase activator as part of a health maintenance program. *Rejuvenation Res.,* **2011**, *14*(1), 45-56.

[http://dx.doi.org/10.1089/rej.2010.1085] [PMID: 20822369]

[91]   Zhao, H.; Zhang, Q.; Zhao, L.; Huang, X.; Wang, J.; Kang, X. Spore Powder of *Ganoderma lucidum* Improves Cancer-Related Fatigue in Breast Cancer Patients Undergoing Endocrine Therapy: A Pilot Clinical Trial. *Evid. Based Complement. Alternat. Med.,* **2012**, *2012*809614 [http://dx.doi.org/10.1155/2012/809614] [PMID: 22203880]

[92]   Martínez-Montemayor, M.M.; Acevedo, R.R.; Otero-Franqui, E.; Cubano, L.A.; Dharmawardhane, S.F. Ganoderma lucidum (Reishi) inhibits cancer cell growth and expression of key molecules in inflammatory breast cancer. *Nutr. Cancer,* **2011**, *63*(7), 1085-1094. [http://dx.doi.org/10.1080/01635581.2011.601845] [PMID: 21888505]

[93]   Yu, G-J.; Wang, M.; Huang, J.; Yin, Y.L.; Chen, Y.J.; Jiang, S.; Jin, Y.X.; Lan, X.Q.; Wong, B.H.; Liang, Y.; Sun, H. Deep insight into the Ganoderma lucidum by comprehensive analysis of its transcriptome. *PLoS One,* **2012**, *7*(8)e44031 [http://dx.doi.org/10.1371/journal.pone.0044031] [PMID: 22952861]

[94]   Suarez-Arroyo, I.J.; Rosario-Acevedo, R.; Aguilar-Perez, A.; Clemente, P.L.; Cubano, L.A.; Serrano, J.; Schneider, R.J.; Martínez-Montemayor, M.M. Anti-tumor effects of Ganoderma lucidum (reishi) in inflammatory breast cancer in *in vivo* and *in vitro* models. *PLoS One,* **2013**, *8*(2)e57431 [http://dx.doi.org/10.1371/journal.pone.0057431] [PMID: 23468988]

[95]   Pawlik, A.; Janusz, G.; Dębska, I.; Siwulski, M.; Frąc, M.; Rogalski, J. Genetic and metabolic intraspecific biodiversity of Ganoderma lucidum. *BioMed Res. Int.,* **2015**, *2015*726149 [http://dx.doi.org/10.1155/2015/726149] [PMID: 25815332]

[96]   Liao, C-H.; Hsiao, Y-M.; Lin, C-H.; Yeh, C.S.; Wang, J.C.; Ni, C.H.; Hsu, C.P.; Ko, J.L. Induction of premature senescence in human lung cancer by fungal immunomodulatory protein from Ganoderma tsugae. *Food Chem. Toxicol.,* **2008**, *46*(5), 1851-1859. [http://dx.doi.org/10.1016/j.fct.2008.01.044] [PMID: 18329152]

[97]   Wang, X.; Su, K.; Bao, T. *IMMUNOMODULATORY EFFECTS of FUNGAL PROTEINS.,* **2012**, *10*(1), 1-12.

[98]   Gutstein, H.B. The biologic basis of fatigue. *Cancer,* **2001**, *92*(6) Suppl., 1678-1683. [http://dx.doi.org/10.1002/1097-0142(20010915)92:6+<1678::AID-CNCR1496>3.0.CO;2-R] [PMID: 11598886]

[99]   Bower, J.E.; Ganz, P.A.; Aziz, N.; Fahey, J.L.; Cole, S.W. T-cell homeostasis in breast cancer survivors with persistent fatigue. *J. Natl. Cancer Inst.,* **2003**, *95*(15), 1165-1168. [http://dx.doi.org/10.1093/jnci/djg0019] [PMID: 12902446]

[100]   Chung, V.C.; Wu, X.; Hui, E.P.; Ziea, E.T.; Ng, B.F.; Ho, R.S.; Tsoi, K.K.; Wong, S.Y.; Wu, J.C. Effectiveness of Chinese herbal medicine for cancer palliative care: overview of systematic reviews with meta-analyses. *Sci. Rep.,* **2015**, *5*(November), 18111. [pii]. [http://dx.doi.org/10.1038/srep18111\rsrep18111] [PMID: 26669761]

[101]   Jeong, J.S.; Ryu, B.H.; Kim, J.S.; Park, J.W.; Choi, W.C.; Yoon, S.W. Bojungikki-tang for cancer-related fatigue: a pilot randomized clinical trial. *Integr. Cancer Ther.,* **2010**, *9*(4), 331-338. [http://dx.doi.org/10.1177/1534735410383170] [PMID: 21059621]

[102]   Pannacci, M.; Lucini, V.; Colleoni, F.; Martucci, C.; Grosso, S.; Sacerdote, P.; Scaglione, F. Panax ginseng C.A. Mayer G115 modulates pro-inflammatory cytokine production in mice throughout the increase of macrophage toll-like receptor 4 expression during physical stress. *Brain Behav. Immun.,* **2006**, *20*(6), 546-551. [http://dx.doi.org/10.1016/j.bbi.2005.11.007] [PMID: 16469481]

[103]   Lee, D.C.W.; Lau, A.S.Y. Effects of Panax ginseng on tumor necrosis factor-α-mediated inflammation: a mini-review. *Molecules,* **2011**, *16*(4), 2802-2816. [http://dx.doi.org/10.3390/molecules16042802] [PMID: 21455094]

[104]   Seruga, B.; Zhang, H.; Bernstein, L.J.; Tannock, I.F. Cytokines and their relationship to the symptoms

and outcome of cancer. *Nat. Rev. Cancer,* **2008**, *8*(11), 887-899.
[http://dx.doi.org/10.1038/nrc2507] [PMID: 18846100]

[105]   Miller, A.H.; Bordeaux, U. *NIH Public Access.,* **2009**, *26*(6), 971-982.
[http://dx.doi.org/10.1200/JCO.2007.10.7805.Neuroendocrine-Immune]

[106]   Bower, J.E.; Ganz, P.A.; Irwin, M.R.; Kwan, L.; Breen, E.C.; Cole, S.W. Inflammation and behavioral symptoms after breast cancer treatment: do fatigue, depression, and sleep disturbance share a common underlying mechanism? *J. Clin. Oncol.,* **2011**, *29*(26), 3517-3522.
[http://dx.doi.org/10.1200/JCO.2011.36.1154] [PMID: 21825266]

[107]   Fearon, K.C.H.; Glass, D.J.; Guttridge, D.C. Cancer cachexia: mediators, signaling, and metabolic pathways. *Cell Metab.,* **2012**, *16*(2), 153-166.
[http://dx.doi.org/10.1016/j.cmet.2012.06.011] [PMID: 22795476]

[108]   Jeong, J.S.; Ryu, B.H.; Kim, J.S.; Park, J.W.; Choi, W.C.; Yoon, S.W. Bojungikki-tang for cancer-related fatigue: a pilot randomized clinical trial. *Integr. Cancer Ther.,* **2010**, *9*(4), 331-338.
[http://dx.doi.org/10.1177/1534735410383170] [PMID: 21059621]

[109]   Zhao, H.; Zhang, Q.; Zhao, L.; Huang, X.; Wang, J.; Kang, X. Spore Powder of *Ganoderma lucidum* Improves Cancer-Related Fatigue in Breast Cancer Patients Undergoing Endocrine Therapy: A Pilot Clinical Trial. *Evid. Based Complement. Alternat. Med.,* **2012**, *2012*809614
[http://dx.doi.org/10.1155/2012/809614] [PMID: 22203880]

[110]   Gao, Z; Wang, W; Kao, J; Ma, X; Zang, J. The effect of Kangai injection on colorectal cancer patients with cancer☐related fatigue receiving adjuvant chemotherapy. *JETCM.,* **2010**, (19), 221-222.

[111]   Su, C-X.; Wang, L-Q.; Grant, S.J.; Liu, J-P. Chinese herbal medicine for cancer-related fatigue: a systematic review of randomized clinical trials. *Complement. Ther. Med.,* **2014**, *22*(3), 567-579.
[http://dx.doi.org/10.1016/j.ctim.2014.04.007] [PMID: 24906595]

[112]   Barton, D.L.; Soori, G.S.; Bauer, B.A.; Sloan, J.A.; Johnson, P.A.; Figueras, C.; Duane, S.; Mattar, B.; Liu, H.; Atherton, P.J.; Christensen, B.; Loprinzi, C.L. Pilot study of Panax quinquefolius (American ginseng) to improve cancer-related fatigue: a randomized, double-blind, dose-finding evaluation: NCCTG trial N03CA. *Support. Care Cancer,* **2010**, *18*(2), 179-187.
[http://dx.doi.org/10.1007/s00520-009-0642-2] [PMID: 19415341]

[113]   Finnegan-John, J.; Molassiotis, A.; Richardson, A.; Ream, E. A systematic review of complementary and alternative medicine interventions for the management of cancer-related fatigue. *Integr. Cancer Ther.,* **2013**, *12*(4), 276-290.
[http://dx.doi.org/10.1177/1534735413485816] [PMID: 23632236]

[114]   Ye, L.; Jia, Y.; Ji, K.E.; Sanders, A.J.; Xue, K.; Ji, J.; Mason, M.D.; Jiang, W.G. Traditional Chinese medicine in the prevention and treatment of cancer and cancer metastasis. *Oncol. Lett.,* **2015**, *10*(3), 1240-1250. [Review].
[http://dx.doi.org/10.3892/ol.2015.3459] [PMID: 26622657]

[115]   Liu, R.; He, S.L.; Zhao, Y.C.; Zheng, H.G.; Li, C.H.; Bao, Y.J.; Qin, Y.G.; Hou, W.; Hua, B.J. Chinese herbal decoction based on syndrome differentiation as maintenance therapy in patients with extensive-stage small-cell lung cancer: an exploratory and small prospective cohort study. *Evid. Based Complement. Alternat. Med.,* **2015**, *2015*601067
[http://dx.doi.org/10.1155/2015/601067] [PMID: 25815038]

[116]   Lin, G.; Li, Y.; Chen, S.; Jiang, H. Integrated Chinese-western therapy versus western therapy alone on survival rate in patients with non-small-cell lung cancer at middle-late stage. *J Tradit Chinese Med = Chung i tsa chih ying wen pan.,* **2013**, *33*(4), 433-438. http://www.ncbi.nlm.nih.gov/pubmed/24187861

[117]   Yang, X-B.; Wu, W-Y.; Long, S-Q.; Deng, H.; Pan, Z-Q. Effect of gefitinib plus Chinese herbal medicine (CHM) in patients with advanced non-small-cell lung cancer: a retrospective case-control study. *Complement. Ther. Med.,* **2014**, *22*(6), 1010-1018.
[http://dx.doi.org/10.1016/j.ctim.2014.10.001] [PMID: 25453521]

[118] Wang, S.; Long, S.; Wu, W. Application of Traditional Chinese Medicines as Personalized Therapy in Human Cancers. *Am. J. Chin. Med.,* **2018**, *46*(5), 953-970.
[http://dx.doi.org/10.1142/S0192415X18500507] [PMID: 29986595]

[119] Wong, V.K.W.; Zhang, M.M.; Zhou, H.; Lam, K.Y.; Chan, P.L.; Law, C.K.; Yue, P.Y.; Liu, L. Saikosaponin-d Enhances the Anticancer Potency of TNF-α via Overcoming Its Undesirable Response of Activating NF-Kappa B Signalling in Cancer Cells. *Evid. Based Complement. Alternat. Med.,* **2013**, *2013*745295
[http://dx.doi.org/10.1155/2013/745295] [PMID: 23573150]

[120] Gao, L; Wang, XD; Niu, YY Molecular targets of Chinese herbs: a clinical study of hepatoma based on network pharmacology. *Sci Rep.,* **2016**, *6*(November 2017), 24944.
[http://dx.doi.org/10.1038/srep24944]

[121] Zhong, L.L.D.; Chen, H-Y.; Cho, W.C.S.; Meng, X.M.; Tong, Y. The efficacy of Chinese herbal medicine as an adjunctive therapy for colorectal cancer: a systematic review and meta-analysis. *Complement. Ther. Med.,* **2012**, *20*(4), 240-252.
[http://dx.doi.org/10.1016/j.ctim.2012.02.004] [PMID: 22579437]

[122] Qi, F.; Li, A.; Inagaki, Y.; Gao, J.; Li, J.; Kokudo, N.; Li, X.K.; Tang, W. Chinese herbal medicines as adjuvant treatment during chemo- or radio-therapy for cancer. *Biosci. Trends,* **2010**, *4*(6), 297-307.
[PMID: 21248427]

CHAPTER 5

Indirubins as Multi-target Anti-Tumor Agents

Yasamin Dabiri[1], Guangqi Song[2] and Xinlai Cheng[1,*]

[1] *Institute of Pharmacy and Molecular Biotechnology, Pharmaceutical Biology, Heidelberg University, Im Neuenheimer Feld 364, D-69120 Heidelberg, Germany*

[2] *Shanghai Institute of Liver Disease, Department of Gastroenterology, Zhongshan Hospital, Fudan University, Building 19, Fenglin Road 179, Shanghai, China*

Abstract: The traditional use of indirubin for the treatment of leukaemia has opened a vast field of research, studying the anti-tumor properties of indirubin and its derivatives (IRDs) against a wide range of malignancies. The cytotoxic effects of indirubin has been primarily attributed to its inhibitory function on a number of protein kinases, including cyclin-dependent kinases (CDKs), glycogen-synthase kinase 3 (GSK-3), and receptor tyrosine kinases (RTKs). In the past few decades, a lot of effort has been directed to the chemical modification of indirubin's backbone towards better pharamcokinetic properties. This has led to the synthesis of various derivatives with new biological activities. We here review from the discovery of indirubin to the development of novel IRDs, and highlight the recent progress on how indirubins influence multiple cancer-associated signaling networks, leading to anti-proliferative and pro-apoptotic effects. Furthermore, we discuss the therapeutic use of indirubins in anti-cancer settings, as well as their potential for future clinical application.

Keywords: Casein Kinases (CKs), Cyclin Dependent Kinase (CDK), Indirubin, Indirubin Derivative (IRD), Insulin-Like Growth Factor Receptor (IGFR), Glycogen Synthase Kinase (GSK), Nuclear Factor-kB (NF-kB), Receptor Tyrosine Kinase (RTK), Transforming Growth Factor β (TGFβ), Ubiquitin-Specific Proteases (USPs).

INTRODUCTION

The successful isolation and identification of Qinghaosu (青蒿素) as an anti-malarial agent from more than 500 recipes of traditional Chinese medicine (TCM) highlights the power of TCM in the clinical application [1, 2]. In general, TCM is an evidence-based approach for the treatment of diseases and consists of all possible medical recourses, including plants, animals and acupuncture [3].

*** Corresponding author Xinlai Cheng:** Institute of Pharmacy and Molecular Biotechnology, Pharmaceutical Biology, Heidelberg University, Im Neuenheimer Feld 364, D-69120 Heidelberg, Germany; E-mail: x.cheng@uni-heidelberg.de

Ferid Murad, Atta-ur-Rahman and Ka Bian (Eds.)

Dangui Luhui Wan (当归芦荟丸) is a mixture of 11 herbal products and was discovered 1000 years ago. In China, *Dangui Luhui Wan* has been used for the treatment of various chronic diseases. Its anti-tumor effect was firstly reported in 1970s in a clinical trial with 22 patients in China with mild side effects [4]. The follow-up studies revealed that indirubin from *Indigofera. tinctoria* L. (青黛, indigo naturalis) was the major active component [5].

Indirubin, indigo and isoindigo are isoforms sharing bis-indole's basic structure (Fig. **1**) [6, 7]. Indirubin and indirubin derivatives (IRDs) have been reported frequently in the literature to induce apoptosis and inhibit cellular growth and proliferation in chronic mylegenous leukaemia (CML) as well as in several other types of solid and soft tumours [8 - 11]. Recent discoveries are increasingly unraveling the molecular basis of such effects. However, the clinical application is largely hampered due to the limited water solubility [12]. Here we will review the known approaches in order to improve water-solubility and bioavailability of indirubin, and highlight the molecular targets as well as the cellular networks that have been proposed as indirubins' mode of action in an anti-cancer setting. Furthermore, we will discuss the clinical perspectives of the use of indirubins in cancer therapy.

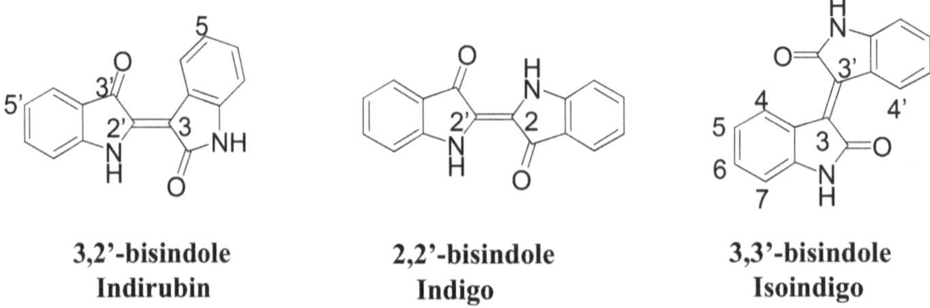

3,2'-bisindole | **2,2'-bisindole** | **3,3'-bisindole**
Indirubin | **Indigo** | **Isoindigo**

Fig. (1). Structures of indirubin, indigo and isoindigo.

TOWARDS BIOAVAILABILITY: CHEMICAL MODIFICATION AND PHARMACEUTICAL FORMULATION

Chemical Modification

Like indigo, indirubin and most derivatives are insoluble in water and also in major organic solvents due to the very stable intramolecular hydrogen bond between 1-NH and 2-CO and intermolecular hydrogen bond between 1'-NH and 2-CO (Fig. **2**) [13]. As a result, the molecule has shown poor bioavailability *in vitro* as well as in mammalian cells and animal models [14 - 16], which became one of the major drawbacks for the clinical application of indirubins. Therefore, several chemical modification approaches were taken in order to improve the water-solubility [12].

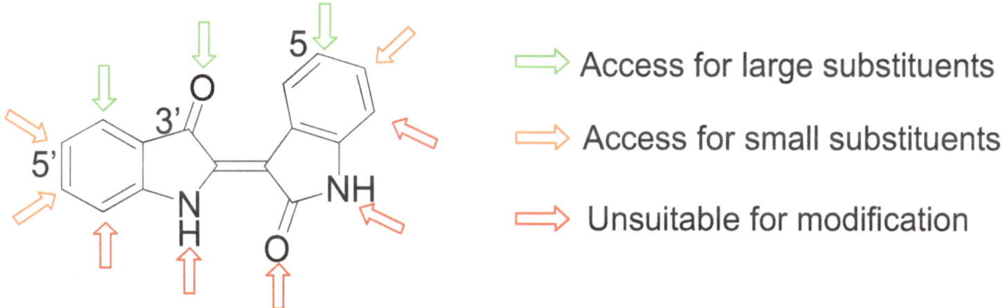

Fig. (2). Strong intra- and inter-molecular H-bridges result in low water-solubility of indirubin.

The study of co-crystal structure of indirubin-3'-oxime and indirubin-5-sulfonate in the ATP-binding pocket of CDK2 [6, 17, 18] pointed out potential positions on the bis-indole moiety of indirubin for chemical medication without negative influence on the biological activity –either using 5- and 3'-positions towards the ribose and triphosphate channels or 5'-position, opening to the solvent Fig. (3).

Fig. (3). Illustration of possible positions for chemical modification towards the ATP-competitive inhibitor pocket. Green: full access; Orange: limited access; Red: not suitable for chemical modification.

The synthesis of indirubin (Fig. **4**) was first reported by Baeyer in 1881 using isatin and indoxyl in MeOH under basic condition [19]. Since the indoxyl is not stable and spontaneously turns to indigo after exposure to air, Russell and Kaupp replaced it with more stable indoxyl acetate in 1969 [20]. This method under mild basic condition is applicable for the synthesis of most indirubin derivatives.

However, 7-aza indoxyl acetate is not stable and degrades under this condition [21]. The synthesis of aza-indirubins were preferentially conducted in acetic acid with 10% concentrated HCl developed by Martinet and Dornier [22].

Fig. (4). Synthesis of indirubin under basic and acidic conditions.

The modification at 3'-position is probably the most successful approach to introduce substituents with basic groups in order to improve the water solubility. Using this position, we and other groups indeed achieved water-soluble indirubin derivatives with improved cytotoxicity [23, 24]. In comparison, 5 and 5'-position can also be applied for synthesis of derivatives, but with more complicated protocol on the basis of producing a stable and active intermediate pentafluorophenyl indirubin-carboxylate [25]. The syntheses have been extensively described in the original article and in our recent review [3].

Pharmaceutical Formulation

A study on the interaction of indirubin with p-glycoprotein revealed that the binding affinity of indirubin to p-glycoprotein is undetectable in the pH 2-11, suggesting that the poor water-solubility is the major factor contributing to low bioavailability of indirubin [16]. Chemical modification led to the synthesis of several water soluble indirubin derivatives, like indirubin-5-sulfonate (sodium salt), which however lost pharmaceutical activity because of its extra hydrophilic property [26]. Thus, pharmaceutical formulation became an alternative to chemical modification towards bioavailability with less influence on the biological activity of drugs. Indeed, both self-microemulsifying and self-nanoemulsifying drug delivery system (SMEDDS and SNEDDS, respectively) have been reported [14, 27]. In SMEDDS, 50 ng/mL indirubin was roughly detected in the plasma after oral administration, while 1800 ng/mL (approximate 10 µM) was achieved using SNEDDS. Considering that the reported IC50-values of indirubin and indirubin derivatives in cellular assays are lower than 10 µM,

SNEDDS could provide a very promising approach to the clinical application of indirubins.

CELLULAR TARGETS OF INDIRUBIN AND DERIVATIVES

Cyclin Dependent Kinases

Indirubins were primarily detected to have a high inhibitory activity towards cyclin-dependent kinases (CDKs) with IC50 values down to the nanomolar range (5-100 nM) [6]. CDKs are serine/threonine protein kinases together with their binding partners, cyclins are responsible for initiating and coordinating the cell cycle progression. There are three transition steps at which the cell cycle regulators including CDKs/cyclins determine passing of cells through the next phase, G1/S, G2/M and during mitosis (M) phase [28]. The first checkpoint, G1/S is mostly regulated by CDK4,6/cyclin D and CDK2/cyclin E complexes, which are responsible for the phosphorylation and inactivation of retinoblastoma protein (Rb). CDK2/cyclin A is required for the S phase progression which is followed by the action of CDK1/cyclin B and CDK2/cyclin B complexes at the G2/M transition, preparing cells for mitotic division [29].

Cell cycle deregulation through the altered activity of CDKs, their activators (cyclins) and/or inhibitors (*e.g.* p21$^{CIP/WAF1}$ and p27^{KIP1}) is a common feature of human malignancies [28]. Therefore, inhibition of CDKs by indirubins and other small molecular inhibitors is most likely to be advantageous in the treatment of cancer, mainly *via* blocking the cell cycle progression at both G1/S and G2/M transition steps (Fig. **5**) [12, 28, 30]. In this respect, indirubin and its derivatives have been reported to bind to and inhibit CDK1/cyclin B [31] CDK2/cyclin A, CDK2/cyclin E [6] and CDK5/p25 [32] complexes.

Crystal structures of CDK2 in complex with IRDs revealed that indirubin occupies the ATP binding pocket of the CDK's catalytic subunit through hydrophobic interactions and hydrogen bonds, thereby inhibiting the activity of the enzyme [6]. Indirubin has poor water solubility and low bioavailability, thus a lot of effort has been put in order to improve these properties by introducing hydrophilic groups in the structure of IRDs [12]. Extent structure-activity relationship studies (SAR) have suggested that chemical modifications at position 3' and/or 5 enhance the absorption as well as the water solubility, while preserving the kinase inhibitory function and anti-tumor properties [6]. In this respect, indirubin-3'-monoxime and indirubin-5-sulphonate have been synthesised, exhibiting higher affinity for CDKs and potent inhibition of the enzymes [6, 18]. While the sulphonate analogue fails to be up-taken by tumor cells, monoxime substituent is cell-permeable and shows high efficacy in several malignancy models [12], making it the most widely-studied derivative of indirubins. Accordingly, Hoessel *et al.* showed that the kinase inhibitory activity of the water soluble IRD, indirubin-3'-oxime is accompanied by reduced phosphorylation of the Rb protein, and subsequently G1 and G2/M cell cycle arrest in the human leukaemia cell line, Jurkat [6]. Additionally, the compound showed growth inhibitory effects in the mammary cancerous cell line, MCF-7 by inducing a G2/M cell cycle arrest through inhibition of CDK 1 [31]. Furthermore, it increased the levels of the CDK inhibitor, p27, and reduced the expression of CDK 2 and cyclin E, leading to a G0/G1 arrest in human neuroblastoma cell lines [33].

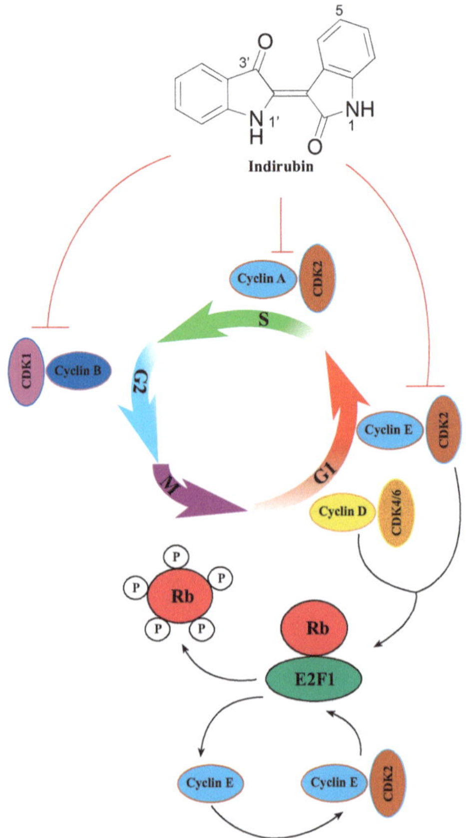

Fig. (5). Regulation of cell cycle by indirubin. The cell cycle machinery is tightly controlled by the action of different cyclin/CDK complexes at three transitional points, G1/S, G2/M and during mitosis as indicated. Indirubin blocks the progression of cells to the next phase by inhibiting the cyclin/CDK activity at both G1/S and G2/M checkpoints, thereby exerting its anti-proliferative effects. In the bottom, the positive feedback loop in which cyclin E/CDK2 and cyclin D/CDK 4/6 complexes promote the release of E2F1 transcription factor is shown. The feedback mechanism ensures that the retinoblastoma protein (Rb) remains hyper-phosphorylated, driving cells into S phase.

Glycogen Synthase Kinase 3

The CDK inhibitory activity of indirubins is normally found together with the inhibition of the related kinase, glycogen synthase kinase 3β (GSK-3β) [12]. GSK-3β is a multifunctional serine/threonine kinase, acting as a key component in the canonical Wnt signalling pathway which plays an essential role in several physiological processes ranging from cell cycle, oncogenesis, metabolism, glucose homeostasis, neuroprotection and dorsal-ventral patterning during embryonic development [34]. Furthermore, it serves as an important enzyme in insulin signaling [34]; over-expression of GSK-3β has been reported in type 2 diabetes and GSK-3β inhibitors have shown anti-diabetic effects in-vitro and in-vivo [35]. GSK-3β along with CDK5 is involved in hyperphosphorylation of the microtubule binding protein, tau which is a diagnostic factor in many neuro-degenerative diseases, particularly Alzheimer's disease [12]. It has been reported that several indirubin derivatives which were initially defined as potent CDK inhibitors, inhibit the GSK-3β enzyme in a ATP-competitive manner similar to their interaction with CDKs, and represent the first class of GSK-3β pharmacological inhibitors that are effective at low nano molar concentrations (5-50 nM) [32, 36, 37]. Leclerc and colleagues showed that the indirubin cell-permeable analogue, indirubin-3'-oxime inhibits tau protein aggregation in-vitro and in-vivo by blocking two protein kinases, CDK5/ p25 and GSK-3β concomitantly. Moreover, indirubin-3'-oxime was able to block the phosphorylation of dopamine- and cyclic adenosine 3'-5'-mono-phosph-te-regulated phospho-protein 32 (DARPP-32) by CDK5 in-vivo, thereby mimicking dopamine effects in the stratum [32]. In an effort to develop new scaffolds that are able to selectively interfere with the GSK-3β function, it has been described by Meijer *et al.* that a simple modification at position 6 increases the GSK-3 specificity over CDKs [32]. In this regard, 6-bromoindirubin derived from "tyrian purple" dye of mollusks and its oxime substituent, 6-bromoindirubi--3'-oxime (6BIO) have been reported as selective pharmacological inhibitors of GSK-3α/β (Fig. **6**) [36]. The compounds mimicked Wnt signaling, reduced phosphorylation of β-catenin in--vivo and showed more than 16 fold higher selectivity for CDK2 as compared to CDK5 [36]. Therefore, indirubin and its derivatives present promising candidates not only in cancer therapy, but also in the treatment of other diseases in which selective GSK-3 inhibition is desired, such as diabetes and Alzheimer's disease. Importantly, the controversial role of GSK-3β in tumorigenesis should be taken into consideration while applying GSK-3β inhibitors for cancer treatment. On one hand, GSK-3β inhibits Wnt signalling by phosphorylation and subsequent proteasomal degradation of β-catenin; in this context GSK-3β acts as a tumour suppressor. On the other hand, it may promote tumorigenesis by stimulating the activity of Wnt/β-catenin signalling through phosphorylation of Wnt co-receptor, LRP 5/6 [38]. The latter effect might explain the anti-proliferative and cytotoxic effects observed with GSK-3β inhibitors, such as indirubins. Apart from the previously mentioned roles for GSK-3β, this kinase is increasingly identified as a modulator of invasion and metastasis which involves the cooperation of both cancer cells and the stroma [39]. Williams and colleagues showed that the GSK-3β inhibitory activity of indirubins suggests a new therapeutic potential by preventing invasion of glioma cells and glioma-initiating cells *in vitro* and in a glioma bearing mouse model. Besides, indirubins were found to reduce cellular migration of endothelial cells, an essential component of tumor angiogenesis [40].

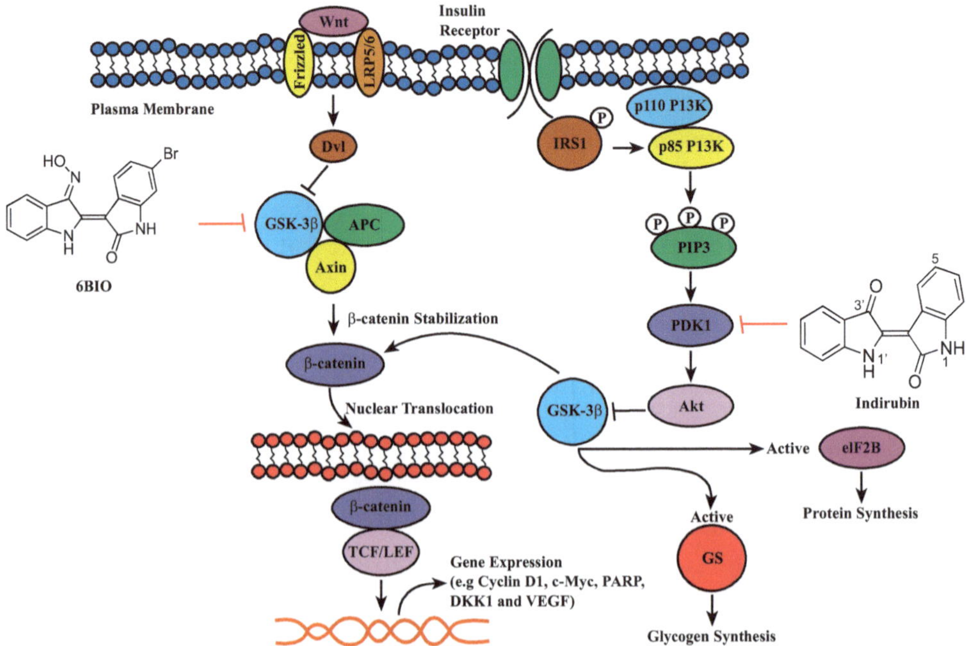

Fig. (6). Indirubin-mediated inhibition of GSK-3β, an essential element of Wnt/β-catenin pathway and insulin signalling. GSK-3β together with APC and Axin forms a multi-protein complex in the cytosol. Upon binding of Wnt to its receptor frizzled and its co-receptor LRP5/6, Dishevelled (Dvl) is activated which in turn deactivates GSK-3β. As a result, GSK-3β inhibition of β-catenin is relieved, leading to its stabilisation and translocation to the nucleus. β-catenin in association with LEF/TCF transcription factors increases the expression of several pro-survival (*e.g.* cyclin D1 and c-Myc) and angiogenic (*e.g.* VEGF) target genes as indicated. As illustrated in the figure at the right side, in the presence of insulin, insulin receptor is activated, followed by phosphorylation and activation of insulin receptor substrate (IRS) and subsequently PI3/PDK1/Akt activation that phosphorylates GSK-3β. Inactive phosphorylation of GSK-3β relieves its inhibitory activity on glycogen synthase (GS) and elF2B, resulting in glycogen and protein synthesis, respectively. GSK-3β, glycogen synthesis kinase-3β; APC, adenomas polyposis coli; LRP5/6, LDL related protein; LEF/TCF, lymphoid enhancer factor/T cell factor; VEGF, vascular endothelial growth factor; PI3K, phosphoinositide 3 kinase; PDK1, phosphoinositide dependent tyrosine kinase 1; elF2B, eukaryotic initiation factor 2B; 6BIO, 6-bromo-indirubin-3'-oxime.

According to their findings, GSK-3β inhibition is accompanied by dephosphorylation thereby stabilisation of β-catenin and subsequently reduced migratory phenotypes [40]. Despite the importance of β-catenin in the proposed mechanism, they showed that silencing this protein does not completely rescue the anti-migratory effects of indirubins in glioma [40], implicating additional targets to GSK-3β in mediating the observed effects. Focusing on the anti-metastatic properties of indirubins, Braig *et al.* reported the IRD 6BIO as a promising chemical tool that significantly diminishes migration of breast cancer cells into the lungs at subtoxic concentrations (1 mg/kg) in an aggressive breast cancer mouse model (4T1) [41]. While the known targets of 6BIO, GSK-3β as well as the phosphoinositide-dependent tyrosine kinase 1 (PDK1) [12] should be granted for the overall anti-migratory effects of 6BIO in this study, they were not found to be the major contributors. Instead, Inhibition of the kinases, Src and janus kinase (JAK) followed by decreasing the activity of their substrate, signal transducer and activator of transcription 3 (STAT3) turned out to play a dominant role [41]. STAT3 inhibition led to decreased levels of C-terminal tension like protein (CTEN) and matrix metalloproteinase 2 (MMP2), both of which are down-stream migration regulators of the Src/JAK/STAT signalling cascade [41]. The combined inhibition of multiple kinases by the IRD 6BIO could be of great benefit in order to target different aspects of cancer simultaneously, ranging from extensive proliferation of cells to migration, invasion, angiogenesis and metastasis.

Aryl Hydrocarbon Receptor

Although the CDK/GSK-3β inhibitory activity of indirubins is possibly the reason behind most of the cytotoxic effects, the interaction of indirubins with the aryl hydrocarbon receptor (AhR, also known as the "dioxin receptor") has to be taken into account especially in terms of indirubin-mediated cytostasis. Reported by Adachi *et al.*, indirubin was for the first time discovered with potent AhR agonist activity [42] which was later connected to the indirubin-mediated cell cycle regulation [43]. Of note, the CDK 2 inhibitor p27^{KIPI}, a known target gene of AhR was shown to be directly linked to the sharp G1/S cell cycle arrest induced by the kinase-inactive yet AhR-active derivatives of indirubins carrying a methyl group on position 1 (1-methyl-indirubins) [43]. In a different study, indirubin-3'-oxime and 1-methyl-indirubin-3'-oxime were reported to suppress centrosome amplification stimulated by ectopic AhR expression in breast cancer cells [44]. This finding suggests the potential application of these derivatives in preventing the malignant progression of tumors with over-expressed AhR. Despite the anti-proliferative effects of AhR ligands including indirubins, translating AhR activation into cancer treatment approaches, should be done cautiously. On one hand, several reports support the advantage of AhR ligands in anti-cancer treatments, particularly human pancreatic cancer [45]. On the other hand, AhR activation has been reported repeatedly in oncogenesis [46]. Understanding the molecular mechanisms and the down-stream targets by which AhR ligands exert their anti-cancer properties can be achieved by designing structures with enhanced selectivity (such as 1-methyl-indirubins) and will be helpful in finding the correct context in which the AhR activators are advantageous.

STAT

Anti-angiogenic activity of indirubins, in particular in case of the IRD E804, is mainly through the inhibition of VEGFR. Upon inhibition of VEGF signaling by indirubins, the downstream molecules, such as STATs, MAPKs and focal adhesion kinase (FAK) are as well inhibited leading to the down-regulation of target genes (*e.g.* MMP 2/9 and VEGF) with key roles in cellular migration.

As shown on the left side of the figure, indirubin-3'-oxime (3IO) blocks the activity of the tyrosine kinase receptor FGFR-1, thus affecting the downstream signaling molecules including STAT and MAPKs, which eventually leads to anti-proliferative and pro-apoptotic effects in FGFR-1-dependent cancerous cell lines.

In search of novel therapeutic targets for indirubins, the anti-tumor activity of a number of IRDs have been attributed at least partially to their inhibition of STAT signalling. The role of STAT family of proteins, particularly STAT3 and to a lesser degree STAT5 has been mentioned repeatedly in tumorigenesis [47 - 49]. STAT3 induces cellular survival and proliferation by up-regulating the anti-apoptotic proteins (*e.g.* Bcl-xL, survivin and Mcl-1) and cell cycle regulators (*e.g.* cyclin D and c-Myc) (Fig. **7**) [48]. Besides, many of its target genes have been implicated in migration, invasion and metastasis in various types of cancer [48, 49]. The up-stream tyrosine kinases, JAK and Src work cooperatively to phosphorylate and activate STAT3 (Fig. **7**) [50, 51]. Elevated expression of Src/JAK tyrosine kinases [52, 53] and their substrate STAT3 [47 - 49] has been found in the majority of cancer types. Therefore, targeting the JAK/Src/STAT signal transduction pathway appears to be a promising option in cancer treatment. It has been reported by Nam and colleagues that a number of IRDs, including E564, E728 and E804 are able to inhibit the constitutively active STAT3 signalling in human breast and prostate tumor cell lines [54]. One of the derivatives, indirubin-3'-(2,3 dihyroxypropyl)-oximether referred to as E804 directly interfered with the Src kinase activity (Fig. **7**) at submicromolar concentrations (IC50 = 0.43 μM), thereby reduced tyrosyl phosphorylation of its substrate, STAT3 in both an in-vitro kinase assay as well as in cultured human breast (MDA-MB-468 and -435) and prostate (DU145) cancer cells. Furthermore, two of the anti-apoptotic target genes of STAT3, Mcl-1 and survivin, were

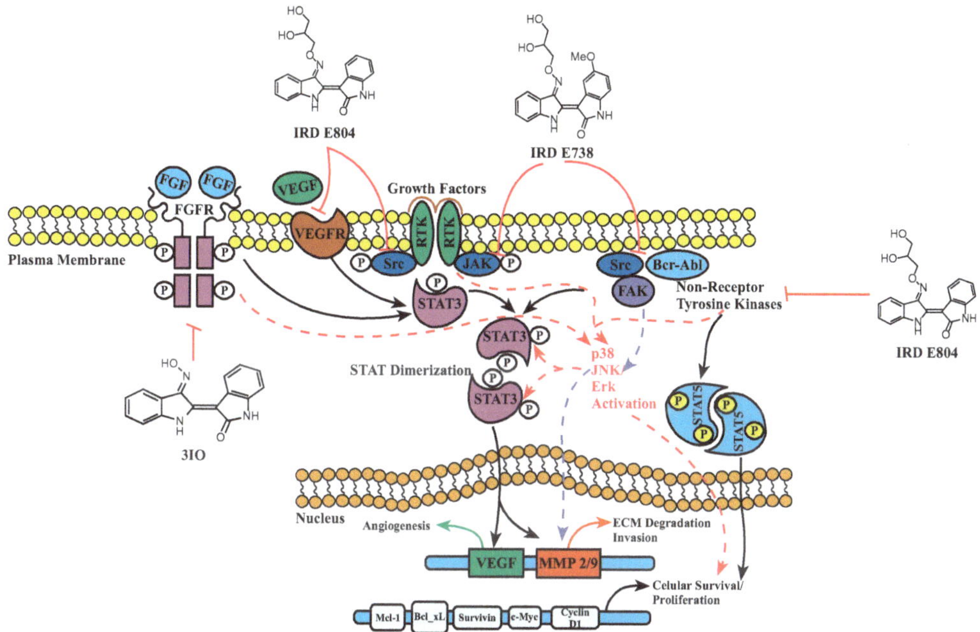

Fig. (7). Indirubins interfere with STAT signalling through inhibiting various kinases. Receptor tyrosine kinases (RTKs) are activated upon ligand binding, which in turn either directly activate STAT or phosphorylate the intermediate kinases, JAK and Src. Phosphorylation of JAK and Src provides docking sites for the recruitment of monomeric STAT molecules and subsequent tyrosyl phosphorylation, which is accompanied by STAT dimerization and nuclear translocation. Additionally, non-receptor tyrosine kinases such as Src and BCR-ABL can directly phosphorylate STAT, in the absence of ligand-induced receptor activation as illustrated on the right side of the figure. Mitogen activated protein kinases (MAPKs), namely p38, JNK, and Erk are stimulated in parallel to STAT activation, enhancing its activity by phosphorylating serine residues at its C-terminal transactivation domain. STAT, signal transducer and activator of transcription factor; JAK, janus kinase; JNK, C-Jun N-terminal kinase; Erka, extracellular signal-regulated kinase; VEGFR; vascular endothelial growth factor receptor; VEGF, vascular endothelial growth factor; MMP 2/9, matrix metaloproteinase 2/9; ECM, extracellular matrix; FGF, fibroblast growth factor; FGFR, fibroblast growth factor receptor.

dramatically down-regulated upon treatment with E804 in breast cancer cells, contributing to the pro-apoptotic effects. Importantly, the induction of apoptosis by E804 was not found in normal cells lacking increased STAT3 activity, which further confirms that the anti-tumoral effects of E804 are at least partially due to the blockage of Src/STAT3 signalling [54]. Another member of the STAT family with a critical role in oncogenesis, in particular hematopoietic malignancies is STAT5 [55 - 57]. Non-receptor tyrosine kinases, BCR-ABL and Src family kinases (SFKs) have been implicated in the constitutive activation of STAT5 thereby in the regulation of oncogenic pathways (Fig. **7**) [56, 58, 59]. Nam *et al.* showed in a different study that among a series of IRDs, compound E804 is the most potent derivative to induce apoptosis in chronic myelogenous leukaemia

(CML) *via* inhibition of SFK/STAT5 signalling down stream of BCR-ABL kinase (Fig. **7**) [60]. This inhibition was followed by the small molecule's pro-apoptotic effects on human K-562 CML cells, imatinib-resistant human KCL-22 CML cells, expressing mutant BCR-ABL as well as CD34 positive primary CML cells from patients. Furthermore, the levels of Mcl-1, known to be a potential therapeutic target for the treatment of CML, was repressed upon E804 treatment [60]. It is worth mentioning here that the IRD E804 is primarily a potent CDK inhibitor, a common quality of most of the indirubin derivatives. In this respect, the compound has shown anti-proliferative effects in different in-vitro cancerous models, namely human HCT116 colon cancer, human MCF-7 breast cancer, as well as human lung carcinoma cell line, LXFL529L [12].

As previously mentioned, JAK and Src kinases work coordinately in order to phosphorylate STAT3 at certain tyrosine residues [50, 51]. It has been reported that prolonged inhibition of Src triggers a compensatory pathway in which STAT3 is alternatively phosphorylated and activated through the JAK/STAT3 interaction, mediating cancer cell survival and proliferation [61, 62]. Therefore, concomitant inhibition of SFKs and JAK appears to have synergistic cytotoxic effects by blocking STAT3 reactivation that happens upon treatment with Src-specific inhibitors (*e.g.* dasatinib) [61]. In this regard, the IRD E738, possessing a propanediol group at 3'-and a methoxy group at 5-position has been introduced by Nam and colleagues as the first dual inhibitor of JAKs and SFKs with IC50 values of 0.7-74.1 nM and 10.7-263.9 nM respectively, which offers pharmacological benefit in the treatment of cancer by interfering with both porto-oncogene kinases simultaneously (Fig. **7**) [63]. As compared to E804, the compound E738 showed 40-fold increase in the Src inhibitory activity [63]. Combined inhibition of the up-stream kinases by IRD E738, resulted in the reduced tyrosyl phosphorylation of STAT3, that was accompanied by down-regulation of the anti-apoptotic protein, Mcl-1 and induction of apoptosis in human pancreatic cancer cells at submicromolar concentrations [63].

Several other studies have identified the JAK/Src/STAT signal transduction as a mechanism by which different bromo-substituents of indirubin exert their anti-cancer effects. It has been reported by Liu and colleagues that the compound, 6BIO induces apoptosis in melanoma by selectively targeting JAK/STAT3 signalling [64]. 6BIO, among a series of IRDs had the most potency in reducing the phosphorylation of JAK and STAT3 and suppressed tumor growth in a human melanoma xenograft mouse model [64]. Another study reported the anti-cancer activity of a 7-bromoindirubin derivative (designated as MLS-2438) in human melanoma cell lines *via* targeting both STAT3 and Akt kinases. The compound also inhibited tumor growth *in vivo* with relatively low toxicity [65]. Investigating the cellular effects of bromoindirubins, the IRD 7BIO, which carries a bromo group at the 7 position and a hydrophilic group at the 3' position, exhibited a very distinct anti-tumor profile. Unlike its close isomers, 5- and 6-bromoindirubins, 7BIO showed insignificant inhibition of the indirubins' classical targets, CDKs and GSK-3β [66]. The anti-cancer effects of indirubins such as apoptosis induction and cell cycle arrest are classically attributed to their kinase inhibitory function [12]. However, this does not seem to be the case for derivatives carrying substitutions on position 7. Accordingly, 7BIO with only marginal kinase inhibition was able to induce a rapid cell death without triggering the typical markers of apoptosis, such as caspsase cleavage or cytochrome c release [66]. In a more recent study, two analogs of bromo-indirubins, 6BIO and 7BIO showed discrete pro-apoptotic effects in five different breast cancer cell lines, with the invasive cell line, MDA-MB-231 being the most responsive model [67]. 6BIO was shown to induce intrinsic apoptotic pathway *via* cleavage of caspase 9, whereas the anti-proliferative effects of 7BIO were associated with p21 up-regulation, cell cycle arrest and eventually activation of both caspase 8-dependent as well as caspase-independent pathways of cell death [67]. With the recent examples in mind, it can be concluded that the nature of cell death triggered by different substituents of indirubins is not necessarily similar. The apoptosis-independent mode of action of 7-substituted indirubins (*e.g.* 7BIO), is of great benefit particularly in tumor cells with intrinsic or acquired resistance to apoptosis, and so to conventional anti-cancer therapies.

Vascular Endothelial Growth Factor Receptor

One of the hallmarks of malignant neoplasia with a fundamental role in every step of tumour development, including cellular survival, invasion and metastasis is angiogenesis [68]. Angiogenesis is a complex process in which new vessels are produced from pre-existing vessels by the harmonious action of different compartments, including endothelial cells, extracellular matrix (ECM) and angiogenic factors [69, 70]. Angiogenic stimulators, namely vascular endothelial growth factor (VEGF), basic fibroblast growth factor (bFGF), angiogenin, transforming growth factor β (TGFβ) and tumor necrosis factor α (TNFα) on one hand and angiogenic inhibitors such as pigment epithelium-derived factor (PEDF) on the other hand work in an opposing manner in order to tightly regulate the process of angiogenesis [71]. VEGF and its primary receptor, vascular endothelial growth factor receptor 2 (VEGFR2, also referred to as Flk2) are particularly of key importance in tumour vasculature [69]. Upon binding to its receptor, VEGF induces several angiogenesis-related pathways, namely STATs [72], mitogen activated protein kinases (MAPKs) and focal adhesion kinase (FAK) [73, 74]. It has been reported frequently that among the activated signalling pathways, Src/STAT signalling and particularly STAT3 is a main player in VEGFR2-targeted angiogenesis Fig. (**7**) [72, 75, 76]. Uncontrolled angiogenesis has been implicated in the pathogenesis of several diseases including solid tumours. Therefore, the anti-angiogenic approach has been increasingly recruited in cancer therapy as well as in other angiogenic diseases [77]. Investigating the molecular mechanisms underlying the indirubin-mediated angio-suppression, it has been shown that the water soluble derivative, indirubin-3'-oxime exerts its anti-angiogenic properties in endothelial cells at least in part through the down regulation of VEGFR-2 [78]. In a comparative approach, several known CDK inhibitors were tested in a novel anti-angiogenic context [79]. Of those, the well studied IRD, indirubin-3'-oxime which was previously mentioned as a powerful CDK/GSK-3β inhibitor, suppressed several angiogenesis-related parameters, including endothelial cell proliferation, migration and tube formation, through CDK-independent mechanisms and possibly by targeting more than one kinase (*e.g.* GSK-3β and Src) simultaneously [79]. It is noteworthy that the IRD indirubin-3'-oxime had been previously linked to angiogenesis in a screening approach, however no mechanistic analysis was performed [80]. Apart from the oxime derivative, indirubin itself has been shown to inhibit tumor angiogenesis in human prostate cancer cell line, PC-3 *via* blocking VEGFR2-mediated JAK/STAT3 signalling in endothelial cells [81]. For the IRD E804, several molecular targets including CDKs, Src/STAT3 and BCR-ABL/STAT5 had been previously suggested [12, 54, 60]. In a different context, Chan *et al.* examined the anti-angiogenic profile of the compound E804 [82]. In comparison to indirubin-3'-oxime, E804 showed more potent *in vitro* angio-suppression, however both compounds significantly reduced the proliferation, migration and tube formation of human umbilical vein endothelial cells (HUVECs) concentration-dependently (0.4-40 μM) [82]. In contrast to indirubin-3'-oxime, E804 (at a concentration of 4 μM) was able to completely inhibit the outgrowth of endothelial cells from the rat aorta observed in the ex-vivo aortic ring assay, as well as the activity of two members of the MMP family, MMP-2 and MMP-9 [82]. The anti-angiogenic activity of the cell permeable derivative, E804 was further confirmed in a different study where the compound inhibited the angiogenic markers in HUVECs and micro-vessel sprouting from the rat aortic ring [83]. Mechanistic analyses revealed *in vitro* inhibition of the kinase activity of purified VEGFR-2 by E804 (Fig. 7)), and subsequently reduced phosphorylation of the receptor and the down stream kinases, Akt as well as extracellular related kinase (Erk) in endothelial cells stimulated by VEGF [83]. The latter finding highlight the importance of VEGFR-2 signalling pathway as a new mode of action for the compound E804 which had not been characterised previously. Comparing indirubin with inidrubin-3'-oxime and IRD E804, it is worth mentioning that the latter derivative has a stronger potential for the inhibition of angiogenesis. Accordingly, the concentrations by which endothelial cell proliferation, migration and tube formation are inhibited, are significantly higher in the case of indirubin and indirubin-3'-oxime (25-100 µM and 2.5-10 µM respectively) as compared to E804 (1-10 µM) [83].

With respect to in-vivo studies, Zhang and colleagues reported that indirubin counteracts neovascularisation, using chick chorioallantoic membrane (CAM) assay and mouse corneal model [81]. Using transgenic zebrafish embryos, expressing enhanced green fluorescent protein (EGFP) in their vasculature, indirubin showed strong in-vivo anti-angiogenic activity by blocking intersegmental blood vessel formation [84]. The IRD E804 showed angio-suppression in two in-vivo assays, Matrigel plug assay and directed in-vivo angiogenesis assay (DIVAA) [82], and led to reduced tumor volume and tumor weight in the allograft CT-26 colorectal cancer model at a concentration of 20 µM [83], further proving the promising anti-angiogenic potential of novel indirubin derivatives. The current examples clearly show that the anti-tumoral properties of indirubin and its derivatives could be at least partially attributable to the small molecules' angio-suppressive ability; indirubins induce apoptosis and cell cycle arrest in endothelial cells which closely resemble their effects on various cancerous cell lines. Therefore, it is most likely that the inhibitory function of indirubin and its analogs on a number of different kinases, such as CDKs, GSK-3β, and the JAK/Src/STAT signalling contributes to the observed angio-suppression thereby anti-cancer effects, especially if the important role of these kinases in angiogenesis is taken into consideration. Furthermore, it is worth mentioning the great potential of anti-angiogenic therapy in the treatment of non-cancerous conditions with up-regulated and uncontrolled angiogenesis such as atherosclerosis, rheumatoid arthritis and diabetic retinopathy [77]. Therefore, indirubins represent a new candidate in the treatment of not only solid tumours, but every angiogenesis-dependent condition, collectively referred to as "angiogenic diseases".

Fibroblast Growth Factor Receptor

Despite a large number of protein kinases, we have mentioned so far, namely CDKs, GSK-3β, STATs, Src, and VEGFR-2, there is still untold molecular targets for indirubin and its derivatives. It has been reported by Zhen and colleagues that the well-studied IRD, indirubin-3'-oxime inhibits the tyrosine kinase receptor, fibroblast growth factor receptor-1 (FGFR-1) strongly and selectively at concentrations lower than needed for CDK2 inhibition (5 µM *vs.* 20 µM, respectively) (Fig. 7) [85]. Furthermore, it triggered Erk1/2 activity as a consequence of p38 MAPK activation which occurred independent of FGFR-1inhibition [85]. Autophosphorylation of the tyrosine residues within the intracellular domain of FGFR-1 is a key element in the fibroblast growth factor (FGF) signal transduction, which acts *via* different signalling molecules such as

Ras/MAPKs, PI3K/Akt and Src/STAT (Fig. **7**) [86, 87]. Blocking FGFR-1 activation, indirubin-3'-oxime led to reduced proliferation of the FGF1-stimulated NIH/3T3 cell line as well as the human acute myelogenous leukaemia (AML) cells, KG-1a [85]. Using 4 times higher concentration (20 µM), the compound exhibited cellular growth inhibitory effects on the FGFR-1-negative leukaemia cell line, K-562 [85]. The latter effect seems to be at least partly attributable to its CDK inhibitory function since it occurs at higher concentrations, highlighting the more specificity of indirubin-3'-oxime towards FGFR-1 as compared to CDKs. This finding is particularly important while treating FGFR-1-dependent cancers (*e.g.* the AML-derived cancer cell line, KG-1a), however as mentioned before (for the FGFR-1-independent K-562 cell line) the anti-cancer properties of indirubin-3'-oxime is not restricted to FGFR-1-sensitive tumour cells due to the multiple molecular targets being associated with this derivative as well as other IRDs.

Nuclear Factor-kB

Another signalling molecule that has been described in literature as the indirubins' molecular target is the nuclear factor-kB (NF-kB). Seth *et al.* reported that the inhibition of IkBα kinase (IKK) caused by indirubin and subsequently inhibiting the activation of NF-kB signalling pathway might be at least partly the mechanism by which indirubins mediate their anti-inflammatory and anti-cancer effects (Fig. **8**) [88]. In the absence of any stimulator, NF-kB retains in the cytoplasm as a heterotrimer consisting of 3 components, namely p50, p65 and IkB. Upon receiving inflammatory or carcinogenic cues, the signalling pathway gets activated through a series of events that leads to phosphorylation, ubiquitination and degradation of IkB by IKK, and subsequent translocation of p65 to the nucleus where NF-kB regulates the expression of several genes involved in inflammation and tumorigenesis (Fig. **8**) [89, 90]. The pro-survival genes (*e.g.* IAP 1/2, Bcl-xL, Bcl-2 and TRAF-1) as well as the molecules involved in the cell cycle machinery (*e.g.* cyclin D1 and c-Myc) and invasion/metastasis (*e.g.* MMP-9 and COX-2) were drastically down-regulated by indirubin as a result of NF-kB suppression [88]. These observations are in consistency with the previously mentioned studies reporting the down regulation of a number of anti-apoptotic/invasive proteins in response to indirubins through pathways other than NF-kB [54, 60, 82], implicating the fact that there is a considerable number of players in mediating the pro-apoptotic, anti-proliferative and anti-cancer properties of indirubins.

Activation of the canonical NF-kB signalling is induced by a number of different ligand-receptor complexes namely IL1/IL-1R, TNF/TNFR, as well as LPS/TLRs, leading to the IkBα kinase (IKK) activation. IKK phosphorylates IkBα at its serine residues, resulting in its poly-ubiquitination and proteasomal degradation.

Consequently, the inhibitory activity of IkBα is relieved, mediating the translocation of NF-kB homo- or hetero- dimers to the nucleus, where the expression of several inflammatory and pro-survival genes is regulated. The kinase inhibitory activity of indirubin on IKK leads to the suppression of NF-kB nuclear translocation, and subsequent down-regulation of its target genes involved in proliferation (*e.g.* cyclin D1 and c-Myc), survival (*e.g.* Bcl-2, Bcl-xL, TRAF-1 and IAP 1/2), and invasion (*e.g.* COX-2 and MMP-9).

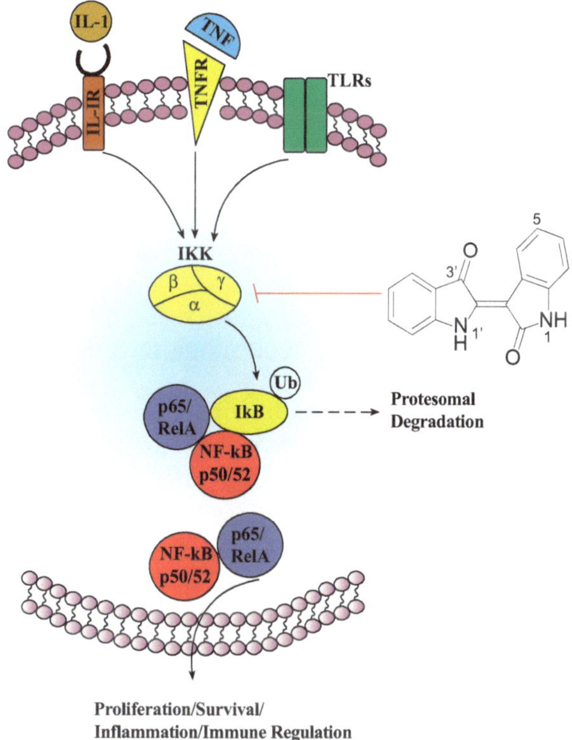

Fig. (8). Indirubin targets NF-kB signalling through blocking the inhibitory kinase, IKK. IL1, interleukin 1; IL-1R, interleukin 1 receptor; TNF, tumour necrosis factor; TNFR, tumor necrosis factor recetor; LPS, lipopolysaccharides; TLRs, Toll-like receptors; NF-kB, nuclear factor-kB.

Casein Kinases

Of the less investigated molecules targeted by indirubins, are casein kinases (CKs). In an attempt to develop more metabolically stable indirubins, several azaindirubins were synthesised, of those 7,7'-diazaindirubin was found to selectively inhibit casein kinases [21]. Using the human breast cancer cell line, MCF-7 the compound showed remarkable anti-proliferative and pro-apoptotic effects which were abolished in the CK-2-deficient MCF-7 cells, highlighting the dependence of this derivative to CK-2 in order to execute its anti-tumour effects [21].

Insulin-like Growth Factor 1 Receptor

Recently, Screening the biological targets of a series of newly synthesised 5'-carboxy substituents led to the identification of a water soluble derivative, indirubin-3'-[2-(4-methylpiperazino)ethyl]oxime ether hydrochloride with strong inhibitory activity towards insulin-like growth factor 1 receptor (IGF-1R) despite having only a marginal inhibition of CDKs and GSK-3β [24]. Additionally, the compound 6ha showed anti-proliferative and cytotoxic effects in the NCI-60 cell line panel at low micro molar concentrations [24]. The IGF1 signalling pathway has a significant role in cell proliferation and survival, accordingly high levels of IGF1 have been implicated in several cancers namely breast, colon, endometrium and prostate [91, 92]. Therefore, pharmacological intervention with the IGF-R1 signalling, using IGF-R1 tyrosine kinase inhibitors such as indirubins appears to be a valuable approach in cancer treatment.

Transforming Growth Factor β/Bone Morphogenetic Protein

Lately, the anti-cancer potential of indirubins was tested in a new context, introducing them as potent modulators of the transforming growth factor β/bone morphogenetic protein (TGFβ/BMP) signal transduction [93]. TGFβ signalling is a complex network of TGFβ and BMP-mediated pathways, exerting its effects by phosphorylating and activating the receptor-regulated SMAD (R-SMAD) proteins which determine the biological outcome of the signalling through transcriptional regulation [94, 95]. Among a series of derivatives, IRD E738 showed the strongest activity in depleting total R-SMAD levels thereby inhibiting TGFβ/BMP signaling [93]. Furthermore, the activity of MAPKs, including p38 and c-Jun NH2-terminal kinase (JNK) was stimulated upon treatment with the compound E738 independent of the TGFβ/BMP suppression [93]. The latter effect is in consistency with the previously reported activation of MAPKs in response to indirubins [85]. Additionally, the activity of ubiquitin specific proteases (USPs), USP 9x and USP 34 was found to be significantly reduced through a direct interaction with IRD E738, adding a novel molecular target to the indirubin's profile: the "ubiquitin proteasome pathway (UPP)" [93]. TGFβ/BMP signaling and its messengers, SMAD proteins have been implicated repeatedly in the pathogenesis of several diseases, including cancer [96]. Given the negative regulation of the signalling pathway at multiple distinct layers by IRD E738 [93], indirubins suggest a new therapeutic potential in order to influence the pro-survival signals of TGFβ/BMP ligands.

Cancer Stem Cell

The dependence of several types of human cancer to the tumour-initiating cells with stem cell-like properties, referred to as cancer stem cells (CSCs) is increasingly being recognised in recent studies, suggesting a new therapeutic paradigm in the treatment of cancer [97 - 99]. Several combinations of cell surface markers have been identified to be selectively expressed in CSCs, such as the CD44+/CD24- [100 - 102], CD44+/CD24+/ESA+ [103] and CD34+/CD133+ [104, 105] phenotypes. In this regards, meisoindigo, a derivative of isoindigo carrying a methyl group at position 1 has been shown to preferentially reduce CSC populations (CD133+ and CD24+/CD44+/ESA+ cells) as well as the self-renewal potential of human pancreatic ductal adenocarcinoma (PDAC) [106]. Furthermore, meisoindigo showed pro-apoptotic effects in gemcitabine-resistant PDAC cells, by disrupting the cellular redox balance [106]. Previous studies had shown meisoindigo to induce apoptosis, inhibit cell proliferation and differentiation as well as angiogenesis in leukaemia both *in-vitro* and *in- vivo* [107, 108]. Of note, meisoindigo unlike its parental molecule, indirubin does not show significant inhibitory activity towards protein kinases [109, 110], implicating other mechanistic pathways than the classical targets (*e.g.* CDKs and GSK-3β) underlying the cytotoxic and anti-proliferative effects of isoindigos. A proposed mechanism involved the AMPK activation through the altered mitochondrial function, followed by the induction of apoptosis in PDAC cell lines [106]. Furthermore, the upstream kinase of AMPK, liver kinase B1 (LKB1) was inhibited in response to meisoindigo, which was accompanied by a reduction in cancer stem cell markers (*e.g.* CD133 and CD44) [106]. This finding provides a deeper insight into the molecular basis underpinning the pro-apoptotic, anti-proliferative as well as anti-cancer stem cell properties of isoindigo derivatives. However, further work needs to be done in order to investigate the involved signalling pathways leading to the anti-tumour effects of the new generation of indirubins.

Indirubin-Mediated Cell Death Through Other Cellular Networks

In many cases, the pro-apoptotic effects of indirubin have been associated with mitochondria-dependent pathways. In this regard, indirubin-3'-oxime was shown to induce apoptosis in human cervical, hepatoma, and colorectal cancer cell lines *via* mitochondria-dependent extrinsic pathway. This was mainly mediated by activation of the pro-apoptotic Bcl-2 family members, Bid and Bax [111]. The influence of this derivative on mitochondrial function was further confirmed in a more recent study, investigating the anti-cancer effects of indirubin on neuroblastoma [33]. Indirubin-3'-oxime was shown to decrease the expression of mitochondrial regulators, ERRγ and PGC-1β. The compound also reduced mitochondrial mass and altered mitochondrial function, as determined by a decrease in mitochondrial membrane potential and an increase in the levels of reactive oxygen species (ROS) in LA-N-1 human neuroblastoma cells [33].

Table 1. Anti-cancer effects of indirubins in animal and clinical studies.

Target (s)	Agent (s)	Stage of development	Key preclinical/clinical findings	Refs
GSK-3	Indirubin-3'-oxime, 6-bromoindirubin-oxime, 6-bromoindirubin acetoxime	Preclinical data only	Growth inhibition anti-invasive, and anti-angiogenic effects in a glioma-bearing mouse model	[38]
JAK/STAT3 signaling	6-bromoindirubin-oxime	Preclinical data only	Inhibition of lung metastasis in a mouse model of aggressive breast cancer (4T1)	[39]
JAK/STAT3 signaling	6-bromoindirubin	Preclinical data only	Growth inhibition in a mouse xenograft model of human melanoma	[62]
JAK/STAT3 and Akt signaling	7-bromoindirubin	Preclinical data only	Growth inhibition in a mouse xenograft model of human melanoma	[63]
VEGFR and JAK/STAT3 signaling	Indirubin	Preclinical data only	Anti-angiogenic effects in mouse corneal model	[79]
-	Indirubin	Preclinical data only	Anti-angiogenic activity in zebrafish embryos	[82]
VEGFR, Akt and Erk signaling	IRD E804	Preclinical data only	Pro-apoptotic and growth inhibitory effects in a syngeneic colorectal cancer (CT26) mouse model	[81]
VEGFR	IRD E804	Preclinical data only	*In vivo* activity against VEGF/bFGF-stimulated neovessel formation, and inhibition of neovascularization in zebrafish embryos	[80]
-	Meisoindigo	Preclinical data only	Anti-tumor activity, characterized by a decrease in spleen size in a mouse model of AML	[106]
Caspase 7, apoptotic pathway	5'-nitro-indirubinoxime 5'fluoro-indirubinoxime 5'-trimethylacetamino-indirubinoxime	Preclinical data only	Inhibition of tumor growth in Sprague-Dawley rats bearing PK3E-ras-induced tumors	[112]

(Table 1) cont.....

Target (s)	Agent (s)	Stage of development	Key preclinical/clinical findings	Refs
-	Indirubin	Comparative clinical study	Similar efficacy in the treatment of CML as compared to the standard agent, busulfan	[116]
-	Indirubin and meisoindigo	Clinical data	Complete cytogenetic response of imatinib in a CML patient previously treated with indirubin and meisoindigo	[118]
-	Indirubin and meisoindigo	Comparative clinical study	Smiliar efficacy in the treatment of CML between indirubin and meisoindigo, with lower adverse effects in case of meisoindigo	[117]
-	Meisoindigo	Comparative clinical study	Similar efficacy in the treatment of CML as compared to busulfan	[117]
-	Meisoindigo	Phase II clinical trial	High remission rates in newly-diagnosed CML patients	[117, 119]
-	Meisoindigo	Phase III clinical trial	Similar remission rates between newly- and previously- diagnosed CML patients	[117, 119]
-	Indirubin and meisoindigo	Retrospective clinical study	Similar anti-cancer efficacy as compared to buslfan and hydroxyurea	[117, 119]

Indirubin-3'-oxime was shown to decrease the expression of mitochondrial regulators, ERRγ and PGC-1β. The compound also reduced mitochondrial mass and altered mitochondrial function, as determined by a decrease in mitochondrial membrane potential and an increase in the levels of reactive oxygen species (ROS) in LA-N-1 human neuroblastoma cells [33]. Another derivative, indirubin-5-nitro-3'-oxime was reported to induce apoptosis in human lung cancer cell lines through a p53- and mitochondria-dependent pathway [112]. A recent study by Song *et al.* introduced the indirubin derivative, 5-diphenylacetamido-indirubin-3'-oxime (also known as LDD398) as a novel mitochondria-targeting agent [113]. LDD398 was shown to induce leukamia cell death through opening the mitochondrial permeability transition pore and a subsequent depletion of ATP, release of cytochrome c and caspase activation [113]. This finding is particularly important when considering the different mode of action of LDD398 from other IRDs as well as conventional chemotherapeutics. Accordingly, the compound was highly effective against both primary leukemia cell lines and malignant cells resistance to anti-lukeamic agents *i.e.* imatinib-resistant K562GR and Ara-C-resistant AML-2/IDAC cell lines [113]. A study on the anti-cancer properties of new indirubin derivatives, 5′-nitro-indirubinoxime, 5′-fluoro-indirubinoxime, and 5′-trimethylacetamino-indirubinoxime revealed the involvement of caspase 7 in the pro-apoptotic effects triggered by the IRDs in PK3E-ras cells [114]. Of note, the derivatives were able to inhibit solid and oral tumor growth in Sprague-Dawley rats harboring RK3E-ras-induced tumors [114].

In addition to apoptotic cell death, indirubin-3′-oxime has been shown to induce autophagy in acute lymphoblastic leukaemia (ALL) and CML cell lines, JM1 and K562, respectively. Importantly, the substance exhibited low or no cytotoxicity on healthy lymphocytes and granulocytes, demonstrating its potential in ALL and CML therapy [115]. In a different study, indirubin-3′-oxime triggered necrosis in human breast cancer cell lines [116]. Moreover, the bromo-substituent derivative, 7BIO was reported to mediate necrotic cell death in human macrophages and mesothelioma cells [117], further proving the ability of indirubins in mediating different modes of cell death.

CLINICAL PERSPECTIVES

The clinical use of indirubin dates back to the 1970-1980s when it was tested in a number of clinical trials for the treatment of CML patients over 50% of which showed partial or complete remission [117]. In a comparative study, indirubin showed similar efficacy to the standard regimen using busulfan, with a higher rate of complete hematologic response (CR) in case of the latter [118]. With regards to toxicity, indirubin caused minor side effects in most of the cases which were limited to abdominal pain, diarrhea and nausea, except for three cases who showed reversible pulmonary hypertension and cardiac insufficiency [10, 119]. Interestingly, a more recent study reported complete cytogenetic response and a long survival of 32 years in a CML patient upon receiving the tyrosine kinase inhibitor, imatininb in combination with indirubin and meisoindigo [120]. Indirubin and meisoindigo have been compared for their anti-tumor activity against CML in a clinical study, showing similar efficacy however with lower adverse effects in case of meisoindigo [119]. In a different clinical study, similar results were obtained between meisoindigo- and busulfan- treated groups, showing comparable rates of complete and partial remission of CML patients upon receiving either of the treatments [119]. A phase II clinical trial of 134 newly diagnosed CML patients receiving meisoindigo (75-150 mg/d) showed a rate of 32.1% and 48.5% of CR and hematological partial response (PR), respectively [119, 121]. The treatment also showed similar CR and PR rates between newly diagnosed and previously treated- CML patients in a phase III clinical trial, with only 14% of the responding patients showing minimal cytogenetic response [119, 121]. A retrospective study on 274 CML patients followed over a period of 5 years revealed no significant difference in terms of hematological response, median duration of chronic phase, median duration of survival and blast crisis rate at 60 months from diagnosis between meisoindigo, hydroxyurea and busulfan [119, 121]. However, combination therapy with meisoindigo and hydroxyurea was able to improve all the above-mentioned criteria significantly as compared to meisoindigo, hydroxyurea and busulfan alone [119, 121], implicating the possible synergistic effects of meisoindigo with hydroxyurea in the treatment of CML. Currently, indirubin is being tested in a multicenter randomized study for improving the outcome of acute promyelocytic leukaemia (APL) in children.

CONCLUDING REMARKS

Indirubin is a lead structure for targeting a number of protein kinases, including CDKs, GSK-3, SFKs, as well as multiple receptor tyrosine kinases, such as VEGFR, FGFR, and IGFR. Given the immense role of these molecules in regulating hallmarks of cancer including cellular survival, cell proliferation and migration, indirubin and its derivatives represent promising candidates in anti-tumor therapy. However, the low water solubility and cellular uptake of indirubin and some derivatives put constraints on their clinical application. Accordingly, a large number of derivatives have been synthesized, such as the well-studied IRD indirubin-3'-oxime and the methyl-substituent of isoindigo, meisoindigo, which exhibit improved physico-chemical properties, as well as remarkable anti-cancer efficacy in-vivo and in clinics.

Although, the kinase inhibitory activity of indirubin appears to be the major contributor to its anti-tumor effects, recent investigations have introduced novel targets, such as components of the ubiquitin proteasome pathway, and cancer stem cells. Using a microRNA reporter assay system, indirubin and its 3'-oxime derivative have been implicated in the regulation of the microRNA let-7, which is known to be a tumor suppressor in ovarian and other cancer types [122]. Furthermore, a different study on the effects of GSK-3 inhibition and microRNA regulation has shown that two GSK-3 inhibitors, CHIR and the IRD 6BIO, lead to a decrease in global microRNA maturation, but an increase in the expression of microRNA-211 in mouse embryonic stem cells [123]. These results are of particular interest due to the emerging role of microRNAs in human malignancies, which could serve as novel therapeutic targets of indirubins, further adding to their multi-facted molecular mechanisms.

CONSENT FOR PUBLICATION

Not applicable.

CONFLICT OF INTEREST

The authors confirm that this chapter content has no conflict of interest.

ACKNOWLEDGEMENT

This work is supported by the DFG grant (CH 1690/2-1) and the 'Landesgraduiertenförderung (LGF) fellowship program for individual doctoral training' from Universität Heidelberg.

REFERENCES

[1]   Tu, Y. The discovery of artemisinin (qinghaosu) and gifts from Chinese medicine. *Nat. Med.,* **2011,** *17*(10), 1217-1220.
        [http://dx.doi.org/10.1038/nm.2471] [PMID: 21989013]

[2]   Miller, L.H.; Su, X. Artemisinin: discovery from the Chinese herbal garden. *Cell,* **2011,** *146*(6), 855-858.
        [http://dx.doi.org/10.1016/j.cell.2011.08.024] [PMID: 21907397]

[3]   Cheng, X.; Merz, K.H. The Role of Indirubins in Inflammation and Associated Tumorigenesis. *Adv. Exp. Med. Biol.,* **2016,** *929,* 269-290.
        [http://dx.doi.org/10.1007/978-3-319-41342-6_12] [PMID: 27771929]

[4]   [Clinical and experimental studies in the treatment of chronic granulocytic leukemia with indirubin (author's transl)] *Zhonghua Nei Ke Za Zhi,* **1979,** *18*(2), 83-8.

[5]   Dai, F.B.; Qiao, C.Z.; Li, L. [Determination of indigo and indirubin in qingdai by HPLC]. *Yao Xue Xue Bao,* **1986,** *21*(11), 868-871. [Determination of indigo and indirubin in qingdai by HPLC].
        [PMID: 3591324]

[6]   Hoessel, R.; Leclerc, S.; Endicott, J.A.; Nobel, M.E.; Lawrie, A.; Tunnah, P.; Leost, M.; Damiens, E.; Marie, D.; Marko, D.; Niederberger, E.; Tang, W.; Eisenbrand, G.; Meijer, L. Indirubin, the active constituent of a Chinese antileukaemia medicine, inhibits cyclin-dependent kinases. *Nat. Cell Biol.,* **1999,** *1*(1), 60-67.
        [http://dx.doi.org/10.1038/9035] [PMID: 10559866]

[7]   Tegethoff, J.; Bischoff, R.; Saleh, S.; Blagojevic, B.; Merz, K-H.; Cheng, X. Methylisoindigo and Its Bromo-Derivatives Are Selective Tyrosine Kinase Inhibitors, Repressing Cellular Stat3 Activity, and Target CD133+ Cancer Stem Cells in PDAC. *Molecules,* **2017,** *22*(9), 1546.
        [http://dx.doi.org/10.3390/molecules22091546]

[8]   Ahn, M.Y.; Kim, T.H.; Kwon, S.M.; Yoon, H.E.; Kim, H.S.; Kim, J.I.; Kim, Y.C.; Kang, K.W.; Ahn, S.G.; Yoon, J.H. 5-Nitro-5′-hydroxy-indirubin-3′-oxime (AGM130), an indirubin-3′-oxime derivative, inhibits tumor growth by inducing apoptosis against non-small cell lung cancer *in vitro* and *in vivo. Eur. J. Pharm. Sci.,* **2015,** *79,* 122-131.
        [http://dx.doi.org/10.1016/j.ejps.2015.08.015] [PMID: 26342773]

[9]   Berger, A.; Quast, S.A.; Plötz, M.; Hein, M.; Kunz, M.; Langer, P.; Eberle, J. Sensitization of melanoma cells for death ligand-induced apoptosis by an indirubin derivative--Enhancement of both extrinsic and intrinsic apoptosis pathways. *Biochem. Pharmacol.,* **2011,** *81*(1), 71-81.
        [http://dx.doi.org/10.1016/j.bcp.2010.09.010] [PMID: 20858462]

[10]   Blažević, T.; Heiss, E.H.; Atanasov, A.G.; Breuss, J.M.; Dirsch, V.M.; Uhrin, P. Indirubin and Indirubin Derivatives for Counteracting Proliferative Diseases. *Evid. Based Complement. Alternat. Med.,* **2015**, *2015*, 654098.
       [http://dx.doi.org/10.1155/2015/654098] [PMID: 26457112]

[11]   Braig, S.; Bischoff, F.; Abhari, B.A.; Meijer, L.; Fulda, S.; Skaltsounis, L.; Vollmar, A.M. The pleiotropic profile of the indirubin derivative 6BIO overcomes TRAIL resistance in cancer. *Biochem. Pharmacol.,* **2014**, *91*(2), 157-167.
       [http://dx.doi.org/10.1016/j.bcp.2014.07.009] [PMID: 25069048]

[12]   Eisenbrand, G.; Hippe, F.; Jakobs, S.; Muehlbeyer, S. Molecular mechanisms of indirubin and its derivatives: novel anticancer molecules with their origin in traditional Chinese phytomedicine. *J. Cancer Res. Clin. Oncol.,* **2004**, *130*(11), 627-635.
       [http://dx.doi.org/10.1007/s00432-004-0579-2] [PMID: 15340840]

[13]   Pandraud, H. Structure Cristalline De Loxindigo. *B Soc Chim Fr,* **1961**, *7*, 1257.

[14]   Heshmati, N.; Cheng, X.; Eisenbrand, G.; Fricker, G. Enhancement of oral bioavailability of E804 by self-nanoemulsifying drug delivery system (SNEDDS) in rats. *J. Pharm. Sci.,* **2013**, *102*(10), 3792-3799.
       [http://dx.doi.org/10.1002/jps.23696] [PMID: 23934779]

[15]   Heshmati, N.; Cheng, X.; Dapat, E.; Sassene, P.; Eisenbrand, G.; Fricker, G.; Müllertz, A. *In vitro* and *in vivo* evaluations of the performance of an indirubin derivative, formulated in four different self-emulsifying drug delivery systems. *J. Pharm. Pharmacol.,* **2014**, *66*(11), 1567-1575.
       [http://dx.doi.org/10.1111/jphp.12286] [PMID: 24961657]

[16]   Heshmati, N.; Wagner, B.; Cheng, X.; Scholz, T.; Kansy, M.; Eisenbrand, G.; Fricker, G. Physicochemical characterization and *in vitro* permeation of an indirubin derivative. *Eur. J. Pharm. Sci.,* **2013**, *50*(3-4), 467-475.
       [http://dx.doi.org/10.1016/j.ejps.2013.08.021] [PMID: 23994641]

[17]   Jautelat, R.; Brumby, T.; Schäfer, M.; Briem, H.; Eisenbrand, G.; Schwahn, S.; Krüger, M.; Lücking, U.; Prien, O.; Siemeister, G. From the insoluble dye indirubin towards highly active, soluble CDK2-inhibitors. *ChemBioChem,* **2005**, *6*(3), 531-540.
       [http://dx.doi.org/10.1002/cbic.200400108] [PMID: 15742375]

[18]   Davies, T.G.; Tunnah, P.; Meijer, L.; Marko, D.; Eisenbrand, G.; Endicott, J.A.; Noble, M.E. Inhibitor binding to active and inactive CDK2: the crystal structure of CDK2-cyclin A/indirubin-5-sulphonate. *Structure,* **2001**, *9*(5), 389-397.
       [http://dx.doi.org/10.1016/S0969-2126(01)00598-6] [PMID: 11377199]

[19]   Baeyer, A. Ueber die Verbindungen der Indigogruppe. *Chem. Ber.,* **1881**, *14*, 1741-1750.
       [http://dx.doi.org/10.1002/cber.18810140238]

[20]   Russell, G.A.; Kaupp, G. Oxidation of Carbanions. 4. Oxidation of Indoxyl to Indigo in Basic Solution. *J. Am. Chem. Soc.,* **1969**, *91*(14), 3851.
       [http://dx.doi.org/10.1021/ja01042a028]

[21]   Cheng, X.; Merz, K.H.; Vatter, S.; Christ, J.; Wölfl, S.; Eisenbrand, G. 7,7′-Diazaindirubin--a small molecule inhibitor of casein kinase 2 *in vitro* and in cells. *Bioorg. Med. Chem.,* **2014**, *22*(1), 247-255.
       [http://dx.doi.org/10.1016/j.bmc.2013.11.031] [PMID: 24326279]

[22]   Martinet, J.; Dornier, O. On the new sulfonated derivatives of oxindol and of isatin. *Cr Hebd Acad Sci,* **1921**, *172*, 1415-1417.

[23]   Vougogiannopoulou, K.; Ferandin, Y.; Bettayeb, K.; Myrianthopoulos, V.; Lozach, O.; Fan, Y.; Johnson, C.H.; Magiatis, P.; Skaltsounis, A.L.; Mikros, E.; Meijer, L. Soluble 3′,6-substituted indirubins with enhanced selectivity toward glycogen synthase kinase -3 alter circadian period. *J. Med. Chem.,* **2008**, *51*(20), 6421-6431.
       [http://dx.doi.org/10.1021/jm800648y] [PMID: 18816110]

[24]   Cheng, X.; Merz, K.H.; Vatter, S.; Zeller, J.; Muehlbeyer, S.; Thommet, A.; Christ, J.; Wölfl, S.; Eisenbrand, G. Identification of a Water-Soluble Indirubin Derivative as Potent Inhibitor of Insulin-like Growth Factor 1 Receptor through Structural Modification of the Parent Natural Molecule. *J. Med. Chem.,* **2017**, *60*(12), 4949-4962.
       [http://dx.doi.org/10.1021/acs.jmedchem.7b00324] [PMID: 28557430]

[25]   Cheng, X.; Rasqué, P.; Vatter, S.; Merz, K.H.; Eisenbrand, G. Synthesis and cytotoxicity of novel indirubin-5-carboxamides. *Bioorg. Med. Chem.,* **2010**, *18*(12), 4509-4515.
       [http://dx.doi.org/10.1016/j.bmc.2010.04.066] [PMID: 20488718]

[26]   Marko, D.; Schätzle, S.; Friedel, A.; Genzlinger, A.; Zankl, H.; Meijer, L.; Eisenbrand, G. Inhibition of cyclin-dependent kinase 1 (CDK1) by indirubin derivatives in human tumour cells. *Br. J. Cancer,* **2001**, *84*(2), 283-289.
       [http://dx.doi.org/10.1054/bjoc.2000.1546] [PMID: 11161389]

[27]   Heshmati, N.; Cheng, X.; Dapat, E.; Sassene, P.; Eisenbrand, G.; Fricker, G.; Müllertz, A. *In vitro* and *in vivo* evaluations of the performance of an indirubin derivative, formulated in four different self-emulsifying drug delivery systems. *J. Pharm. Pharmacol.,* **2014**, *66*(11), 1567-1575.
       [http://dx.doi.org/10.1111/jphp.12286] [PMID: 24961657]

[28]   Malumbres, M.; Barbacid, M. Cell cycle, CDKs and cancer: a changing paradigm. *Nat. Rev. Cancer,* **2009**, *9*(3), 153-166.
       [http://dx.doi.org/10.1038/nrc2602] [PMID: 19238148]

[29]   Iliakis, G.; Wang, Y.; Guan, J.; Wang, H. DNA damage checkpoint control in cells exposed to ionizing radiation. *Oncogene,* **2003**, *22*(37), 5834-5847.
       [http://dx.doi.org/10.1038/sj.onc.1206682] [PMID: 12947390]

[30]   Meijer, L. Chemical inhibitors of cyclin-dependent kinases. *Trends Cell Biol.,* **1996**, *6*(10), 393-397.
       [http://dx.doi.org/10.1016/0962-8924(96)10034-9] [PMID: 15157522]

[31]   Marko, D.; Schätzle, S.; Friedel, A.; Genzlinger, A.; Zankl, H.; Meijer, L.; Eisenbrand, G. Inhibition of cyclin-dependent kinase 1 (CDK1) by indirubin derivatives in human tumour cells. *Br. J. Cancer,* **2001**, *84*(2), 283-289.
       [http://dx.doi.org/10.1054/bjoc.2000.1546] [PMID: 11161389]

[32]   Leclerc, S.; Garnier, M.; Hoessel, R.; Marko, D.; Bibb, J.A.; Snyder, G.L.; Greengard, P.; Biernat, J.; Wu, Y.Z.; Mandelkow, E.M.; Eisenbrand, G.; Meijer, L. Indirubins inhibit glycogen synthase kinase-3 beta and CDK5/p25, two protein kinases involved in abnormal tau phosphorylation in Alzheimer's disease. A property common to most cyclin-dependent kinase inhibitors? *J. Biol. Chem.,* **2001**, *276*(1), 251-260.
       [http://dx.doi.org/10.1074/jbc.M002466200] [PMID: 11013232]

[33]   Liao, X.M.; Leung, K.N. Indirubin-3'-oxime induces mitochondrial dysfunction and triggers growth inhibition and cell cycle arrest in human neuroblastoma cells. *Oncol. Rep.,* **2013**, *29*(1), 371-379.
       [http://dx.doi.org/10.3892/or.2012.2094] [PMID: 23117445]

[34]   Cohen, P.; Frame, S. The renaissance of GSK3. *Nat. Rev. Mol. Cell Biol.,* **2001**, *2*(10), 769-776.
       [http://dx.doi.org/10.1038/35096075] [PMID: 11584304]

[35]   Henriksen, E.J. Dysregulation of glycogen synthase kinase-3 in skeletal muscle and the etiology of insulin resistance and type 2 diabetes. *Curr. Diabetes Rev.,* **2010**, *6*(5), 285-293.
       [http://dx.doi.org/10.2174/157339910793360888] [PMID: 20594161]

[36]   Meijer, L.; Skaltsounis, A.L.; Magiatis, P.; Polychronopoulos, P.; Knockaert, M.; Leost, M.; Ryan, X.P.; Vonica, C.A.; Brivanlou, A.; Dajani, R.; Crovace, C.; Tarricone, C.; Musacchio, A.; Roe, S.M.; Pearl, L.; Greengard, P. GSK-3-selective inhibitors derived from Tyrian purple indirubins. *Chem. Biol.,* **2003**, *10*(12), 1255-1266.
       [http://dx.doi.org/10.1016/j.chembiol.2003.11.010] [PMID: 14700633]

[37]   Polychronopoulos, P.; Magiatis, P.; Skaltsounis, A.L.; Myrianthopoulos, V.; Mikros, E.; Tarricone, A.;

Musacchio, A.; Roe, S.M.; Pearl, L.; Leost, M.; Greengard, P.; Meijer, L. Structural basis for the synthesis of indirubins as potent and selective inhibitors of glycogen synthase kinase-3 and cyclin-dependent kinases. *J. Med. Chem.,* **2004**, *47*(4), 935-946.
[http://dx.doi.org/10.1021/jm031016d] [PMID: 14761195]

[38]   McCubrey, J.A.; Steelman, L.S.; Bertrand, F.E.; Davis, N.M.; Sokolosky, M.; Abrams, S.L.; Montalto, G.; D'Assoro, A.B.; Libra, M.; Nicoletti, F.; Maestro, R.; Basecke, J.; Rakus, D.; Gizak, A.; Demidenko, Z.N.; Cocco, L.; Martelli, A.M.; Cervello, M. GSK-3 as potential target for therapeutic intervention in cancer. *Oncotarget,* **2014**, *5*(10), 2881-2911.
[http://dx.doi.org/10.18632/oncotarget.2037] [PMID: 24931005]

[39]   Domoto, T.; Pyko, I.V.; Furuta, T.; Miyashita, K.; Uehara, M.; Shimasaki, T.; Nakada, M.; Minamoto, T. Glycogen synthase kinase-3β is a pivotal mediator of cancer invasion and resistance to therapy. *Cancer Sci.,* **2016**, *107*(10), 1363-1372.
[http://dx.doi.org/10.1111/cas.13028] [PMID: 27486911]

[40]   Williams, S.P.; Nowicki, M.O.; Liu, F.; Press, R.; Godlewski, J.; Abdel-Rasoul, M.; Kaur, B.; Fernandez, S.A.; Chiocca, E.A.; Lawler, S.E. Indirubins decrease glioma invasion by blocking migratory phenotypes in both the tumor and stromal endothelial cell compartments. *Cancer Res.,* **2011**, *71*(16), 5374-5380.
[http://dx.doi.org/10.1158/0008-5472.CAN-10-3026] [PMID: 21697283]

[41]   Braig, S.; Kressirer, C.A.; Liebl, J.; Bischoff, F.; Zahler, S.; Meijer, L.; Vollmar, A.M. Indirubin derivative 6BIO suppresses metastasis. *Cancer Res.,* **2013**, *73*(19), 6004-6012.
[http://dx.doi.org/10.1158/0008-5472.CAN-12-4358] [PMID: 23946383]

[42]   Adachi, J.; Mori, Y.; Matsui, S.; Takigami, H.; Fujino, J.; Kitagawa, H.; Miller, C.A., III; Kato, T.; Saeki, K.; Matsuda, T. Indirubin and indigo are potent aryl hydrocarbon receptor ligands present in human urine. *J. Biol. Chem.,* **2001**, *276*(34), 31475-31478.
[http://dx.doi.org/10.1074/jbc.c500238200] [PMID: 11425848]

[43]   Knockaert, M.; Blondel, M.; Bach, S.; Leost, M.; Elbi, C.; Hager, G.L.; Nagy, S.R.; Han, D.; Denison, M.; Ffrench, M.; Ryan, X.P.; Magiatis, P.; Polychronopoulos, P.; Greengard, P.; Skaltsounis, L.; Meijer, L. Independent actions on cyclin-dependent kinases and aryl hydrocarbon receptor mediate the antiproliferative effects of indirubins. *Oncogene,* **2004**, *23*(25), 4400-4412.
[http://dx.doi.org/10.1038/sj.onc.1207535] [PMID: 15077192]

[44]   Korzeniewski, N.; Wheeler, S.; Chatterjee, P.; Duensing, A.; Duensing, S. A novel role of the aryl hydrocarbon receptor (AhR) in centrosome amplification - implications for chemoprevention. *Mol. Cancer,* **2010**, *9*, 153.
[http://dx.doi.org/10.1186/1476-4598-9-153] [PMID: 20565777]

[45]   Koliopanos, A.; Kleeff, J.; Xiao, Y.; Safe, S.; Zimmermann, A.; Büchler, M.W.; Friess, H. Increased arylhydrocarbon receptor expression offers a potential therapeutic target for pancreatic cancer. *Oncogene,* **2002**, *21*(39), 6059-6070.
[http://dx.doi.org/10.1038/sj.onc.1205633] [PMID: 12203118]

[46]   Murray, I.A.; Patterson, A.D.; Perdew, G.H. Aryl hydrocarbon receptor ligands in cancer: friend and foe. *Nat. Rev. Cancer,* **2014**, *14*(12), 801-814.
[http://dx.doi.org/10.1038/nrc3846] [PMID: 25568920]

[47]   Bowman, T.; Garcia, R.; Turkson, J.; Jove, R. STATs in oncogenesis. *Oncogene,* **2000**, *19*(21), 2474-2488.
[http://dx.doi.org/10.1038/sj.onc.1203527] [PMID: 10851046]

[48]   Buettner, R.; Mora, L.B.; Jove, R. Activated STAT signaling in human tumors provides novel molecular targets for therapeutic intervention. *Clin. Cancer Res.,* **2002**, *8*(4), 945-954.
[PMID: 11948098]

[49]   Yu, H.; Pardoll, D.; Jove, R. STATs in cancer inflammation and immunity: a leading role for STAT3. *Nat. Rev. Cancer,* **2009**, *9*(11), 798-809.

[http://dx.doi.org/10.1038/nrc2734] [PMID: 19851315]

[50] Erpel, T.; Courtneidge, S.A. Src family protein tyrosine kinases and cellular signal transduction pathways. *Curr. Opin. Cell Biol.,* **1995**, *7*(2), 176-182.
[http://dx.doi.org/10.1016/0955-0674(95)80025-5] [PMID: 7612268]

[51] Yeatman, T.J. A renaissance for SRC. *Nat. Rev. Cancer,* **2004**, *4*(6), 470-480.
[http://dx.doi.org/10.1038/nrc5366] [PMID: 15170449]

[52] Irby, R.B.; Yeatman, T.J. Role of Src expression and activation in human cancer. *Oncogene,* **2000**, *19*(49), 5636-5642.
[http://dx.doi.org/10.1038/sj.onc.1203912] [PMID: 11114744]

[53] Thomas, S.J.; Snowden, J.A.; Zeidler, M.P.; Danson, S.J. The role of JAK/STAT signalling in the pathogenesis, prognosis and treatment of solid tumours. *Br. J. Cancer,* **2015**, *113*(3), 365-371.
[http://dx.doi.org/10.1038/bjc.2015.233] [PMID: 26151455]

[54] Nam, S.; Buettner, R.; Turkson, J.; Kim, D.; Cheng, J.Q.; Muehlbeyer, S.; Hippe, F.; Vatter, S.; Merz, K.H.; Eisenbrand, G.; Jove, R. Indirubin derivatives inhibit Stat3 signaling and induce apoptosis in human cancer cells. *Proc. Natl. Acad. Sci. USA,* **2005**, *102*(17), 5998-6003.
[http://dx.doi.org/10.1073/pnas.0409467102] [PMID: 15837920]

[55] Gesbert, F.; Griffin, J.D. Bcr/Abl activates transcription of the Bcl-X gene through STAT5. *Blood,* **2000**, *96*(6), 2269-2276.
[PMID: 10979976]

[56] Yu, H.; Jove, R. The STATs of cancer--new molecular targets come of age. *Nat. Rev. Cancer,* **2004**, *4*(2), 97-105.
[http://dx.doi.org/10.1038/nrc5275] [PMID: 14964307]

[57] Hoelbl, A.; Schuster, C.; Kovacic, B.; Zhu, B.; Wickre, M.; Hoelzl, M.A.; Fajmann, S.; Grebien, F.; Warsch, W.; Stengl, G.; Hennighausen, L.; Poli, V.; Beug, H.; Moriggl, R.; Sexl, V. Stat5 is indispensable for the maintenance of bcr/abl-positive leukaemia. *EMBO Mol. Med.,* **2010**, *2*(3), 98-110.
[http://dx.doi.org/10.1002/emmm.201000062] [PMID: 20201032]

[58] Klejman, A.; Schreiner, S.J.; Nieborowska-Skorska, M.; Slupianek, A.; Wilson, M.; Smithgall, T.E.; Skorski, T. The Src family kinase Hck couples BCR/ABL to STAT5 activation in myeloid leukemia cells. *EMBO J.,* **2002**, *21*(21), 5766-5774.
[http://dx.doi.org/10.1093/emboj/cdf562] [PMID: 12411494]

[59] Wilson, M.B.; Schreiner, S.J.; Choi, H.J.; Kamens, J.; Smithgall, T.E. Selective pyrrolo-pyrimidine inhibitors reveal a necessary role for Src family kinases in Bcr-Abl signal transduction and oncogenesis. *Oncogene,* **2002**, *21*(53), 8075-8088.
[http://dx.doi.org/10.1038/sj.onc.1206008] [PMID: 12444544]

[60] Nam, S.; Scuto, A.; Yang, F.; Chen, W.; Park, S.; Yoo, H.S.; Konig, H.; Bhatia, R.; Cheng, X.; Merz, K.H.; Eisenbrand, G.; Jove, R. Indirubin derivatives induce apoptosis of chronic myelogenous leukemia cells involving inhibition of Stat5 signaling. *Mol. Oncol.,* **2012**, *6*(3), 276-283.
[http://dx.doi.org/10.1016/j.molonc.2012.02.002] [PMID: 22387217]

[61] Johnson, F.M.; Saigal, B.; Tran, H.; Donato, N.J. Abrogation of signal transducer and activator of transcription 3 reactivation after Src kinase inhibition results in synergistic antitumor effects. *Clin. Cancer Res.,* **2007**, *13*(14), 4233-4244.
[http://dx.doi.org/10.1158/1078-0432.CCR-06-2981] [PMID: 17634553]

[62] Sen, B.; Saigal, B.; Parikh, N.; Gallick, G.; Johnson, F.M. Sustained Src inhibition results in signal transducer and activator of transcription 3 (STAT3) activation and cancer cell survival *via* altered Janus-activated kinase-STAT3 binding. *Cancer Res.,* **2009**, *69*(5), 1958-1965.
[http://dx.doi.org/10.1158/0008-5472.CAN-08-2944] [PMID: 19223541]

[63] Nam, S.; Wen, W.; Schroeder, A.; Herrmann, A.; Yu, H.; Cheng, X.; Merz, K.H.; Eisenbrand, G.; Li,

H.; Yuan, Y.C.; Jove, R. Dual inhibition of Janus and Src family kinases by novel indirubin derivative blocks constitutively-activated Stat3 signaling associated with apoptosis of human pancreatic cancer cells. *Mol. Oncol.,* **2013**, *7*(3), 369-378.
[http://dx.doi.org/10.1016/j.molonc.2012.10.013] [PMID: 23206899]

[64]   Liu, L.; Nam, S.; Tian, Y.; Yang, F.; Wu, J.; Wang, Y.; Scuto, A.; Polychronopoulos, P.; Magiatis, P.; Skaltsounis, L.; Jove, R. 6-Bromoindirubin-3′-oxime inhibits JAK/STAT3 signaling and induces apoptosis of human melanoma cells. *Cancer Res.,* **2011**, *71*(11), 3972-3979.
[http://dx.doi.org/10.1158/0008-5472.CAN-10-3852] [PMID: 21610112]

[65]   Liu, L.; Kritsanida, M.; Magiatis, P.; Gaboriaud, N.; Wang, Y.; Wu, J.; Buettner, R.; Yang, F.; Nam, S.; Skaltsounis, L.; Jove, R. A novel 7-bromoindirubin with potent anticancer activity suppresses survival of human melanoma cells associated with inhibition of STAT3 and Akt signaling. *Cancer Biol. Ther.,* **2012**, *13*(13), 1255-1261.
[http://dx.doi.org/10.4161/cbt.21781] [PMID: 22895078]

[66]   Ribas, J.; Bettayeb, K.; Ferandin, Y.; Knockaert, M.; Garrofé-Ochoa, X.; Totzke, F.; Schächtele, C.; Mester, J.; Polychronopoulos, P.; Magiatis, P.; Skaltsounis, A.L.; Boix, J.; Meijer, L. 7-Bromoindirubin-3′-oxime induces caspase-independent cell death. *Oncogene,* **2006**, *25*(47), 6304-6318.
[http://dx.doi.org/10.1038/sj.onc.1209648] [PMID: 16702956]

[67]   Nicolaou, K.A.; Liapis, V.; Evdokiou, A.; Constantinou, C.; Magiatis, P.; Skaltsounis, A.L.; Koumas, L.; Costeas, P.A.; Constantinou, A.I. Induction of discrete apoptotic pathways by bromo-substituted indirubin derivatives in invasive breast cancer cells. *Biochem. Biophys. Res. Commun.,* **2012**, *425*(1), 76-82.
[http://dx.doi.org/10.1016/j.bbrc.2012.07.053] [PMID: 22820195]

[68]   Carmeliet, P.; Jain, R.K. Angiogenesis in cancer and other diseases. *Nature,* **2000**, *407*(6801), 249-257.
[http://dx.doi.org/10.1038/35025220] [PMID: 11001068]

[69]   Coultas, L.; Chawengsaksophak, K.; Rossant, J. Endothelial cells and VEGF in vascular development. *Nature,* **2005**, *438*(7070), 937-945.
[http://dx.doi.org/10.1038/nature04479] [PMID: 16355211]

[70]   Potente, M.; Gerhardt, H.; Carmeliet, P. Basic and therapeutic aspects of angiogenesis. *Cell,* **2011**, *146*(6), 873-887.
[http://dx.doi.org/10.1016/j.cell.2011.08.039] [PMID: 21925313]

[71]   Folkman, J. Angiogenesis--retrospect and outlook. *EXS,* **1992**, *61*, 4-13.
[http://dx.doi.org/10.1007/978-3-0348-7001-6_2] [PMID: 1377561]

[72]   Chen, Z.; Han, Z.C. STAT3: a critical transcription activator in angiogenesis. *Med. Res. Rev.,* **2008**, *28*(2), 185-200.
[http://dx.doi.org/10.1002/med.20101] [PMID: 17457812]

[73]   Masson-Gadais, B.; Houle, F.; Laferrière, J.; Huot, J. Integrin alphavbeta3, requirement for VEGFR2-mediated activation of SAPK2/p38 and for Hsp90-dependent phosphorylation of focal adhesion kinase in endothelial cells activated by VEGF. *Cell Stress Chaperones,* **2003**, *8*(1), 37-52.
[http://dx.doi.org/10.1379/1466-1268(2003)8<37:IVRFVA>2.0.CO;2] [PMID: 12820653]

[74]   Holmes, K.; Roberts, O.L.; Thomas, A.M.; Cross, M.J. Vascular endothelial growth factor receptor-2: structure, function, intracellular signalling and therapeutic inhibition. *Cell. Signal.,* **2007**, *19*(10), 2003-2012.
[http://dx.doi.org/10.1016/j.cellsig.2007.05.013] [PMID: 17658244]

[75]   Niu, G.; Wright, K.L.; Huang, M.; Song, L.; Haura, E.; Turkson, J.; Zhang, S.; Wang, T.; Sinibaldi, D.; Coppola, D.; Heller, R.; Ellis, L.M.; Karras, J.; Bromberg, J.; Pardoll, D.; Jove, R.; Yu, H. Constitutive Stat3 activity up-regulates VEGF expression and tumor angiogenesis. *Oncogene,* **2002**, *21*(13), 2000-2008.

[http://dx.doi.org/10.1038/sj.onc.1205260] [PMID: 11960372]

[76]   Kujawski, M.; Kortylewski, M.; Lee, H.; Herrmann, A.; Kay, H.; Yu, H. Stat3 mediates myeloid cell-dependent tumor angiogenesis in mice. *J. Clin. Invest.,* **2008**, *118*(10), 3367-3377.
[http://dx.doi.org/10.1172/JCI35213] [PMID: 18776941]

[77]   Carmeliet, P. Angiogenesis in life, disease and medicine. *Nature,* **2005**, *438*(7070), 932-936.
[http://dx.doi.org/10.1038/nature04478] [PMID: 16355210]

[78]   Kim, J.K.; Shin, E.K.; Kang, Y.H.; Park, J.H. Indirubin-3'-monoxime, a derivative of a chinese antileukemia medicine, inhibits angiogenesis. *J. Cell. Biochem.,* **2011**, *112*(5), 1384-1391.
[http://dx.doi.org/10.1002/jcb.23055] [PMID: 21337385]

[79]   Zahler, S.; Liebl, J.; Fürst, R.; Vollmar, A.M. Anti-angiogenic potential of small molecular inhibitors of cyclin dependent kinases *in vitro. Angiogenesis,* **2010**, *13*(3), 239-249.
[http://dx.doi.org/10.1007/s10456-010-9181-1] [PMID: 20706783]

[80]   Tran, T.C.; Sneed, B.; Haider, J.; Blavo, D.; White, A.; Aiyejorun, T.; Baranowski, T.C.; Rubinstein, A.L.; Doan, T.N.; Dingledine, R.; Sandberg, E.M. Automated, quantitative screening assay for antiangiogenic compounds using transgenic zebrafish. *Cancer Res.,* **2007**, *67*(23), 11386-11392.
[http://dx.doi.org/10.1158/0008-5472.CAN-07-3126] [PMID: 18056466]

[81]   Zhang, X.; Song, Y.; Wu, Y.; Dong, Y.; Lai, L.; Zhang, J.; Lu, B.; Dai, F.; He, L.; Liu, M.; Yi, Z. Indirubin inhibits tumor growth by antitumor angiogenesis *via* blocking VEGFR2-mediated JAK/STAT3 signaling in endothelial cell. *Int. J. Cancer,* **2011**, *129*(10), 2502-2511.
[http://dx.doi.org/10.1002/ijc.25909] [PMID: 21207415]

[82]   Chan, Y.K.; Kwok, H.H.; Chan, L.S.; Leung, K.S.; Shi, J.; Mak, N.K.; Wong, R.N.; Yue, P.Y. An indirubin derivative, E804, exhibits potent angiosuppressive activity. *Biochem. Pharmacol.,* **2012**, *83*(5), 598-607.
[http://dx.doi.org/10.1016/j.bcp.2011.12.003] [PMID: 22178720]

[83]   Shin, E.K.; Kim, J.K. Indirubin derivative E804 inhibits angiogenesis. *BMC Cancer,* **2012**, *12*, 164.
[http://dx.doi.org/10.1186/1471-2407-12-164] [PMID: 22554053]

[84]   Alex, D.; Lam, I.K.; Lin, Z.; Lee, S.M. Indirubin shows anti-angiogenic activity in an *in vivo* zebrafish model and an *in vitro* HUVEC model. *J. Ethnopharmacol.,* **2010**, *131*(2), 242-247.
[http://dx.doi.org/10.1016/j.jep.2010.05.016] [PMID: 20488232]

[85]   Zhen, Y.; Sørensen, V.; Jin, Y.; Suo, Z.; Wiedłocha, A. Indirubin-3'-monoxime inhibits autophosphorylation of FGFR1 and stimulates ERK1/2 activity *via* p38 MAPK. *Oncogene,* **2007**, *26*(44), 6372-6385.
[http://dx.doi.org/10.1038/sj.onc.1210473] [PMID: 17533378]

[86]   Boilly, B.; Vercoutter-Edouart, A.S.; Hondermarck, H.; Nurcombe, V.; Le Bourhis, X. FGF signals for cell proliferation and migration through different pathways. *Cytokine Growth Factor Rev.,* **2000**, *11*(4), 295-302.
[http://dx.doi.org/10.1016/S1359-6101(00)00014-9] [PMID: 10959077]

[87]   Eswarakumar, V.P.; Lax, I.; Schlessinger, J. Cellular signaling by fibroblast growth factor receptors. *Cytokine Growth Factor Rev.,* **2005**, *16*(2), 139-149.
[http://dx.doi.org/10.1016/j.cytogfr.2005.01.001] [PMID: 15863030]

[88]   Sethi, G.; Ahn, K.S.; Sandur, S.K.; Lin, X.; Chaturvedi, M.M.; Aggarwal, B.B. Indirubin enhances tumor necrosis factor-induced apoptosis through modulation of nuclear factor-kappa B signaling pathway. *J. Biol. Chem.,* **2006**, *281*(33), 23425-23435.
[http://dx.doi.org/10.1074/jbc.M602627200] [PMID: 16785236]

[89]   Aggarwal, B.B. Nuclear factor-kappaB: the enemy within. *Cancer Cell,* **2004**, *6*(3), 203-208.
[http://dx.doi.org/10.1016/j.ccr.2004.09.003] [PMID: 15380510]

[90]   Karin, M. Nuclear factor-kappaB in cancer development and progression. *Nature,* **2006**, *441*(7092), 431-436.

[http://dx.doi.org/10.1038/nature04870] [PMID: 16724054]

[91] Pollak, M. Insulin and insulin-like growth factor signalling in neoplasia. *Nat. Rev. Cancer,* **2008**, *8*(12), 915-928.
[http://dx.doi.org/10.1038/nrc2536] [PMID: 19029956]

[92] Pollak, M. N. Insulin-like growth factors and neoplasia *Novartis Found Symp,* **2004**, *262,*, 84-98. discussion 98-107, 265-8
[http://dx.doi.org/10.1002/0470869976.ch6]

[93] Cheng, X.; Alborzinia, H.; Merz, K.H.; Steinbeisser, H.; Mrowka, R.; Scholl, C.; Kitanovic, I.; Eisenbrand, G.; Wölfl, S. Indirubin derivatives modulate TGFβ/BMP signaling at different levels and trigger ubiquitin-mediated depletion of nonactivated R-Smads. *Chem. Biol.,* **2012**, *19*(11), 1423-1436.
[http://dx.doi.org/10.1016/j.chembiol.2012.09.008] [PMID: 23177197]

[94] Schmierer, B.; Hill, C.S. TGFbeta-SMAD signal transduction: molecular specificity and functional flexibility. *Nat. Rev. Mol. Cell Biol.,* **2007**, *8*(12), 970-982.
[http://dx.doi.org/10.1038/nrm2297] [PMID: 18000526]

[95] Massagué, J. TGFβ signalling in context. *Nat. Rev. Mol. Cell Biol.,* **2012**, *13*(10), 616-630.
[http://dx.doi.org/10.1038/nrm3434] [PMID: 22992590]

[96] Massagué, J. TGFbeta in Cancer. *Cell,* **2008**, *134*(2), 215-230.
[http://dx.doi.org/10.1016/j.cell.2008.07.001] [PMID: 18662538]

[97] Pardal, R.; Clarke, M.F.; Morrison, S.J. Applying the principles of stem-cell biology to cancer. *Nat. Rev. Cancer,* **2003**, *3*(12), 895-902.
[http://dx.doi.org/10.1038/nrc5232] [PMID: 14737120]

[98] McDonald, S.A.; Preston, S.L.; Lovell, M.J.; Wright, N.A.; Jankowski, J.A. Mechanisms of disease: from stem cells to colorectal cancer. *Nat. Clin. Pract. Gastroenterol. Hepatol.,* **2006**, *3*(5), 267-274.
[http://dx.doi.org/10.1038/ncpgasthep0473] [PMID: 16673006]

[99] Kreso, A.; Dick, J.E. Evolution of the cancer stem cell model. *Cell Stem Cell,* **2014**, *14*(3), 275-291.
[http://dx.doi.org/10.1016/j.stem.2014.02.006] [PMID: 24607403]

[100] Al-Hajj, M.; Wicha, M.S.; Benito-Hernandez, A.; Morrison, S.J.; Clarke, M.F. Prospective identification of tumorigenic breast cancer cells. *Proc. Natl. Acad. Sci. USA,* **2003**, *100*(7), 3983-3988.
[http://dx.doi.org/10.1073/pnas.0530291100] [PMID: 12629218]

[101] Mani, S.A.; Guo, W.; Liao, M.J.; Eaton, E.N.; Ayyanan, A.; Zhou, A.Y.; Brooks, M.; Reinhard, F.; Zhang, C.C.; Shipitsin, M.; Campbell, L.L.; Polyak, K.; Brisken, C.; Yang, J.; Weinberg, R.A. The epithelial-mesenchymal transition generates cells with properties of stem cells. *Cell,* **2008**, *133*(4), 704-715.
[http://dx.doi.org/10.1016/j.cell.2008.03.027] [PMID: 18485877]

[102] Hirsch, H.A.; Iliopoulos, D.; Tsichlis, P.N.; Struhl, K. Metformin selectively targets cancer stem cells, and acts together with chemotherapy to block tumor growth and prolong remission. *Cancer Res.,* **2009**, *69*(19), 7507-7511.
[http://dx.doi.org/10.1158/0008-5472.CAN-09-2994] [PMID: 19752085]

[103] Li, C.; Heidt, D.G.; Dalerba, P.; Burant, C.F.; Zhang, L.; Adsay, V.; Wicha, M.; Clarke, M.F.; Simeone, D.M. Identification of pancreatic cancer stem cells. *Cancer Res.,* **2007**, *67*(3), 1030-1037.
[http://dx.doi.org/10.1158/0008-5472.CAN-06-2030] [PMID: 17283135]

[104] Moriyama, T.; Ohuchida, K.; Mizumoto, K.; Cui, L.; Ikenaga, N.; Sato, N.; Tanaka, M. Enhanced cell migration and invasion of CD133+ pancreatic cancer cells cocultured with pancreatic stromal cells. *Cancer,* **2010**, *116*(14), 3357-3368.
[http://dx.doi.org/10.1002/cncr.25121] [PMID: 20564084]

[105] Abraham, S.A.; Hopcroft, L.E.; Carrick, E.; Drotar, M.E.; Dunn, K.; Williamson, A.J.; Korfi, K.; Baquero, P.; Park, L.E.; Scott, M.T.; Pellicano, F.; Pierce, A.; Copland, M.; Nourse, C.; Grimmond, S.M.; Vetrie, D.; Whetton, A.D.; Holyoake, T.L. Dual targeting of p53 and c-MYC selectively

eliminates leukaemic stem cells. *Nature,* **2016**, *534*(7607), 341-346.
[http://dx.doi.org/10.1038/nature18288] [PMID: 27281222]

[106] Cheng, X.; Kim, J.Y.; Ghafoory, S.; Duvaci, T.; Rafiee, R.; Theobald, J.; Alborzinia, H.; Holenya, P.; Fredebohm, J.; Merz, K.H.; Mehrabi, A.; Hafezi, M.; Saffari, A.; Eisenbrand, G.; Hoheisel, J.D.; Wölfl, S. Methylisoindigo preferentially kills cancer stem cells by interfering cell metabolism *via* inhibition of LKB1 and activation of AMPK in PDACs. *Mol. Oncol.,* **2016**, *10*(6), 806-824.
[http://dx.doi.org/10.1016/j.molonc.2016.01.008] [PMID: 26887594]

[107] Xiao, Z.; Wang, Y.; Lu, L.; Li, Z.; Peng, Z.; Han, Z.; Hao, Y. Anti-angiogenesis effects of meisoindigo on chronic myelogenous leukemia *in vitro. Leuk. Res.,* **2006**, *30*(1), 54-59.
[http://dx.doi.org/10.1016/j.leukres.2005.05.012] [PMID: 15982734]

[108] Lee, C.C.; Lin, C.P.; Lee, Y.L.; Wang, G.C.; Cheng, Y.C.; Liu, H.E. Meisoindigo is a promising agent with *in vitro* and *in vivo* activity against human acute myeloid leukemia. *Leuk. Lymphoma,* **2010**, *51*(5), 897-905.
[http://dx.doi.org/10.3109/10428191003672115] [PMID: 20233051]

[109] Bouchikhi, F.; Anizon, F.; Moreau, P. Synthesis and antiproliferative activities of isoindigo and azaisoindigo derivatives. *Eur. J. Med. Chem.,* **2008**, *43*(4), 755-762.
[http://dx.doi.org/10.1016/j.ejmech.2007.05.012] [PMID: 17628214]

[110] Wee, X.K.; Yeo, W.K.; Zhang, B.; Tan, V.B.; Lim, K.M.; Tay, T.E.; Go, M.L. Synthesis and evaluation of functionalized isoindigos as antiproliferative agents. *Bioorg. Med. Chem.,* **2009**, *17*(21), 7562-7571.
[http://dx.doi.org/10.1016/j.bmc.2009.09.008] [PMID: 19783149]

[111] Shi, J.; Shen, H.M. Critical role of Bid and Bax in indirubin-3'-monoxime-induced apoptosis in human cancer cells. *Biochem. Pharmacol.,* **2008**, *75*(9), 1729-1742.
[http://dx.doi.org/10.1016/j.bcp.2008.01.021] [PMID: 18377873]

[112] Lee, J.W.; Moon, M.J.; Min, H.Y.; Chung, H.J.; Park, E.J.; Park, H.J.; Hong, J.Y.; Kim, Y.C.; Lee, S.K. Induction of apoptosis by a novel indirubin-5-nitro-3'-monoxime, a CDK inhibitor, in human lung cancer cells. *Bioorg. Med. Chem. Lett.,* **2005**, *15*(17), 3948-3952.
[http://dx.doi.org/10.1016/j.bmcl.2005.05.105] [PMID: 15993584]

[113] Song, J.H.; Lee, J.E.; Cho, K.M.; Park, S.H.; Kim, H.J.; Kim, Y.C.; Kim, T.S. 5-diphenylacetamid-indirubin-3'-oxime as a novel mitochondria-targeting agent with anti-leukemic activities. *Mol. Carcinog.,* **2016**, *55*(5), 611-621.
[http://dx.doi.org/10.1002/mc.22307] [PMID: 25788004]

[114] Kim, S.A.; Kim, Y.C.; Kim, S.W.; Lee, S.H.; Min, J.J.; Ahn, S.G.; Yoon, J.H. Antitumor activity of novel indirubin derivatives in rat tumor model. *Clin. Cancer Res.,* **2007**, *13*(1), 253-259.
[http://dx.doi.org/10.1158/1078-0432.CCR-06-1154] [PMID: 17200363]

[115] Lee, M.Y.; Liu, Y.W.; Chen, M.H.; Wu, J.Y.; Ho, H.Y.; Wang, Q.F.; Chuang, J.J. Indirubin-3-monoxime promotes autophagic and apoptotic death in JM1 human acute lymphoblastic leukemia cells and K562 human chronic myelogenous leukemia cells. *Oncol. Rep.,* **2013**, *29*(5), 2072-2078.
[http://dx.doi.org/10.3892/or.2013.2334] [PMID: 23468088]

[116] Damiens, E.; Baratte, B.; Marie, D.; Eisenbrand, G.; Meijer, L. Anti-mitotic properties of indirubin-3-monoxime, a CDK/GSK-3 inhibitor: induction of endoreplication following prophase arrest. *Oncogene,* **2001**, *20*(29), 3786-3797.
[http://dx.doi.org/10.1038/sj.onc.1204503] [PMID: 11439342]

[117] Li, H.; Ambade, A.; Re, F. Cutting edge: Necrosis activates the NLRP3 inflammasome. *J. Immunol.,* **2009**, *183*(3), 1528-1532.
[http://dx.doi.org/10.4049/jimmunol.0901080] [PMID: 19596994]

[118] Zhang, Z.N.; Liu, E.K.; Zheng, T.L.; Li, D.G. Treatment of chronic myelocytic leukemia (CML) by traditional Chinese medicine and Western medicine alternately. *J. Tradit. Chin. Med.,* **1985**, *5*(4), 246-248.

[PMID: 3869272]

[119] Xiao, Z.; Hao, Y.; Liu, B.; Qian, L. Indirubin and meisoindigo in the treatment of chronic myelogenous leukemia in China. *Leuk. Lymphoma,* **2002**, *43*(9), 1763-1768.
[http://dx.doi.org/10.1080/1042819021000006295] [PMID: 12685829]

[120] Chen, F.; Li, L.; Ma, D.; Yan, S.; Sun, J.; Zhang, M.; Ji, C.; Hou, M. Imatinib achieved complete cytogenetic response in a CML patient received 32-year indirubin and its derivative treatment. *Leuk. Res.,* **2010**, *34*(2), e75-e77.
[http://dx.doi.org/10.1016/j.leukres.2009.09.001] [PMID: 19773083]

[121] Xiao, Z.; Qian, L.; Liu, B.; Hao, Y. Meisoindigo for the treatment of chronic myelogenous leukaemia. *Br. J. Haematol.,* **2000**, *111*(2), 711-712.
[http://dx.doi.org/10.1046/j.1365-2141.2000.02357.x] [PMID: 11122126]

[122] Guo, R.; Abdelmohsen, K.; Morin, P.J.; Gorospe, M. Novel MicroRNA Reporter Uncovers Repression of Let-7 by GSK-3β. *PLoS One,* **2013**, *8*(6), e66330.
[http://dx.doi.org/10.1371/journal.pone.0066330] [PMID: 23840442]

CHAPTER 6

Anticancer Agents: Plants Used in Ayurveda

Uma Ranjan Lal, Dharmik Joshi and **Sugato Banerjee**[*]

Department of Pharmaceutical Sciences and Technology, Birla Institute of Technology, Mesra, Ranchi, India

Abstract: Cancer is one of the deadliest diseases of the century. Though a lot is known about its pathogenesis, a cure for the disease is not yet available. The present therapies for cancer lack specificity and show various toxicities. Ayurveda is one of the oldest traditional systems of medicine along with the Chinese system of medicine, Siddha, and Unani. Cancer has been described as clinical entities arbuda and granthi in the famous ayurvedic text Sushrutha samhita centuries before the detection of cancer by modern medicine. In this chapter, we discuss the phytoconstituents of medicinal plants with anticancer properties as described in Ayurveda from ethnopharmacology and experimental pharmacology perspective. The chapter summarizes and emphasizes the importance of Ayurveda, a traditional system of medicine in the treatment of cancer.

Keywords: Ayurveda, Ayurvedic formulation, cancer, natural compounds, extract, plant, phytopharmacology.

INTRODUCTION

Cancer is a pathological condition which results when abnormal cells divide in an uncontrolled way and eventually spreads to different tissues. By 2020, fifteen billion new cases of cancer are expected with a mortality rate of 12 billion worldwide [1]. It is a disease with a complex etiology and cure may still be a distant future due to its complex pathogenesis and biochemical complications arising due to side effects of conventional therapy.

Medicine from plant sources has provided us with numerous lead compounds with high efficacy and low toxicity. Thus compounds isolated from natural sources may provide us with promising anti-cancer agents. Ayurveda is one of the ancient Indian systems of medicine along with Siddha and Unani. In Ayurvedic formulations, a combination of plants is being used for treating any specific ailment. It is based on the principle that additive or synergistic effects of the

[*] **Corresponding Author Sugato Banerjee**: Department of Pharmaceutical Sciences and Technology, Birla Institute of Technology, Mesra, Ranchi, India; Tel: 7250001584; Email: sbanerjee@bitmesra.ac.in

Ferid Murad, Atta-ur-Rahman and Ka Bian (Eds.)

secondary metabolites present in those plants may enhance the therapeutic efficacy of these formulations compared to single plant extracts. Ayurveda has been involved in treating complex diseases such as cancer, diabetes, arthritis, and asthma for centuries, which may be managed but cannot be cured by modern medicine [2]. The system uses a complex combination of plants and minerals, with doses based on the physiology of patient and stage of the disease. Thus, to develop therapeutics for cancer from the Ayurvedic perspective, several factors need to be considered:

- Authentication of the plant species traditionally used for the treatment of cancer like diseases;
- Traditional techniques employed for such therapies;
- Consideration of adverse drug reactions and relevant interactions of such products
- Method development and validation of efficient manufacturing processes for such health products.

According to Ayurveda, our physiology is primarily controlled by Vata or air and space, Pitta or fire and water, and Kapha or water and earth. According to Ayurveda when one or two of the above gets dysregulated a person may develop solid benign tumors also referred to as Vataja, Pittaja or Kaphaja, however, the body is still trying to balance the dysregulation. However, when vata, pitta, and kapha lose their mutual coordination it may lead to malignant tumors (Tridosaja) where tissue damage and morbidity become inevitable. Various external factors or diet may be responsible for the above loss of coordination. Vata may get aggravated by excessive intake of bitter, spicy, astringent food and stress. Excessive intake of sour tasting food, salt, oil or fried foods and excessive anger may aggravate Pitta, while sweet and oily diet and lack of exercise may act as Kapha aggravating factors. Another approach in Ayurveda explains the pathogenesis of cancer from the cell metabolism perspective. According to Ayurveda, Agni or Pitta is responsible for human metabolism. Thus the decrease in Agni in cells of a particular tissue will result in Dhatwagni (deranged metabolism) producing Arbuda, or tumor growth. Cancer is a multifactorial disorder with metabolic abnormalities playing a predominant role, this may be due to disequilibrium between the Vata, Pitta and Kapha forces, resulting in uncontrolled growth and proliferation and reduction in apoptotic functions of cells.

Ama may be described as impurities and toxins, which originates from digestive waste due to impaired metabolism. It may build up in individuals with the weak digestive system or due to an unhealthy diet. A weakened Agni may usually lead to accumulation of Ama which is regarded as a risk factor for various diseases. The Ama may obstruct micro channels resulting in loss of homeostasis and potentiating inflammation, and degeneration. Circulating Ama may also produce reactive and toxic forms with antigenic and pro-inflammatory properties. This may disrupt immune function and affect disease states. In the context of cancer and inflammation, the concept of Ama becomes important because of its antigenic and pro-inflammatory properties [3]. While Ojas is the vital essence of the body. It is the essence of the Dhatus which make up the tissues and is likened to the immune system. Excess accumulation of Ama may also lead to depleted Ojas. Lack or depletion of ojas may lead to cancer while chemotherapy may also deplete the Ojas resulting in Dhatukshaya which may lead to tissue degeneration [4]. The review on cancer from the Ayurvedic perspective by Balachandran P and Govindrajan R 2005 gives a detailed description of cancer management strategies by Ayurvedic practitioners [5]. However, they have limited themselves to the pharmacological aspects of the Ayurvedic plants without correlating them with the chemical structures of isolated compounds. This chapter aims to review the chemistry of various plants used in Ayurveda in the area of cancer therapy.

CANCER THERAPIES AND THEIR LIMITATIONS

The conventional treatment of cancer revolves around the premise that all somatic cells contain a similar malignant potential. The deficiency of the particularity in these strategies has rendered them ineffective to provide long-lasting protection against cancer. On the contrary, the drugs which are more target specific can cause the regression of the bulk of the tumor but is unable to accomplish the complete elimination of the cancer stem cells. The results that are observed are quite devastating considering the atavism of cancer after discontinuation of the administered drug.

Genetic Approach- The genetic approach in cancer research was centralized on the identification and determination of the genetic pattern and genetic abnormalities caused by the mutational or another chromosomal anomaly. However, only a fistful amount of genetic mutations associated with cancer has been recognized in patients that are unable to explain the large genetic deviation that eventually manifests in the malignant phenotype of the tumor. It has been depicted that epigenetic mechanisms can boost the foundation of tumorigenesis and can facilitate the continuity of the malignant phenotype in cancer cells. Methylation of the CpG domain residing in the promoter region of various genes such as Rb, p16, and p53 which are responsible for tumor suppression could produce a devastating effect on cell cycle regulation. The silencing of these genes can lead to the unrestrained proliferation of cells. The enzyme which is responsible for the methylation of CpG dinucleotide is DNA methyltransferase (DNMT). But the idea of targeting the DNMT has concerns regarding its lack of specificity. This is because the inhibiting agents are not particularized for the affected hypermethylated genes (*e.g.*, Tumor suppressor genes), they can lead to the hypomethylation of the whole genome. This may randomly activate some other genes which are supposed to be silenced in an adult individual.

Stem cell transplant – This approach is particularly fruitful against lymphomas and leukemia but may also be used against neuroblastoma and multiple myeloma. In this type of therapy, pluripotent stem cells are injected into the blood which later differentiates into blood components which have been destroyed by high doses of chemotherapy and radiation therapy, or both. However, the primary toxicity associated with an allogeneic transplant is graft-*versus*-host response which may eventually lead to hepatic, intestinal and other vital organ damage.

Hormone therapy – Also known as hormonal therapy, hormone treatment or endocrine therapy is treatment strategy against cancers where hormones play a significant role like prostate or breast cancer. The underlying principle behind hormone therapy is to down-regulate the release of hormones involved in cancer growth. However by preventing the regular release of hormones the treatment leads to many undesirable side effects. Hormonal therapy against prostate cancer may cause undue side effects like hot flashes, loss of libido, loss of bone strength, diarrhea, nausea, and lack of energy. Hormonal therapy in women with breast cancer also shows side effects like hot flashes, vaginal dryness, infrequent period, loss of libido, nausea, mood swings, lack of energy. All the above results lead to the significant decadence in quality of life.

Immunotherapy – The underlying principle behind the immune therapy is to stimulate the immune cells so that they may be able to fight out the cancer-causing cells. One of the reasons for cancer cells extended longevity is their ability to go unnoticed by the immune system. Antibodies help to mark the cancerous cells, which are then targeted and destroyed by the immune cell. However, this type of biological treatment has its limitations. Side effects are similar to allergic and inflammatory reactions which may include mild skin rash, pain, swelling, tenderness, rubor, itchiness to flu-like symptoms which may be associated with fever, chills, weakness, dizziness, nausea or vomiting. It may be related to moderate toxicities like muscle or joint pain, chronic fatigue, trouble breathing, hypertension, heart palpitations, the risk of infection *etc*. Immunotherapies may also cause severe or even fatal allergic reaction in certain individuals. Thus the conventional therapeutics against cancer is accompanied by its many ill side effects demanding the development of alternate less toxic therapeutic approaches [6].

PRINCIPLES OF DRAVYA GUNA

Dravya' means a drug in this context. It has a substratum of properties and actions. In this connection, two broad propositions are established:

1. Ayurveda says each and every substance in the world has therapeutic value.
2. All drugs are composed of five bhutas namely (Panchabhutas *i.e.* Akasha, Vayu, Agni, Jala, and Prithivi) which are regarded as the physicochemical basis of all material objects.

When life came into being from the above five three of them namely Vata, Pitta and Kapha regulated biological functions and are known as Tridhatu responsible for the following functions namely Vikshepa (movement), Adana (assimilation) and Visarga (growth) respectively.

Gunas: Guna (quality or property) is defined as that which is inherently existent in substance and is the inherent cause (of its effect). Gunas are forty-one in number and are classified into four groups somatic, psychic, physical and applicative.

Rasa is the object of gustatory sense organ and is located in dravya. Rasa is perceived through nipata (contact with the gustatory sense organ). Rasas are six in number – madhura (sweet), amla (sour), lavana (salty), katu (pungent), tikta (bitter) and kashaya (astringent). Rasas affect vata, pitta and kapha.

Vipaka' is the term for the final transformed state of drugs after metabolism. In most cases, the rasas pass on as such, and there is no change in their nature, but in some instances, there is a definite change with a different vipaka which determines the future course and action of the drug. For example, Shunthi (dry ginger) is pungent (katu) in taste but is transformed to madhura vipaka which determines its action. It is of three types according to taste and effect on doshas – madhura (sweet), amla (sour) and katu (pungent) and two types according to properties-guru (heavy) and laghu (light). Vipaka has a similar effect on doshas as do rasa.

Virya: Virya is the Shakti or the potency of a substance. So virya is the instrument of the drug responsible for its prabhava or action. It may be represented as the active fraction of the drug which is again made up of the five bhutas and its quality determines its action like the pacification of the doshas.

Prabhava: This specific power is based on the particular nature (bhautika composition) and exerts specific action. It is known from the particular kind initiated by specific combination (of bhutas). This specific nature leads to particular action like emesis, purgation, *etc*. Vagbhata also follows the same line – 'The specific action in spite of the similarity in rasa, *etc*. is caused by prabhava' [7].

DEVELOPMENT OF ANTICANCER AGENTS FROM PLANT SOURCES

Ayurvedic formulations include arka, asavas, aristas, churna, taila, vati, gutika, bhasma which have been part of the health care system since ancient times.

Arka is a liquid formulation obtained by aqueous distillation.

Aasava or Aristas- are fermented formulations from the plant source.

Avaleha- is a semi-solid preparation in the form of a thick paste primarily meant for licking.

Churnas are finely powdered drugs. Usually, the plant materials are dried cleaned size reduced and finely sieved to get this formulation.

Ghana is a dried aqueous extract of kwatha. The aqueous portion is evaporated from 'kwaaha,' and then the dried extract is solidified.

Tailas (Medicated oils) and Ghritas (Medicated Ghee) are prepared by mixing and boiling oil (taila) or ghee with the decoction or drug paste.

Vati and Gutikas are drug forms prepared in the way of tablet or pills.

Bhasma means an ash obtained through incineration. The starting material (Herbo-mineral/metals/non-metals preparations) undergoes an elaborate process of purification and this process is followed by the reaction phase, which involves incorporation of some other minerals and/or herbal extract and exposing to certain quantum of heat as per puta system of Ayurveda [8].

Metabolites of diverse chemical compounds have been isolated from the rhizomes, stems, leaves and other parts of medicinal plants. Lead molecules like vincristine, vinblastine, taxol, podophyllotoxin, camptothecin with potent cytotoxic activity have been isolated from various plant sources. Various functional groups have been incorporated or altered with the parent backbone to produce analogues with better efficacy, lower toxicity, and higher permeability. Successful anticancer molecules like topotecan, irinotecan, taxotere, etoposide, teniposide have emerged after modifications from their natural leads [9]. A number of molecular targets have been identified and high throughput screening of compounds both *in silico* and *in vitro* against such targets has been the basis of modern day drug discovery.

In the area of cancer biology cyclin-dependent kinases play an important role in the regulation of cell cycle, thus inhibition of their activity interferes with specific stages of the cell cycle resulting in cell cycle arrest [10]. Quercetin, a moderately anti-tumor active flavonoid may mimic ATP since its planar bicyclic chromone ring system is an isostere of adenine. It exerts its anti-tumor effects by inhibiting cell cycle progression by inhibition of Cdk. Flavopiridol was developed as a highly selective CDK inhibitor showing 100-fold greater selectivity for Cdks over tyrosine kinases. Flavopiridol is a synthetic moiety based on flavonoid structure of rohitukine isolated from *Dysoxylum binectariferum* Hook. f. (Meliaceae) a phylogenic relative of *Dysoxylum malabaricum* Bedd. It may prevent inflammation and may also modulate the immune system and hence used against rheumatoid arthritis [11]. Another synthetic derivative roscovitine has been derived from its natural compound olomucine. Olomucine isolated initially from the cotyledons of radish, *Raphanus sativus* L. (Brassicaceae) may act as a cyclin-dependent kinases (Cdk) inhibitor. Chemical modifications of Olomucine resulted in the synthesis of roscovitine a more potent analogue currently undergoing Phase II clinical trials. Purvalanols were also developed in the same line [12]. The combretastatins are also showing promising results. These are stilbenes isolated from the South African "bush willow", *Combretum caffrum* (Eckl. & Zeyh.) Kuntze (Combretaceae) [13]. They act as anti-angiogenic agents thus reducing vasculature around tumors resulting in necrosis of tumor cells. Its water-soluble analog, combretastatin A4 phosphate (CA4), is undergoing clinical trials. The combretastatins species of the Combretum and Terminalia genera, of Combretaceae family, is popularly used in the treatment of hepatitis and malaria. However, several Terminalia species have also been used ethologically in the treatment of different cancers [14].

The above examples are compounds which are promising drug candidates in clinical trials and have been derived from the traditional medicine template. The parent molecules from which they have been developed were isolated from medicinal plants which were used for treating "cancer", and all have some linkage to Ayurveda. If we critically see the therapeutic techniques used in Ayurveda for the treatment and management of cancer and the above- mentioned molecules some correlation can be made. Ayurvedic methods used are; preparation of herbal decoctions, paste formation, extraction with alkali, extraction with sugar, taking herbs with butter milk preparations, all employing water as solvent except butter milk preparations [14]. The gaining importance of water-soluble constituents these days also underline the importance of traditional preparations. Flavonoids (bicyclic chromane ring) and polyphenolics form the primary class of components which are readily decocted by water. Some of the polyphenolics of Terminalia genus have anticancer properties too. This genus is also well exploited traditionally in Ayurveda. Detailed chemistry of various plants has been discussed in next sections (summarized in Table **1**) while chemical structures of compounds isolated from them with anticancer activity have been depicted in Fig. (**1**).

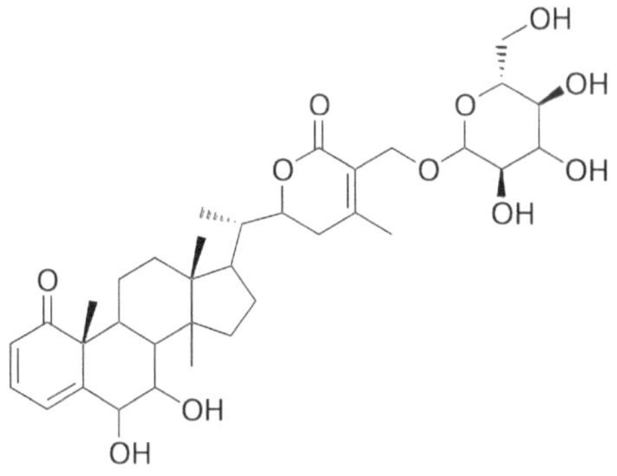

daturametelins J

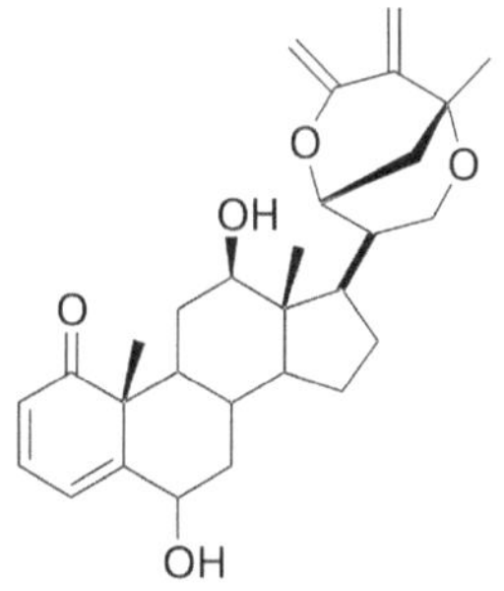

7,27-dihydroxy-1-oxowitha-2,5,24-trienolide

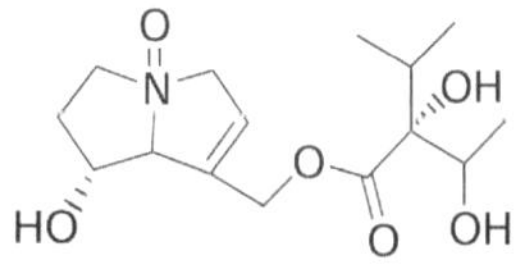

. indicine N-oxide

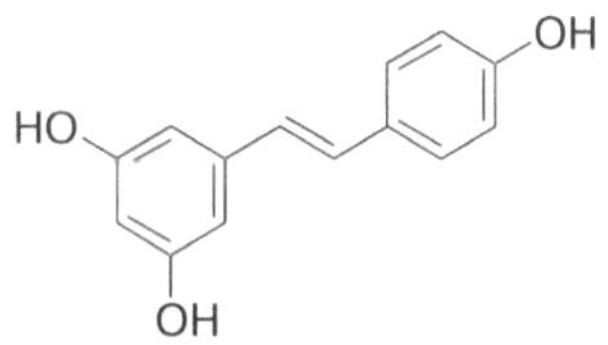

Resveratrol

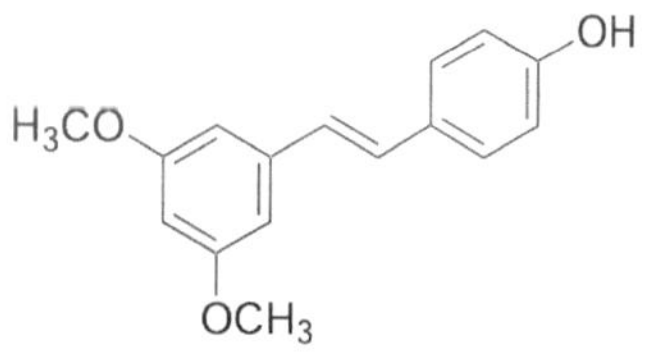

pterostilbene.

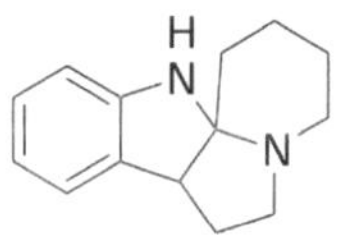

Echitamine chloride

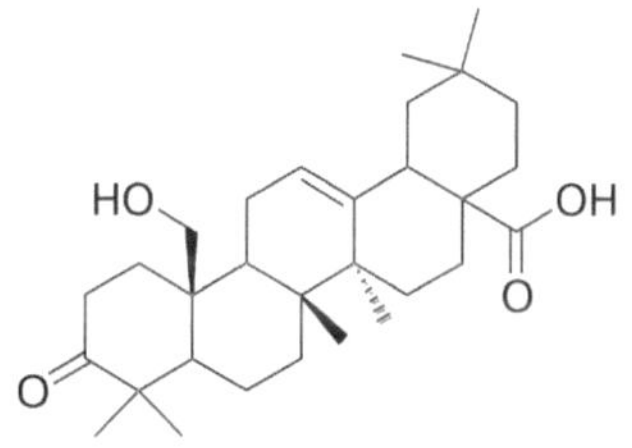

Amooranin

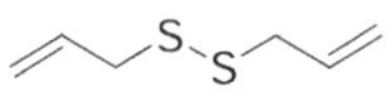

diallyl disulfide

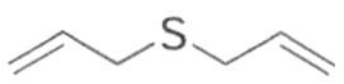

Diallyl sulfide

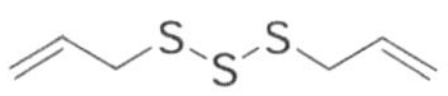

Diallyl trisulfide

Fig. 1 cont.....

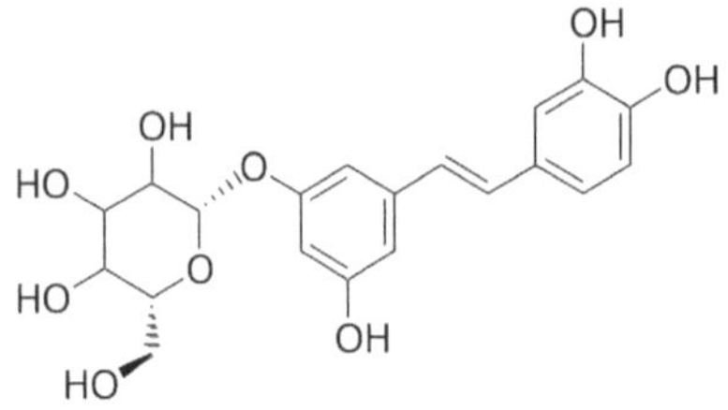

trans-astringin

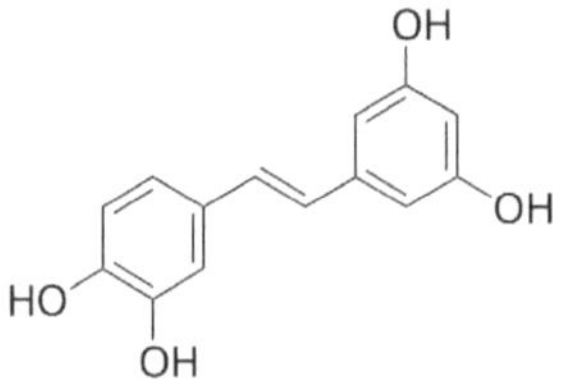

trans-piceatannol

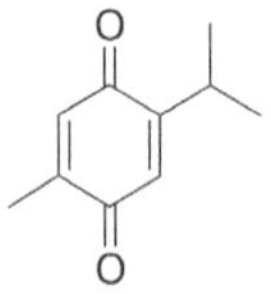

Thymoquinone

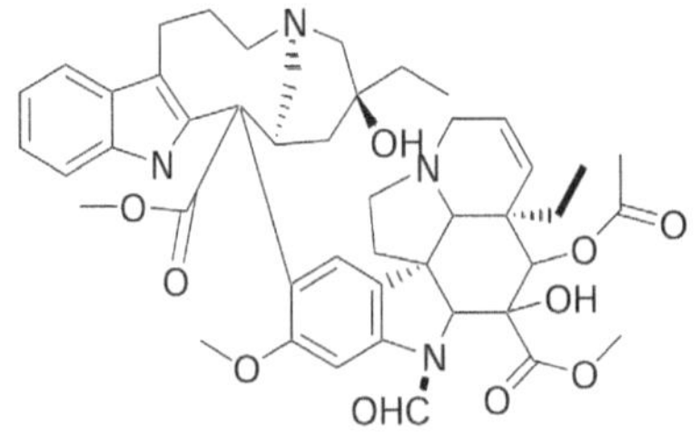

Vincristine

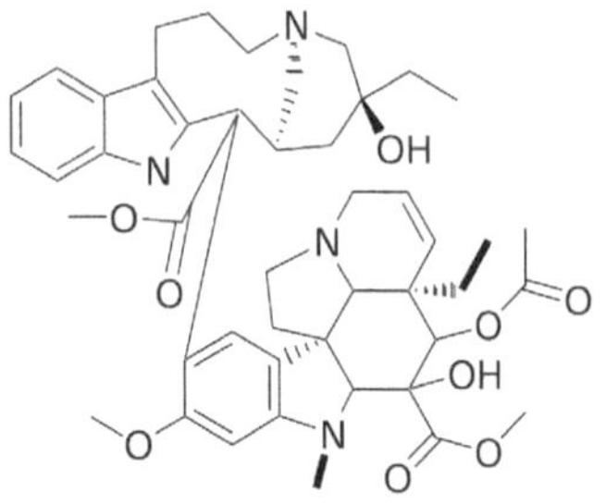

Vinblatine

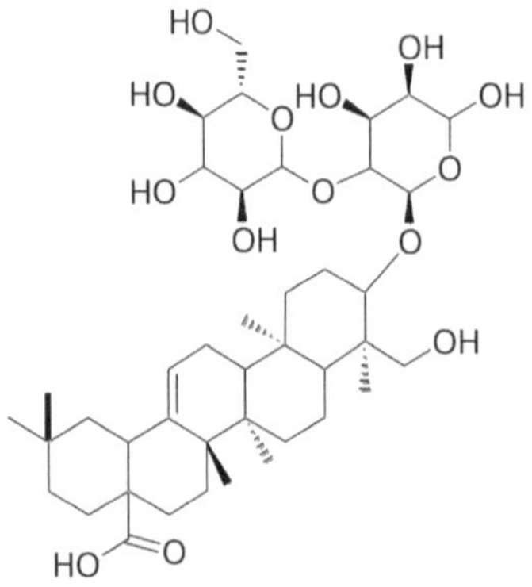

hederin

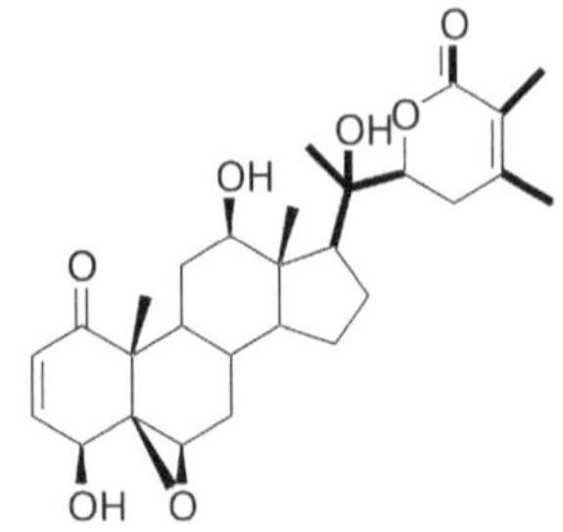

Withanolide D

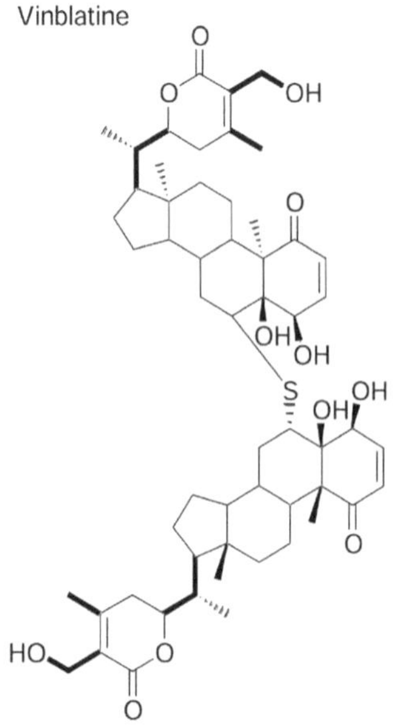

Ashwagandhanolide

Fig. (1). Chemical structures of phytoconstituents with anticancer activity.

Table 1. Anticancer agents from plants mentioned in ayurveda.

Plants	Active Chemical Constituents	Chemical Class	Indication and Mechanism of Action	References
Abrus precatorius	Abrin and Abrus agglutinin	Glycoprotein lectin	Yoshida sarcoma (rats) Fibrosarcoma (mice) Protein Synthesis Inhibition	[18]
Allium sativum	Diallyl disulfide, Diallyl sulfide and Diallyl trisulfide *etc.*	Organosulfur compounds (OSCs)	Mammary, Colon, Esophagus, Lung & Forestomach, Skin and Liver cancer (cell cycle arrest, induced apoptosis, inhibition of DNA-AAF adducts formation)	[24, 25]
Aloe vera	Aloin	Anthraquinone	Human uterine carcinoma. Cell cycle arrest and induction of apoptosis	[32]
	Aloe emodin	Anthraquinone	Gastric carcinoma cells T24 human bladder cancer cells inhibit proliferation of U-373MG glioma cells Merkel cell carcinoma (induction of apoptosis)	[29, 33, 37]
	PAC-I	mannose rich polysaccharide	A potent stimulator of murine macrophage	
	Aloctin I	Lectin	Ehrlich ascites tumors in mice (Immunomodulatory and mitogenic effects)	
Alstonia scholaries	Echitamine chloride (EC),	Indole alkaloid	Sarcoma-180 bearing mice (Modulation of the impaired drug metabolism) Fibrosarcoma in rats by reduced glycolysis in Ehrlich ascites carcinoma cells	[40, 41]
Amoora rohitaka	Amooranin-AMR	Triterpene acid	Human breast carcinoma (cell growth was suppressed by cell cycle arrest and increase in caspase mediated apoptosis, overcomes multidrug resistance in human leukemia and colon carcinoma	[46]

(Table 1) cont.....

Plants	Active Chemical Constituents	Chemical Class	Indication and Mechanism of Action	References
Anacardium occidentale	Anacardic acids	Pentadecane aliphatic chain containing. Hydroxyl carboxylic acid	Breast and cervix carcinoma cells.	[50]
Andrographis paniculata	Andrographolide	Diterpenoid lactone	Inhibits human hematoma derived Hep3B cell growth. Prevents activation of JNK	[51]
Annona atemoya/muricata	Bullatacin	Bis fatty acid lactone	It induces cell death by reducing cellular energy sources like cAMP and cGMP in hepatocarcinoma.	[56, 57]
Berberis aristata	Berberine	Alkaloid	Inhibits 20-methylcholanthrene or N-nitrosodiethylamine induced carcinogenesis in mice.	[61]
Calotropis gigantea	19-Nor- and 18,20-Epox--cardenolides	Glycosides; Steroid	Cytotoxic activity against KB, BC, and NCI-H187 cancer cell lines	[64]
Datura metel	Withanolides	Glycoside	Human colorectal carcinoma (HCT-116) cell line A549 (lung), BGC-823 (gastric), and K562 (leukemia) cancer cell lines	[67, 68]
Heliotropium indicum	Indicine N-oxide	Pyrrolizidine alkaloid	Ehrlich ascites carcinoma and sarcoma in mice	[70, 72]
Nigella sativa	Thymoquinone (TQ)		p53-dependent apoptosis in human colon cancer cells and activation of caspase-8 in leukemia cells	[70]
	α- hederin		Elicits necrosis and apoptosis	
	3-O-[β-D-xyl(p)(13)-α-L-rham(p)(1→2)-α-L-ara(p)]-28-O-[α-L-rham(p)(1→2)-(1→4)-β-D-glu(p)-(1→6)-β-D-glu(p)]-hederagenin	Saponin	Tumor inhibition properties	

(Table 1) cont.....

Plants	Active Chemical Constituents	Chemical Class	Indication and Mechanism of Action	References
	3-O-[β-D- xyl(p)(1→3)-α-L-rham(p)(1→2)-α-L-ara(p)]-hederagenin.	Saponin	Tumor inhibition properties	
	kaempferol 3-O-[β-D-glucosyl-(1→2)-O-β-D-glucosyl(1→2)]glucoside	Flavonoid glucoside	Tumor inhibition properties	
Phyllanthus niruri/amarus			*In vitro* anticancer activity and antimutagenic activity while chemopreventive against hepatic carcinoma in rats	[74 - 77]
Picrorrhiza kurroa			Protects from hepatocarcinogenesis and sarcoma in mice	[80, 81]
Piper longum	Piperine	Piperidine Alkaloid	Chemopreventive activity of piperine in oral cancer is probably due to its antioxidant and prevention of lipid peroxidation properties. Piperine may act as an anticancer agent by balancing the protein bound carbohydrate levels in various tissues	[82, 84]
Podophyllum hexandrum linn. (Podophyllin)	Podophyllotoxin	Aryltetralin-type lignin	It is a powerful anticancer agent acting through mitotic inhibition, nuclear fragmentation, and impaired spindle formation, causing necrosis.	[90]
Semecarpus anacardium	Biflavone	Bioflavonoid	Normalizes glycoprotein and mineral content in cancerous tissues and prevents carcinogen activation by inducing phase I and phase II biotransformation enzymes.	[91]

(Table 1) cont.....

Plants	Active Chemical Constituents	Chemical Class	Indication and Mechanism of Action	References
Tinospora cordifolia	Syringin and cordiol cordioside and cordiofolioside A	Glycosides	It exerts its anticancer potential by various mechanisms like induction of caspase-3 activated DNase mediated apoptosis in EAT cells, reducing the GSH concentration and increasing in lipid peroxidation in tumor cells in Ehrlich ascites carcinoma bearing mice, augmenting proliferation of thymocytes with a concomitant decrease in thymocyte apoptosis thus retarding tumor growth and prolonging survival of tumor-bearing mice, activating tumor-associated macrophages and showing the antitumor effect on the spontaneous T-cell lymphoma.	[96 - 100]
Vinca rosea	Vincristine and Vinblatine	Indole alkaloid	Depolymerization of microtubules.	[9]
Vitis vinifera	Trans-Astringin Trans-piceatannol	Stilbenoid	Cancer chemoprevention activity in mouse mammary gland organ culture assay.	[109]
Withania somnifera	Withanferin A	Steroidal lactone	Mouse Ehrlich ascites carcinoma, induced vacuolation of the cytoplasm. A Potential inhibitor of angiogenesis. Par-4-dependent apoptosis in prostate cancer cells I-kappa-β- kinase hyperphosphorylation inhibition.	[110 - 112]

(Table 1) cont.....

Plants	Active Chemical Constituents	Chemical Class	Indication and Mechanism of Action	References
Withania somnifera	Withanolides Withanolide D Ashwagandholide	Steroidal Lactones Steroidal lactone Dimeric thiowithanolide	Growth inhibition of human tumor cell lines.	
			Potentiates apoptosis, inhibits metastasis, by suppression of NF-κB activation and associated gene expression.	
			Significant antitumor activity *in vivo* against Sarcoma and Ehrlich ascites carcinoma. Lipid peroxidation and cyclooxygenase inhibition.	
	Palmitic Acid and its esters	Fatty acid	Gastric carcinoma cells	
	WSG	Acidic Glycoprotien	Phospholipase inhibitor	

PLANTS MENTIONED IN AYURVEDA WITH ANTI-CANCER POTENTIAL

Abrus Precatorius

Antitumor activity of *Abrus precatorius* was first reported in 1966 when the seed extract of *Abrus precatorius* L. was tested on mitotic and meiotic chromosomes in the testes of the grasshopper. Poecilocera pieta was found to causes chromosomal abnormalities [15], later on, protein extract of a this plant was found active *in vivo* when tested on Yoshida sarcoma (solid and ascites forms) in rats and a fibrosarcoma in mice [16]. Since then various studies have been carried out on the antitumor activity of *Abrus precatorius*. Chin Hsuan et.al purified two toxic proteins namely Abrin A and Abrin C. Abrin C was found to be more toxic than Abrin A on mice [17]. Till date, three toxins, Abrin-I, -II, and -III, and two agglutinins, APA-I and -II, were isolated and purified from the seeds of *Abrus precatorius* [18, 19]. Abrus agglutinin derived peptides were also studied for their anticancer activity and the underlying mechanism of action was the induction of mitochondria-dependent apoptosis [20]. Antitumor activity of Abrin in mice at a sublethal dose was carried out by intralesional and intraperitoneal administration of abrin and found effective in reducing solid tumor development [21]. Abrin showed extended immunomodulatory property by enhancing the proliferation of splenocytes and thymocytes (lymphocytes in general) in response to mitogens with subsequent enhancement of the natural killer cell activity [22]. Abrus seeds contain a toxic lectin, abrin (an albumotoxin), a fat-splitting enzyme, a glucoside (abrussic acid), urease, abarnin, trigonelline, choline, hypaphorine, and steroidal oil which have abortive effects.

In Śodhana of abrus seeds, they are subjected to the svedana in dolā yantra with Godugdha or Kāñji for 3–6 h. The Śodhita material is then subjected to washing with hot water and drying under shade [23].

Allium Sativum

Garlic (*Allium sativum* L.) is cultivated all over the world and is used as a vegetable and condiment. Traditionally ethnoveterinary practitioners used garlic as an excellent natural product that has immense therapeutic potential in many pathological conditions. It has antimicrobial, antithrombotic, hypolipidemic, antiarthritic, hypoglycemic and antitumor activity. The bulb of garlic is used as an antirheumatic and stimulant. It is also used in conditions like paralysis, forgetfulness, tremor colicky pain and chronic fever [24]. Garlic and its organosulfur compounds (OSCs) namely diallyl disulfide, diallyl sulfide, and diallyl trisulfide have chemopreventive properties. OSCs may show anticarcinogenic action through various mechanisms which include reduction of oxidative stress thus preventing DNA damage, reduced cell proliferation, regulation of carcinogen metabolism and induction of apoptosis [25]. Diallyl sulfide has been shown to protect against mammary adenocarcinomas in rats while benzyl selenocyanate inhibited mammary adenocarcinomas, colon cancer in rats and stomach tumors in mice [25 - 27]. Diallyl trisulfide, a constituent of processed garlic is found effective in chemoprevention [28].

Aloe Vera

Aloe vera, or Ghrit Kumari in Sanskrit has been one of the most important plants used in folk medicine. The healing benefits of the gel obtained from the plant's leaves were recognized in the ancient Indian, Chinese, Greek, and Roman civilizations. It has been traditionally used for wound healing, relieving itching and swelling [29], for treating constipation and protecting the skin from sunburn. Aloe-emodin is an anthraquinone and one of the major constituents present in the leaves of Aloe vera [30]. Aloe-emodin, has shown promising activity against AGS and NCI-N87 gastric carcinoma cells while the cytotoxic mechanism is through the induction of apoptosis [31, 32]. Aloe-emodin was found to modulate PKC isozymes and inhibits proliferation of U-373MG glioma cells inhibiting cancer by apoptosis [33]. Aloe-emodin significantly inhibited the growth of merkel carcinoma cell line isolated from the Merkel cell carcinoma (MCC) patient. It has been shown to be nontoxic for normal cells but to possess specific toxicity for neuroectodermal tumor cells [34]. Aloin another anthraquinone form Aloe vera showed the antiproliferative and cytotoxic effect on HeLaS3 cells. This was due to S phase cell cycle arrest and a marked increase in cell apoptosis [35].

Another active constituents of Aloe vera gel is a mannose-rich polysaccharide (acemannan) a potent stimulator of murine macrophage *in vitro* [36]. Tumoricidal properties of activated macrophage might account for the *in vivo* antitumor properties of PAC-I (active fraction of a polysaccharide) [37, 38], Aloctin I is a lectin isolated from Aloe vera leaf pulp extract showing good anticancer activity in Ehrlich ascites tumors in mice due to its immunomodulatory and mitogenic effects [39].

Alstonia Scholaris

It is commonly known as blackboard tree, devil tree, ditabark, and is an evergreen tropical tree native to India, Malesia and Australia. Echitamine chloride, an indole alkaloid from *Alstonia scholaris*, bark have been shown to have both *in vitro* and *in vivo* anticancer potential. Echitamine chloride may reduce fibrosarcoma in rats. It has been shown to reduce mitochondrial respiration resulting in reduced cellular energy and loss of S-180 sarcoma cell viability [40]. Echitamine chloride may also affect drug metabolizing enzymes thus reducing the toxicity associated with anticancer drugs [41]. A combination study of Echitamine chloride with vitamin A and Adriamycin has an enhanced cytotoxic effect on Ehrlich Ascites carcinoma cell culture [42 - 44].

Amoora Rohituka

A. rohituka stem bark contains Amooranin (AMR), is a novel triterpene acid and is one of the components of medicinal preparations used in Ayurveda against human malignancies [45]. AMR has been shown to induce p53 independent caspase-mediated apoptosis in human breast carcinoma cells [46]. It may also induce apoptosis in adenocarcinoma cells. In another study by Ramchandran *et al.* Amooranin (AMR) was cytotoxic to SW620 human colon carcinoma cell line with an IC_{50} value of 2.9µg/mL. This novel compound causes depolarization of the mitochondrial membrane thus decreasing membrane potential, indicating an initial signal for apoptosis induction [47]. Multidrug resistance in human leukemia and colon carcinoma cell lines could be overcome by application of amooranin [48].

Anacardium Occidentale

The cashew tree *Anacardium occidentale* is a tropical evergreen tree that produces the cashew seed and the cashew apple. The fruit bark juice and the nut oil have been used traditionally against calluses, corns, warts and cancerous ulcers. Anacardol and anacardic acid have been shown to be active against sarcoma [49].

Three anacardic acids have been isolated from cashew as cytotoxic agents against BT-20 breast carcinoma cells and epithelioid cervix carcinoma cells [50].

Andrographis Paniculata

Andrographis paniculata also known as kalmegh or kalamegha has been traditionally used by Indian and Chinese practitioners in the treatment of infection and inflammation. Andrographolide, a diterpenoid lactone from kalmegha has been shown to increase the apoptosis of hepatomas by the activation of different mitogen-activated protein kinases [49]. Andrographolide may downregulate VEGF, proinflammatory cytokines and NO while increasing levels of anti-angiogenic molecules preventing angiogenesis, thus may be helpful in preventing tumor growth and metastasis [52, 53]. The further immunostimulatory activity of *Andrographis paniculata* extract and andrographolides in human immune cells and cancer cells was evidenced by increased production of interleukin-2 resulting in the proliferation of lymphocytes [54]. Andrographolide has also been shown to increase the tumor necrosis factor-α production in cytotoxic T cells, resulting in the destruction of cancer cells by these T cells thus, contributing to its anticancer activity [55].

Annona Atemoya/Muricata

Bullatacin, isolated from the seeds of *Annona atemoya*, has potential antitumor activity. Annonaceous acetogenin induces cell death by reducing cellular energy sources like cAMP and cGMP in hepatocarcinoma [56, 57], Several other annonaceous acetogenins like atemoyacin-B, acetogenin 89-2 have been shown to reduce the multidrug resistance of resistant KBv200 and KB cells, which has been associated with the decrease of P-glycoprotein function in these cells [58, 59].

Berberis Aristata

Berberis aristata also known as Indian barberry or tree turmeric is often found in the hilly slopes. All its parts have some medicinal value and are used in Ayurveda. Rasaut, a preparation made by boiling in water the bark of the root and the lower part of the stem is a beneficial preparation that has been traditionally used in curing various disorders [60]. Berberine, a bitter alkaloid isolated from the plant has been shown to inhibit 20-methylcholanthrene or N-nitrosodiethylamine induced carcinogenesis in mice [61].

Calotropis Gigantean

Calotropis gigantean is called Madar in English and Akra in Sanskrit. The whole plant is useful and may be used as a tonic, expectorant, depurative, and anthelmintic. The dried root bark may act as a laxative along with the above uses. The powdered root has been used in Ayurveda against respiratory disorders including asthma and bronchitis. Its leaves may treat paralysis, arthralegia, and inflammation. The flowers may be used as bitter thus helping in digestion and stomachic [62, 63]. Two new cardenolides along with 12 known compounds isolated from the leaves of *Calotropis gigantea* were found to be cytotoxic against KB, BC, and NCI-H187 cancer cell lines [64].

Datura Metel

Datura metel is a shrub-like annual herb commonly known as devil's trumpet and metel. It is native to India, China, and South Asia. Tropane alkaloids namely atropine, hyoscyamine, scopolamine and withanolide glycosides are the main constituents of Datura metal. It has been used in Ayurveda for relaxation of bronchial muscles in asthma, also to treat intoxicatication and as emetic and digestive [65]. The first report of *Datura metal* as an anticancer agent came in 1968 when an alcoholic extract of the whole plant was found active against the human epidermal carcinoma of the nasopharynx in tissue culture [66]. Datura metal's withanolide glycosides have shown promising activity towards human colorectal carcinoma and K562 (leukemia) cell lines. Three new withanolide glycosides namely daturametelins H-J, daturataturin A and 7, 27-dihydroxy-1-oxowitha-2, 5, 24-trienolide have been tested for their antiproliferative activity in colorectal cancer cell lines. The nonglycosidic compound exhibited the highest activity in this study (IC_{50}= 0.2 to 3.2 µM) [67]. In another report, four withanolides exhibited potent cytotoxic activities against lung, gastric, and leukemia cell lines [68]. Datura seeds are highly toxic and may be fatal. Most of the side-effects (dryness of the mouth, excessive thirst, cramps, unconsciousness, and giddiness) are due to the anticholinergic property of the alkaloids present in this plant.

In the purification process the Dhattūra, seeds are soaked in freshly collected Gomūtra and kept aside for 12 h. After washing, the seeds are transferred to the dolā yantra for svedana process for 3 h. The seeds are again washed with lukewarm water, allowed to dry, and the testa is removed before use [23].

Heliotropium Indicum

Commonly known as Indian heliotrope, it is one of the widely used herbs in Ayurveda mainly found in southern India. The main chemical constituent of this plant are tumorigenic pyrrolizidine alkaloids. The juice from the pounded leaves is used on wounds, skin ulcers, and furuncles. Extracts of *Heliotropium indicum* Linn. (Boraginaceae) showed significant activity in several experimental tumor systems. The first report of anticancer activity came in 1976 when Kugelman *et al*. isolated the active principle N-oxide of the alkaloid, indicine. Later on, it was found to be effective against Ehrlich ascites carcinoma and sarcoma in mice when given orally. Indicine N-oxide has been used in clinical trials against leukemia and solid tumors [69 - 71].

Nigella Sativa

Commonly known as kalonji or black-caraway, seeds of *Nigella sativa*, a dicotyledon of the Ranunculaceae family, has been employed for thousands of years as a spice and food preservative. The oil and seed contain conjugated linoleic acid, nigellone, nigilline, and thymoquinine (TQ), the later in particular has shown potential medicinal properties in traditional medicine. Thymoquinine activates intracellular nonenzymatic metabolism dependent on GSH, NADH or NADPH that may modulate cellular antioxidant defenses. Further Nigella sativa has also shown NO-mediated alterations in dimethylhydrazine-induced colon cancer in rats. Saponins and flavonoid glycosides have also shown antitumor properties in cancer cell lines [72].

Phyllanthus Niruri/Amarus

Phyllanthus amarus Schum and Thonn (syn. *Phyllanthus niruri*) commonly known by the names of gale of the winds, stonebreaker or seed-under-leaf is an important plant of the Indian Ayurvedic system that is mainly used as an anti-viral agent in association with secondary hepatitis. It is also used for jaundice, gonorrhea, frequent menstruation, and diabetes and blocking the formation of kidney stones. It is typically used as a poultice for skin ulcer, sores, swelling, and itchiness [73]. *In vitro* studies show the antitumor, anti-mutagenic and anti-carcinogenic effects of *Phyllanthus amarus*. Aqueous extract from *P. amarus* has been shown to prevent N-nitrosodiethylamine mediated hepatic tumor development in rats and increased the lifespan of these animal [74, 75]. In another report, the aqueous extract has been proved to be chemoprotective and anticarcinogenic in cyclophosphamide and 20-methylcholanthrene (20-MC) induced toxicity [76, 77]. The Aqueous extract of *P. amarus* may also inhibit the P450 enzyme, aniline hydroxylase. The extract also inhibited mutant DNA topoisomerase II of Saccharomyces cerevisiae and inhibited cdc25 tyrosine phosphatase, known to be involved in cell cycle progression [75]. Multidrug resistance, one of the major obstacles in cancer therapy is primarily mediated by high levels of P-glycoprotein, a cellular transporter responsible for removal of various cytotoxic drugs resulting in drug-resistance. *P. amarus* lignans like nirtetralin, niranthin, phyllanthin have been shown to reduce doxorubicin resistance [78].

Picrorrhiza Kurroa

Known as Kutki. It is a perennial herb and is used as a substitute for Indian gentian (Gentiana kurroo). It has been reported to possess potent pharmacological activity against bronchial infections, asthma, hepatotoxicity, diabetes, inflammation, cancer, *etc* [79]. Extract of *Emblica officinalis* (EO), *Phyllanthus amarus* (P. amarus) and *Picrorrhiza kurroa* (P. kurroa) significantly inhibited hepatocarcinogenesis induced by N-nitrosodiethylamine (NDEA) in a dose-dependent manner [80]. Anti-tumour and anti-carcinogenic activity of *Picrorrhiza kurroa* extract was studied in mice. Administration of 20-methylcholanthrene (20 MC) produced 100% induction of sarcoma in control mice, whereas the tumor incidence and tumor related deaths were significantly inhibited by the oral administration of *P. kurroa* extract [81].

Piper Longum

Piperine, an alkaloid extracted from black pepper (*Piper nigrum* Linn) and long pepper (*Piper longum* Linn), widely used in the Ayurvedic system of medicine is a major ingredient in ayurvedic anticancer formulations. Piperine is found to be excellent chemopreventive and immunomodulatory agent in various *in vivo* anticancer assays. The chemopreventive activity of piperine in oral cancer is probably due to its antioxidant and prevention of lipid peroxidation properties [82]. Piperine is being evaluated for its anticancer potential in Benzo(a)pyrene mediated experimental carcinogenesis in mice. Activities of mitochondrial enzymes in lung cancer-bearing mice decreased significantly and there was a rise in glutathione-metabolizing enzymes indicating antitumor activity [83]. Piperine reduced DNA damage by enhancing the detoxification of enzymes [84] and also reduced the protein bound carbohydrate in serum, lung and liver tissues which are regarded as a primary indicator of tumorigenesis. Thus piperine may act as an anticancer agent by balancing the protein bound carbohydrate levels in various tissues [85]. The cell-mediated immune response of piperine increased the Natural Killer (NK) cell-mediated cytolysis in normal as well as tumor-bearing BALB/c mice [86]. Piperine may also inhibit nodule formation and reduce metastasis of lung melanoma cells [87]. Piperine and its methanolic extract have shown pronounced antitumor and immunomodulatory effect *in vitro* in Dalton's lymphoma ascites and Ehrlich ascites carcinoma cells [88, 89].

Podophyllum Hexandrum linn. (Podophyllin)

Podophyllum hexandrum commonly known as the Himalayan May apple and bantrapushi/giriparpat in Ayurveda is a rich source of podophyllum resin, which can be processed to extract podophyllin. *Podophyllum peltatum* L. or *P. emodi* Wall (syn. *P. hexandnum* Royle) is a good source for the aryltetralin-type lignin, podophyllotoxin. It is a powerful anticancer agent acting through mitotic inhibition, nuclear fragmentation, and impaired spindle formation, causing necrosis. Podophyllotoxin derivatives like etoposide, etopophos (etoposide phosphate), and teniposide may have anti-viral and antineoplastic properties [90]. Current research on these compounds is focused on structural optimization of podo and developing derivate with superior anticancer activity with minimal side effect and development of alternative and renewable sources of podophyllotoxin.

Semecarpus Anacardium

Semecarpus anacardium is a native of India and is known as Bhallaatak. It is closely related to cashew. Crude extract from *Semecarpus anacardium* (chloroform fraction) has been shown to possess anti-tumor activity against various leukemia, lymphomas, and gliomas. The extract showed protection from hepatocarcinoma due to its immune stimulant action and also normalized alpha-fetoprotein levels. It normalized glycoprotein and mineral content in cancerous tissues and prevented carcinogen activation by inducing phase I and phase II biotransformation enzymes. A regression was observed and cell necrosis prevention was seen on administration of *S. anacardium* extract to hepatocarcinoma in animals. Several Ayurvedic formulations containing *Semecarpus anacardium* have been shown to be beneficial against oesophageal, urinary bladder, liver, breast cancer and chronic myeloid leukaemia. Semecarpus nuts are rich in bioflavonoids which are proven cytotoxic agents [91]. Bhilawanol and anacardic acids are the phytoconstituents responsible for the irritation, blisters, toxicity and contact dermatitis.

The Śodhana procedure of Bhallātaka includes soaking the fruits in Gomūtra, Godugdha and rubbing it on brick gravels. After removing the thalamus portions, the fruits are kept either in Gomūtra (for 7 days) or Godugdha (for 7 days), which are finally washed with water. The seeds are then shifted to a bag containing brick gravels (for 3 days), rubbed thoroughly and dried. During the process of Śodhana of Bhāllataka, coconut oil is applied to the exposed body parts of the persons involved in the processing to reduce the chances of dermatitis [23].

Tinospora Cordifolia

Tinospora cordifolia (WILLD.) is commonly known as Guduchi, Giloy or Amritha. Also known as heart-leaved moonseed, it is a large, glabrous, deciduous climbing shrub belonging to the family Menispermaceae. It is distributed throughout tropical Indian subcontinent and China, ascending to an altitude of 300 m. Guduchi has various therapeutic properties like general tonic, antiperiodic, anti-spasmodic, anti-inflammatory, antiarthritic, anti-allergic and antidiabetic and widely used in veterinary folk medicine and Ayurvedic system of medicine [92 -

94]. Guduchi has been shown to be effective against throat cancer with little side effects [95].

To date, a lot of work has been done on anticancer potential of *T. cordifolia* but very few active constituents have been isolated from the extracts and evaluated for anticancer activity. It exerts its anticancer potential by various mechanisms like induction of caspase-3 activated DNase mediated apoptosis in EAT cells [96], reducing the GSH concentration and increasing the lipid peroxidation in tumor cells in Ehrlich ascites carcinoma bearing mice [97], augmenting proliferation of thymocytes with a concomitant decrease in thymocyte apoptosis thus retarding tumor growth and prolonging survival of tumor-bearing mice [96], activating tumor-associated macrophages and showing the antitumor effect on the spontaneous T-cell lymphoma [99, 100]. Recently, a polysaccharide-rich fraction and Octacosanol a long-chain aliphatic alcohol isolated from of *T. cordifolia* have been shown to decrease metastatic potential of B16F-10 melanoma cells and angiogenesis, respectively [101 - 103]. *T. cordifolia* constitutes many immunomodulatory principles like syringin and cordiol cordioside and cordiofolioside A, which enhance the host immune system by increasing immunoglobulin and blood leukocyte levels and by the stimulation of stem cell proliferation. This may prevent the development of tumor cells and immunosuppression in various cancers [104].

Vinca Rosea

It is commonly known as the Madagascar periwinkle [*Catharanthus roseus* (L.) G. Don]. It is the only source of the monoterpenoid indole alkaloids (MIAs), vinblastine and vincristine. Microtubules in the spindle fibers are depolymerized by vinblastine and vincristine thus combating a wide range of cancers [9].

Vitis Vinifera

Vitis vinifera L. (Vitaceae) [common grape vine] Turkish name, "Asma", is a perennial liana, climber. It is native to Asia which was later introduced in Europe and Mediterranean region. Several traditional medications have been derived from various parts of the plant especially the fruit [105]. "Darakchasava", an Indian preparation dating almost 2000 years ago was prepared from *Vitis vinifera* L. was the first known grape extract for human use. It was used as a health tonic as well as a cardiotonic. This formulation contains polyphenols like resveratrol and pterostilbene known for their antioxidant and anticancer activities [106]. Resveratrol is an established antioxidant and antimutagen; it inhibits cyclooxygenase and hydroperoxidase functions to mediate anti-inflammatory effects and induces human promyelocytic leukemia cell differentiation [107]. Ayurvedic (Indian) medicine uses Grapes, its seeds and leaves as a diuretic to soothe the digestive tract by reducing constipation, improving circulation, reducing inflammation and bleeding, preventing diarrhea, and detoxifying the body [108]. Reports showed that trans-astringent, a plant stilbenoid and its aglycon trans-piceatannol found in wine, was found to be active against mouse mammary carcinoma. It functioned differently from that of trans-resveratrol, a known antioxidant [109].

Withania Somnifera

Ashwagandha (*Withania somnifera* L. Dunal) roots and dried leaves are commonly used in Ayurveda for different health-promoting effects. Various extracts have shown promising antitumor activities *in vivo* and *in vitro*. Its extract showed synergistic effects and potentiates the immunomodulating properties of other anticancer agents. Water extract of ashwagandha leaves have also been shown to have cytotoxic and tumor suppression potential in human osteosarcoma, breast carcinoma and fibrocarcinoma cell lines [110]. The major withanolide, Withaferin A has also been found to inhibit proliferation of various cancer cell lines. Apoptosis occurs through reactive oxygen generation, mitochondrial dysfunction, kinase inhibition and inhibition of hyperphosphorylation. Other withanolides have also shown protective effects on various cancer cell lines and may have a similar mechanism of action owing to their structure similarity [111].

AYURVEDIC FORMULATIONS WITH ANTICANCER AND RADIO PROTECTIVE POTENTIAL

Amritaprasham contains *Holstemma annulare, Vigna vexilata, Phaseolus adenanthus, Glycyrrhiza glabra, Zingiber officinale, Asparagus recemosus, Boerhaavia diffusa, Sida retusa, Clerodendrum serratum, Macuna pruriens, Hedychium spicatium, Phylanthus niruri, Piper longum, Vitis viniferra, Embelica officinalis, Purerira tuberose, Saccharum officinalum, Piper nigrum, Cinnamomum zeylanica, Elettaria cardamomum, Garcinia Morella*, and *Mesua ferrea* It has been shown to reduce radiotoxic effects [112].

Arkeshwara Rasa is a mixture of mercuric sulfide was then powdered and mixed with latex of *C. procera* and decoction of *Triphala* with *Plumbago. zeylanica* whole plants. It showed anti- proliferative activity in pancreatic (MIA-PaCa-2) cancer cells [113].

Ashwagandha rasayana contains *Withania sominifera, Purerira tuberosa, Hemidesmus indicus, Ciminum cuminum, Aloe barbidensis, Vitis vinifera, Elettaria cardamomum, Zingiber officinale, Piper nigrum*, and *Piper*. It has been shown to reduce radiotoxic effects [112].

Brahma Rasayana is a mixture of *Emblica officinalis* (20%), *Terminalia chebula* (6.67%), *Urarira pitca, Desmodium gangeticum, Gmelina arborea, Solanum nigrum, Tribulus terrestris, Aegle marmelos, Premna tomentosa, Stereospermum suvaeolens, Sida rhombilfolia, Boerhaavia diffusa, Ricinus communis, Vigna vexilata, Phaseolus adenanthus, Asperagus racemosus, Holostemma annulare, Leptadenia reticulate, Desmostachya bipinnata, Saccharum officinarum, Oryza malampuzhensis, Cinnamomum iners, Elettaria cardamomum, Cyperus rotundus, Curcuma longa, Piper longum, Aquilaria agallocha, Santalum album, Centella asciatica, Mesua ferrea, Clitoria ternate, Acorus calamus, Scirpus crossus, Glycyrrhiza glabra* and *Embelia ribes*. It has been shown to reduce radiotoxic effects [112].

Chyawanprash contains *Emblica officinalis, Bambusa arundinacea, Agele marmelos, Clerodendrum phlomidis, Oroxylum indicum, Gmelina arborea, Stereospermum suaveolens, Sida cordifolia, Desmodium gangeticum, Uraria picta, Teramnus labialis, Piper longum, Tribulus terrestris, Solanum indicum, Solanum xanthocarpum, Pistacia integerrima, Phaseolus trilobus, Phyllanthus niruri, Vitis vinifera, Leptadenia reticulata, Inula racemosa, Aquilaria agallocha, Tinospora cordifolia, Terminalia chebula, Ellettaria cardamomum, Cinnamom cassia, Cinnamom iners, Habenaria intermedia, Microstylis walichii, Microstylis museifera, Mesua ferra, Hedychium spicatum, Cyperus rotundus, Boerhaavia diffusa, Polygonatum verticillatum, Nymphaea alba, Santalum album, Pueraria tuberosa, Adhatoda vasica, Roscoea alpina, Martynia diandra*, and *Sesamum indicum*. It has been shown to reduce radiotoxic effects [112].

Indukantha Ghritha contains *Zingiber officinale* (Dried rhizome), *Plumbago zeylanica* (Root) *Plumbago rosea* (Root), *Piper chaba* (Root), *Piper longum* (Fruit & Root), *Tribulus terrestris* (Fruit & Root), *Desmodium gangeticum* (Root), *Pseudarthria viscida* (Root), *Solanum melongena* (Root), *Solanum xanthocarpum* (Root), *Oroxylum indicum* (Root), *Stereospermum suaveolens* (Root), *Premna serratifolia* (Root), *Gmelina arborea* (Root), *Aegle marmelos* (Root), *Cedrus deodara* (Heartwood), *Holoptelea integrifolia* (Bark). It shows anticancer potential by stimulating the immune system [114].

Maharishi Amrit Kalash (MAK) is an ayurvedic polyherbal formulation. The ingredients of MAK-4 are T*erminalia chebula, Phyllanthus emblica, Elettaria cardamomum, Cyperus rotundus, Curcuma longa, Piper longum, Santalum album, Cyperus scariosus, Mesuaferrea, Convolvulus pluricaulis, Glycyrrhiza glabra, Embelia ribes, Centella asiatica*, ghee, honey, and sugar.

The ingredients of MAK-5 are *Withania somnifera, Glycyrrhiza glabra, Ipomoea digitata, Asparagus adescendens, Emblica officinalis, Tinospora cordifolia,*

Asparagus racemosus, Convolvulus pluricaulis, Vitex trifolia, Argyreia speciosa, Curculigo orchioides, Capparis aphylla, Acacia arabica. Both MAK4 and 5 have been shown to have anticancer activity in both human and murine melanoma and neuroblastoma cells [115, 116, 117]. MAK-4 may enhance lymphocyte proliferation, while MAK-5 may have both lymphocyte responsiveness as well as macrophage function, thus acting as immune modulators [118]. It has been shown that MAK-5 may potentiate macrophages in killing tumor cells. These macrophages may also produce more NO upon activation with LPS- or IFN-than macrophages from animals not on MAK-5 supplemented diet [119]. MAK-4-supplement may significantly reduce metastatic lung nodules in Lewis lung carcinoma [120]. While MAK-4 has also been shown to reduce 7,12-dimethylbenz(a)anthracene and DMBA-induced mammary tumors in rats [121, 122]. Based on a clinical trial on 214 patients suffering from breast cancer MAK if administered with cyclophosphamide, methotrexate and 5-flourouracil may reduce the toxicities of the above chemotherapeutic agents and improve their quality of life [123].

Narasimha Rasayana contains *Acacia catechu, Plumbago xylanica, Xylia dolabriformis, Pterocarpus marsupium, Embelia ribes, Semecarpus anacardium, Eclipta alba, Terminalia chebula, Embelica officinalis*, and *Terminalia belerica*. It has been shown to reduce radiotoxic effects [124].

Panchakola, is an herbal formulation. Pippali (*Piper longum*), Pippalimula (root of the *Piper longum*), Chavya (*Piper chaba*), Chitraka (*Plumbago zeylanica*), and Sunthi (*Zingiber officinale*) are the ingredients of panchakol. It has been shown to have cytotoxic potential in MCF-7 breast cancer cell lines [125].

Triphala is an Ayurvedic herbal rasayana formula consisting of equal parts of three myrobalans, taken without seed: Amalaki (*Emblica officinalis*), Bibhitaki (*Terminalia bellirica*), and Haritaki (*Terminalia chebula*). It has shown cytotoxic potential in breast cancer cell lines [126].

CONCLUSION

Cancer, one of the deadliest and rapidly spreading disease is the leading cause of deaths throughout the world. Scientists and clinicians are making their best efforts to fight this disease but effective treatment is still awaited. Modern medications are associated with various side effects so clinicians throughout the world are turning to Ayurveda and alternate and complementary (CAM) therapy. Many herbs incorporated in different formulations work on different biological pathways and help to prevent cancer or reduce the side effects of conventional anti-cancer therapy. Nine plant-derived compounds including vinblastine, vincristine, etoposide, teniposide, taxol, navelbine, taxotere, topotecan and irinotecan are in clinical use as anticancer drugs and many other compounds are under investigation. Each herb contains multiple active phytoconstituents that often operate synergistically producing therapeutic benefits and lowering the risks of adverse effects, and avoids the need for supplemental therapy to manage cancer cachexia. Thus, it is now essential to raise awareness and encourage randomized clinical trials on promising phytochemicals as well as Ayurvedic formulations so that new alternate medicine therapies may be integrated with current treatment approaches for successful management and treatment of cancer.

CONSENT FOR PUBLICATION

Not applicable.

CONFLICT OF INTEREST

The author(s) confirm that this chapter content has no conflict of interest.

ACKNOWLEDGEMENT

Declared none.

REFERENCES

[1]   Anand, P.; Kunnumakkara, A.B.; Sundaram, C.; Harikumar, K.B.; Tharakan, S.T.; Lai, O.S.; Sung, B.; Aggarwal, B.B. Cancer is a preventable disease that requires major lifestyle changes. *Pharm. Res.,* **2008**, *25*(9), 2097-2116.
[http://dx.doi.org/10.1007/s11095-008-9661-9] [PMID: 18626751]

[2]   Chauhan, A.; Semwal, D.K.; Mishra, S.P.; Semwal, R.B. Ayurvedic research and methodology: Present status and future strategies. *Ayu,* **2015**, *36*(4), 364-369.
[http://dx.doi.org/10.4103/0974-8520.190699] [PMID: 27833362]

[3]   Sumantran, V.N.; Tillu, G. Cancer, inflammation, and insights from ayurveda. *Evid. Based Complement. Alternat. Med.,* **2012**, *2012*, 306346.
[http://dx.doi.org/10.1155/2012/306346] [PMID: 22829853]

[4]   Dhruva, A.; Hecht, F.M.; Miaskowski, C.; Kaptchuk, T.J.; Bodeker, G.; Abrams, D.; Lad, V.; Adler, S.R. Correlating traditional Ayurvedic and modern medical perspectives on cancer: results of a qualitative study. *J. Altern. Complement. Med.,* **2014**, *20*(5), 364-370.
[http://dx.doi.org/10.1089/acm.2013.0259] [PMID: 24341342]

[5]   Balachandran, P.; Govindarajan, R. Cancer--an ayurvedic perspective. *Pharmacol. Res.,* **2005**, *51*(1), 19-30.
[http://dx.doi.org/10.1016/j.phrs.2004.04.010] [PMID: 15519531]

[6]   National Cancer Institute. *Cancer treatment,* https://www.cancer.gov/about-cancer/treatment

[7]   Kumar, A.; Dubey, S.D.; Prakas, S.; Singh, P. Principle of Dravyaguna (Ayurvedic Pharmacology). *Biomed. Pharmacol. J.,* **2011**, *4*(1), 147-152.
[http://dx.doi.org/10.13005/bpj/273]

[8]   Savrikar, S.S.; Ravishankar, B. Bhaishajya Kalpanaa - the Ayurvedic pharmaceutics - an overview. *Afr. J. Tradit. Complement. Altern. Med.,* **2010**, *7*(3), 174-184.
[http://dx.doi.org/10.4314/ajtcam.v7i3.54773] [PMID: 21461144]

[9]   Srivastava, V.; Negi, A.S.; Kumar, J.K.; Gupta, M.M.; Khanuja, S.P. Plant-based anticancer molecules: a chemical and biological profile of some important leads. *Bioorg. Med. Chem.,* **2005,** *13*(21), 5892-5908.
        [http://dx.doi.org/10.1016/j.bmc.2005.05.066] [PMID: 16129603]

[10]   Newman, D.J.; Cragg, G.M.; Holbeck, S.; Sausville, E.A. Natural products and derivatives as leads to cell cycle pathway targets in cancer chemotherapy. *Curr. Cancer Drug Targets,* **2002,** *2*(4), 279-308.
        [http://dx.doi.org/10.2174/1568009023333791] [PMID: 12470208]

[11]   Kumara, P.M.; Soujanya, K.N.; Ravikanth, G.; Vasudeva, R.; Ganeshaiah, K.N.; Shaanker, R.U. Rohitukine, a chromone alkaloid and a precursor of flavopiridol, is produced by endophytic fungi isolated from Dysoxylum binectariferum Hook.f and Amoora rohituka (Roxb).Wight & Arn. *Phytomedicine,* **2014,** *21*(4), 541-546.
        [http://dx.doi.org/10.1016/j.phymed.2013.09.019] [PMID: 24215673]

[12]   Meijer, L.; Raymond, E. Roscovitine and other purines as kinase inhibitors. From starfish oocytes to clinical trials. *Acc. Chem. Res.,* **2003,** *36*(6), 417-425.
        [http://dx.doi.org/10.1021/ar0201198] [PMID: 12809528]

[13]   Chang, Y.T.; Gray, N.S.; Rosania, G.R.; Sutherlin, D.P.; Kwon, S.; Norman, T.C.; Sarohia, R.; Leost, M.; Meijer, L.; Schultz, P.G. Synthesis and application of functionally diverse 2,6,9-trisubstituted purine libraries as CDK inhibitors. *Chem. Biol.,* **1999,** *6*(6), 361-375.
        [http://dx.doi.org/10.1016/S1074-5521(99)80048-9] [PMID: 10375538]

[14]   Reddy, L.; Odhav, B.; Bhoola, K.D. Natural products for cancer prevention: a global perspective. *Pharmacol. Ther.,* **2003,** *99*(1), 1-13.
        [http://dx.doi.org/10.1016/S0163-7258(03)00042-1] [PMID: 12804695]

[15]   Desai, V.B.; Sirsi, M.; Shankarappa, M.; Kasturibai, A.R. Studies on the toxicity of Abrus precatorius L. I. Effect of aqueous extracts of seeds on mitosis and meiosis in grasshopper, Poecilocera picta. *Indian J. Exp. Biol.,* **1966,** *4*(3), 164-166.
        [PMID: 5966956]

[16]   Reddy, V.V.S.; Sirsi, M. Effect of Abrus precatorius L. on experimental tumors. *Cancer Res.,* **1969,** *29*(7), 1447-1451.
        [PMID: 5799161]

[17]   Wei, C.H.; Hartman, F.C.; Pfuderer, P.; Yang, W.K. Purification and characterization of two major toxic proteins from seeds of Abrus precatorius. *J. Biol. Chem.,* **1974,** *249*(10), 3061-3067.
        [PMID: 4830236]

[18]   Lin, J.Y.; Lee, T.C.; Tung, T.C. Isolation of antitumor proteins abrin-A and abrin-B from Abrus precatorius. *Int. J. Pept. Protein Res.,* **1978,** *12*(5), 311-317.
        [http://dx.doi.org/10.1111/j.1399-3011.1978.tb02902.x] [PMID: 744690]

[19]   Absar, N.; Funatsu, G. Purification and characterization of Abrus precatorius agglutinin. *Nihon Shokuhin Kogakkaishi,* **1984,** *29*(2-3), 103-115.

[20]   Bhutia, S.K.; Mallick, S.K.; Stevens, S.M.; Prokai, L.; Vishwanatha, J.K.; Maiti, T.K. Induction of mitochondria-dependent apoptosis by Abrus agglutinin derived peptides in human cervical cancer cell. *Toxicol. In Vitro,* **2008,** *22*(2), 344-351.
        [http://dx.doi.org/10.1016/j.tiv.2007.09.016] [PMID: 18024076]

[21]   Ramnath, V.; Kuttan, G.; Kuttan, R. Antitumour effect of abrin on transplanted tumours in mice. *Indian J. Physiol. Pharmacol.,* **2002,** *46*(1), 69-77.
        [PMID: 12024960]

[22]   Ramnath, V.; Kuttan, G.; Kuttan, R. Effect of abrin on cell-mediated immune responses in mice. *Immunopharmacol. Immunotoxicol.,* **2006,** *28*(2), 259-268.
        [http://dx.doi.org/10.1080/08923970600816764] [PMID: 16873094]

[23]   Maurya, S.K.; Seth, A.; Laloo, D.; Singh, N.K.; Gautam, D.N.; Singh, A.K. Śodhana: An Ayurvedic

process for detoxification and modification of therapeutic activities of poisonous medicinal plants. *Anc. Sci. Life,* **2015**, *34*(4), 188-197.
[http://dx.doi.org/10.4103/0257-7941.160862] [PMID: 26283803]

[24] Senapati, S.K.; Dey, S.; Dwivedi, S.K.; Swarup, D. Effect of garlic (Allium sativum L.) extract on tissue lead level in rats. *J. Ethnopharmacol.,* **2001**, *76*(3), 229-232.
[http://dx.doi.org/10.1016/S0378-8741(01)00237-9] [PMID: 11448543]

[25] Nagini, S. Cancer chemoprevention by garlic and its organosulfur compounds-panacea or promise? *Anticancer. Agents Med. Chem.,* **2008**, *8*(3), 313-321.
[http://dx.doi.org/10.2174/187152008783961879] [PMID: 18393790]

[26] Wargovich, M.J. Diallyl sulfide, a flavor component of garlic (Allium sativum), inhibits dimethylhydrazine-induced colon cancer. *Carcinogenesis,* **1987**, *8*(3), 487-489.
[http://dx.doi.org/10.1093/carcin/8.3.487] [PMID: 3815744]

[27] El-Bayoumy, K.; Sinha, R.; Pinto, J.T.; Rivlin, R.S. Cancer chemoprevention by garlic and garlic-containing sulfur and selenium compounds. *J. Nutr.,* **2006**, *136*(3) Suppl., 864S-869S.
[http://dx.doi.org/10.1093/jn/136.3.864S] [PMID: 16484582]

[28] Shukla, Y.; Kalra, N. Cancer chemoprevention with garlic and its constituents. *Cancer Lett.,* **2007**, *247*(2), 167-181.
[http://dx.doi.org/10.1016/j.canlet.2006.05.009] [PMID: 16793203]

[29] Capasso, F.; Borrelli, F.; Capasso, R. Aloe and its therapeutic use. *Phytother. Res.,* **1998**, *12*, S124-S127.
[http://dx.doi.org/10.1002/(SICI)1099-1573(1998)12:1+<S124::AID-PTR271>3.0.CO;2-X]

[30] Reynold, T. The compounds in Aloe leaf exudates: a review. *Bot. J. Linn. Soc.,* **1985**, (90), 157-177.
[http://dx.doi.org/10.1111/j.1095-8339.1985.tb00377.x]

[31] Chen, S.H.; Lin, K.Y.; Chang, C.C.; Fang, C.L.; Lin, C.P. Aloe-emodin-induced apoptosis in human gastric carcinoma cells. *Food Chem. Toxicol.,* **2007**, *45*(11), 2296-2303.
[http://dx.doi.org/10.1016/j.fct.2007.06.005] [PMID: 17637488]

[32] Lin, J.G.; Chen, G.W.; Li, T.M.; Chouh, S.T.; Tan, T.W.; Chung, J.G. Aloe-emodin induces apoptosis in T24 human bladder cancer cells through the p53 dependent apoptotic pathway. *J. Urol.,* **2006**, *175*(1), 343-347.
[http://dx.doi.org/10.1016/S0022-5347(05)00005-4] [PMID: 16406939]

[33] Acevedo-Duncan, M.; Russell, C.; Patel, S.; Patel, R. Aloe-emodin modulates PKC isozymes, inhibits proliferation, and induces apoptosis in U-373MG glioma cells. *Int. Immunopharmacol.,* **2004**, *4*(14), 1775-1784.
[http://dx.doi.org/10.1016/j.intimp.2004.07.012] [PMID: 15531293]

[34] Wasserman, L.; Avigad, S.; Beery, E.; Nordenberg, J.; Fenig, E. The effect of aloe emodin on the proliferation of a new merkel carcinoma cell line. *Am. J. Dermatopathol.,* **2002**, *24*(1), 17-22.
[http://dx.doi.org/10.1097/00000372-200202000-00003] [PMID: 11803275]

[35] Nićiforović, A.; Adzić, M.; Spasić, S.D.; Radojcić, M.B. Antitumor effects of a natural anthracycline analog (Aloin) involve altered activity of antioxidant enzymes in HeLaS3 cells. *Cancer Biol. Ther.,* **2007**, *6*(8), 1200-1205.
[http://dx.doi.org/10.4161/cbt.6.8.4383] [PMID: 17726368]

[36] Im, S.A.; Oh, S.T.; Song, S.; Kim, M.R.; Kim, D.S.; Woo, S.S.; Jo, T.H.; Park, Y.I.; Lee, C.K. Identification of optimal molecular size of modified Aloe polysaccharides with maximum immunomodulatory activity. *Int. Immunopharmacol.,* **2005**, *5*(2), 271-279.
[http://dx.doi.org/10.1016/j.intimp.2004.09.031] [PMID: 15652758]

[37] Liu, C.; Leung, M.Y.K.; Koon, J.C.M.; Zhu, L.F.; Hui, Y.Z.; Yu, B.; Fung, K.P. Macrophage activation by polysaccharide biological response modifier isolated from Aloe vera L. var. chinensis (Haw.) Berg. *Int. Immunopharmacol.,* **2006**, *6*(11), 1634-1641.

[http://dx.doi.org/10.1016/j.intimp.2006.04.013] [PMID: 16979117]

[38]   Zhang, L.; Tizard, I.R. Activation of a mouse macrophage cell line by acemannan: the major carbohydrate fraction from Aloe vera gel. *Immunopharmacology,* **1996**, *35*(2), 119-128.
[http://dx.doi.org/10.1016/S0162-3109(96)00135-X] [PMID: 8956975]

[39]   Akev, N.; Turkay, G.; Can, A.; Gurel, A.; Yildiz, F.; Yardibi, H.; Ekiz, E.E.; Uzun, H. Tumour preventive effect of Aloe vera leaf pulp lectin (Aloctin I) on Ehrlich ascites tumours in mice. *Phytother. Res.,* **2007**, *21*(11), 1070-1075.
[http://dx.doi.org/10.1002/ptr.2215] [PMID: 17685385]

[40]   Saraswathi, V.; Ramamoorthy, N.; Subramaniam, S.; Mathuram, V.; Gunasekaran, P.; Govindasamy, S. Inhibition of glycolysis and respiration of sarcoma-180 cells by echitamine chloride. *Chemotherapy,* **1998**, *44*(3), 198-205.
[http://dx.doi.org/10.1159/000007115] [PMID: 9612610]

[41]   Saraswathi, V.; Mathuram, V.; Subramanian, S.; Govindasamy, S. Modulation of the impaired drug metabolism in sarcoma-180-bearing mice by echitamine chloride. *Cancer Biochem. Biophys.,* **1999**, *17*(1-2), 79-88.
[PMID: 10738904]

[42]   Viswanathan, S.; Ramamoorthy, N.; Subramaniam, S.; Mathuram, V.; Govindasamy, S. Enhancement of the cytotoxic effects of Echitamine chloride by vitamin A: an *in vitro* study on Ehrlich ascites carcinoma cell culture. *Indian J. Pharmacol.,* **1997**, *29*(4), 244-249.

[43]   Saraswathi, V.; Subramanian, S.; Ramamoorthy, N. Mathuram. V.; Govindasamy, S. *In vitro* cytotoxicity of echitamine chloride and Adriamycin on Ehrlich ascites carcinoma cell cultures. *Med. Sci. Res.,* **1997**, *25*(3), 167-170.

[44]   Jagetia, G.C.; Baliga, M.S. Evaluation of anticancer activity of the alkaloid fraction of Alstonia scholaris (Sapthaparna) *in vitro* and *in vivo. Phytother. Res.,* **2006**, *20*(2), 103-109.
[http://dx.doi.org/10.1002/ptr.1810] [PMID: 16444661]

[45]   Rabi, T.; Wang, L.; Banerjee, S. Novel triterpenoid 25-hydroxy-3-oxoolean-12-en-28-oic acid induces growth arrest and apoptosis in breast cancer cells. *Breast Cancer Res. Treat.,* **2007**, *101*(1), 27-36.
[http://dx.doi.org/10.1007/s10549-006-9275-z] [PMID: 17028990]

[46]   Rabi, T.; Ramachandran, C.; Fonseca, H.B.; Nair, R.P.K.; Alamo, A.; Melnick, S.J.; Escalon, E. Novel drug amooranin induces apoptosis through caspase activity in human breast carcinoma cell lines. *Breast Cancer Res. Treat.,* **2003**, *80*(3), 321-330.
[http://dx.doi.org/10.1023/A:1024911925623] [PMID: 14503804]

[47]   Ramachandran, C.; Nair, P.K.; Alamo, A.; Cochrane, C.B.; Escalon, E.; Melnick, S.J. Anticancer effects of amooranin in human colon carcinoma cell line *in vitro* and in nude mice xenografts. *Int. J. Cancer,* **2006**, *119*(10), 2443-2454.
[http://dx.doi.org/10.1002/ijc.22174] [PMID: 16894569]

[48]   Ramachandran, C.; Rabi, T.; Fonseca, H.B.; Melnick, S.J.; Escalon, E.A. Novel plant triterpenoid drug amooranin overcomes multidrug resistance in human leukemia and colon carcinoma cell lines. *Int. J. Cancer,* **2003**, *105*(6), 784-789.
[http://dx.doi.org/10.1002/ijc.11180] [PMID: 12767063]

[49]   *Anacardium   occidentale*   L.   http://   www.hort.purdue.edu/newcrop/duke_energy/Anacardium_occidentale.html **2018**.

[50]   Kubo, I.; Ochi, M.; Vieir, A.; Komatsu, P.C. Antitumor agents from the cashew (Anacardium occidentale) apple juice. Sakae. *J. Agric. Food Chem.,* **1993**, *41*(6), 1012-1015.
[http://dx.doi.org/10.1021/jf00030a035]

[51]   Ji, L.; Liu, T.; Liu, J.; Chen, Y.; Wang, Z. Andrographolide inhibits human hepatoma-derived Hep3B cell growth through the activation of c-Jun N-terminal kinase. *Planta Med.,* **2007**, *73*(13), 1397-1401.
[http://dx.doi.org/10.1055/s-2007-990230] [PMID: 17918040]

[52]   Jiang, C.G.; Li, J.B.; Liu, F.R.; Wu, T.; Yu, M.; Xu, H.M. Andrographolide inhibits the adhesion of gastric cancer cells to endothelial cells by blocking E-selectin expression. *Anticancer Res.,* **2007**, *27*(4B), 2439-2447.
[PMID: 17695536]

[53]   Sheeja, K.; Guruvayoorappan, C.; Kuttan, G. Antiangiogenic activity of Andrographis paniculata extract and andrographolide. *Int. Immunopharmacol.,* **2007**, *7*(2), 211-221.
[http://dx.doi.org/10.1016/j.intimp.2006.10.002] [PMID: 17178389]

[54]   Kumar, R.A.; Sridevi, K.; Kumar, N.V.; Nanduri, S.; Rajagopal, S. Anticancer and immunostimulatory compounds from Andrographis paniculata. *J. Ethnopharmacol.,* **2004**, *92*(2-3), 291-295.
[http://dx.doi.org/10.1016/j.jep.2004.03.004] [PMID: 15138014]

[55]   Rajagopal, S.; Kumar, R.A.; Deevi, D.S.; Satyanarayana, C.; Rajagopalan, R. Andrographolide, a potential cancer therapeutic agent isolated from Andrographis paniculata. *J. Exp. Ther. Oncol.,* **2003**, *3*(3), 147-158.
[http://dx.doi.org/10.1046/j.1359-4117.2003.01090.x] [PMID: 14641821]

[56]   Chiu, H.F.; Chih, T.T.; Hsian, Y.M.; Tseng, C.H.; Wu, M.J.; Wu, Y.C. Bullatacin, a potent antitumor Annonaceous acetogenin, induces apoptosis through a reduction of intracellular cAMP and cGMP levels in human hepatoma 2.2.15 cells. *Biochem. Pharmacol.,* **2003**, *65*(3), 319-327.
[http://dx.doi.org/10.1016/S0006-2952(02)01554-X] [PMID: 12527325]

[57]   Chih, H.W.; Chiu, H.F.; Tang, K.S.; Chang, F.R.; Wu, Y.C. Bullatacin, a potent antitumor annonaceous acetogenin, inhibits proliferation of human hepatocarcinoma cell line 2.2.15 by apoptosis induction. *Life Sci.,* **2001**, *69*(11), 1321-1331.
[http://dx.doi.org/10.1016/S0024-3205(01)01209-7] [PMID: 11521756]

[58]   Fu, L.W.; Pan, Q.C.; Liang, Y.J.; Huang, H.B. Circumvention of tumor multidrug resistance by a new annonaceous acetogenin: atemoyacin-B. *Zhongguo Yao Li Xue Bao,* **1999**, *20*(5), 435-439.
[PMID: 10678092]

[59]   Fu, L.W.; He, L.R.; Liang, Y.J.; Chen, L.M.; Xiong, H.Y.; Yang, X.P.; Pan, Q.C. Experimental chemotherapy against xenografts derived from multidrug resistant KBv200 cells and parental drug-sensitive KB cells in nude mice by annonaceous acetogenin 89-2. *Yao Xue Xue Bao,* **2003**, *38*(8), 565-570.
[PMID: 14628443]

[60]   Parmar, C.; Kaushal, M.K. Berberis aristata.*Wild Fruits*; Kalyani Publishers: New Delhi, **1982**, pp. 10-14.

[61]   Anis, K.V.; Rajeshkumar, N.V.; Kuttan, R. Inhibition of chemical carcinogenesis by berberine in rats and mice. *J. Pharm. Pharmacol.,* **2001**, *53*(5), 763-768.
[http://dx.doi.org/10.1211/0022357011775901] [PMID: 11370717]

[62]   Agharkar, S.P. *Medicinal plants of Bombay presidency*; Scientific Publ India, **1991**, pp. 48-49.

[63]   Warrier, P.K.; Nambiar, V.P.K.; Mankutty, C. *Indian Medicinal Plants*; Orient Longman: Chennai, **1994**, pp. 341-345.

[64]   Lhinhatrakool, T.; Sutthivaiyakit, S. 19-Nor- and 18,20-epoxy-cardenolides from the leaves of Calotropis gigantea. *J. Nat. Prod.,* **2006**, *69*(8), 1249-1251.
[http://dx.doi.org/10.1021/np060249f] [PMID: 16933890]

[65]   Kapoor, L.D. Ed Handbook of ayurvedic medicinal plants: herbal reference library. **1990**; p. 157.

[66]   Dhar, M.L.; Dhar, M.M.; Dhawan, B.N.; Mehrotra, B.N.; Ray, C. Screening of Indian plants for biological activity: I. *Indian J. Exp. Biol.,* **1968**, *6*(4), 232-247.
[PMID: 5720682]

[67]   Ma, L. Xie, C.; Li, J.; Lou, F.; Hu, L.; Daturametelins, H. I, and J: 3 new withanolide glycosides from Datura metel L. *Chem. Biodivers.,* **2006**, *3*(2), 180-186.

[http://dx.doi.org/10.1002/cbdv.200690021] [PMID: 17193256]

[68] Pan, Y.; Wang, X.; Hu, X. Cytotoxic withanolides from the flowers of Datura metel. *J. Nat. Prod.,* **2007**, *70*(7), 1127-1132.
[http://dx.doi.org/10.1021/np070096b] [PMID: 17583953]

[69] Dutta, S.K.; Sanyal, U.P.; Chakraborty, S.K. A modified method of isolation of indicine N-oxide from Heliotropium indicum and its antitumor activity against Ehrlich ascites carcinoma and sarcoma 180. *Indian Journal of Cancer Chemotherapy,* **1987**, *9*(2), 73-77.

[70] Kugelman, M.; Liu, W.C.; Axelrod, M.; McBride, T.J.; Rao, K.V. Indicine-N-oxide: the antitumor principle of Heliotropium indicum. *Lloydia,* **1976**, *39*(2-3), 125-128.
[PMID: 948236]

[71] Ohnuma, T.; Sridhar, K.S.; Ratner, L.H.; Holland, J.F. Phase I study of indicine N-oxide in patients with advanced cancer. *Cancer Treat. Rep.,* **1982**, *66*(7), 1509-1515.
[PMID: 7093966]

[72] Khan, M.A.; Chen, H.C.; Tania, M.; Zhang, D.Z. Anticancer activities of *Nigella sativa* (black cumin). *Afr. J. Tradit. Complement. Altern. Med.,* **2011**, *8*(5) Suppl., 226-232.
[PMID: 22754079]

[73] Thyagarajan, S.P.; Subramanian, S.; Thirunalasundari, T.; Venkateswaran, P.S.; Blumberg, B.S. Effect of Phyllanthus amarus on chronic carriers of hepatitis B virus. *Lancet,* **1988**, *2*(8614), 764-766.
[http://dx.doi.org/10.1016/S0140-6736(88)92416-6] [PMID: 2901611]

[74] Joy, K.L.; Kuttan, R. Inhibition by Phyllanthus amarus of hepatocarcinogenesis induced by N-nitrosodiethylamine. *J. Clin. Biochem. Nutr.,* **1998**, (24), 133-139.
[http://dx.doi.org/10.3164/jcbn.24.133]

[75] Jeena, K.J.; Joy, K.L.; Kuttan, R. Effect of Emblica officinalis, Phyllanthus amarus and Picrorrhiza kurroa on N-nitrosodiethylamine induced hepatocarcinogenesis. *Cancer Lett.,* **1999**, *136*(1), 11-16.
[http://dx.doi.org/10.1016/S0304-3835(98)00294-8] [PMID: 10211933]

[76] Rajeshkumar, N.V.; Joy, K.L.; Kuttan, G.; Ramsewak, R.S.; Nair, M.G.; Kuttan, R. Antitumour and anticarcinogenic activity of Phyllanthus amarus extract. *J. Ethnopharmacol.,* **2002**, *81*(1), 17-22.
[http://dx.doi.org/10.1016/S0378-8741(01)00419-6] [PMID: 12020923]

[77] Kumar, K.B.H.; Kuttan, R. Chemoprotective activity of an extract of Phyllanthus amarus against cyclophosphamide induced toxicity in mice. *Phytomedicine: International Journal of Phytotherapy and Phytopharmacology,* **2005**, *12*(6-7), 494-500.

[78] Leite, D.F.; Kassuya, C.A.; Mazzuco, T.L.; Silvestre, A.; de Melo, L.V.; Rehder, V.L.; Rumjanek, V.M.; Calixto, J.B. The cytotoxic effect and the multidrug resistance reversing action of lignans from Phyllanthus amarus. *Planta Med.,* **2006**, *72*(15), 1353-1358.
[http://dx.doi.org/10.1055/s-2006-951708] [PMID: 17054045]

[79] Ahmed, B.; Masoodi, M.H.; Khan, S. Pharmacological and phytochemical review on picrorrhiza kurroa. *Indian Journal of Natural Products,* **2007**, *23*(2), 3-13.

[80] Jeena, K.J.; Joy, K.L.; Kuttan, R. Effect of Emblica officinalis, Phyllanthus amarus and Picrorrhiza kurroa on N-nitrosodiethylamine induced hepatocarcinogenesis. *Cancer Lett.,* **1999**, *136*(1), 11-16.
[http://dx.doi.org/10.1016/S0304-3835(98)00294-8] [PMID: 10211933]

[81] Joy, K.L.; Rajeshkumar, N.V.; Kuttan, G.; Kuttan, R. Effect of Picrorrhiza kurroa extract on transplanted tumours and chemical carcinogenesis in mice. *J. Ethnopharmacol.,* **2000**, *71*(1-2), 261-266.
[http://dx.doi.org/10.1016/S0378-8741(00)00168-9] [PMID: 10904172]

[82] Senthil, N.; Manoharan, S.; Balakrishnan, S.; Ramachandran, C.R.M.; Radhakrishnan, M. Chemopreventive and antilipidperoxidative efficacy of Piper longum (Linn.) on 7, 12-dimethylbenz (a) anthracene (DMBA) induced hamster buccal pouch carcinogenesis. *J. Appl. Sci. (Faisalabad),* **2007**, *7*(7), 1036-1042.

[http://dx.doi.org/10.3923/jas.2007.1036.1042]

[83]   Selvendiran, K.; Thirunavukkarasu, C.; Singh, J.P.; Padmavathi, R.; Sakthisekaran, D.; Sakthisekaran, D. Chemopreventive effect of piperine on mitochondrial TCA cycle and phase-I and glutathione-metabolizing enzymes in benzo(a)pyrene induced lung carcinogenesis in Swiss albino mice. *Mol. Cell. Biochem.,* **2005**, *271*(1-2), 101-106.
        [http://dx.doi.org/10.1007/s11010-005-5615-2] [PMID: 15881660]

[84]   Selvendiran, K.; Banu, S.M.; Sakthisekaran, D. Oral supplementation of piperine leads to altered phase II enzymes and reduced DNA damage and DNA-protein cross links in Benzo(a)pyrene induced experimental lung carcinogenesis. *Mol. Cell. Biochem.,* **2005**, *268*(1-2), 141-147.
        [http://dx.doi.org/10.1007/s11010-005-3702-z] [PMID: 15724447]

[85]   Selvendiran, K.; Prince Vijeya Singh, J.; Sakthisekaran, D. *In vivo* effect of piperine on serum and tissue glycoprotein levels in benzo(a)pyrene induced lung carcinogenesis in Swiss albino mice. *Pulm. Pharmacol. Ther.,* **2006**, *19*(2), 107-111.
        [http://dx.doi.org/10.1016/j.pupt.2005.04.002] [PMID: 15975841]

[86]   Sunila, E.S.; Kuttan, G. Effect of Piper longum and piperine in cell mediated immune response. *Amala Research Bulletin,* **2005**, *25*, 188-195.

[87]   Pradeep, C.R.; Kuttan, G. Effect of piperine on the inhibition of lung metastasis induced B16F-10 melanoma cells in mice. *Clin. Exp. Metastasis,* **2002**, *19*(8), 703-708.
        [http://dx.doi.org/10.1023/A.1021398601388] [PMID: 12553376]

[88]   Sunila, E.S.; Kuttan, G. Immunomodulatory and antitumor activity of Piper longum Linn. and piperine. *J. Ethnopharmacol.,* **2004**, *90*(2-3), 339-346.
        [http://dx.doi.org/10.1016/j.jep.2003.10.016] [PMID: 15013199]

[89]   Sunila, E.S.; Kuttan, G. Antitumor activity of Piper longum and piperine. *Amala Research Bulletin,* **2002**, *22*, 9-14.

[90]   Canel, C.; Moraes, R.M.; Dayan, F.E.; Ferreira, D. Podophyllotoxin. *Phytochemistry,* **2000**, *54*(2), 115-120.
        [http://dx.doi.org/10.1016/S0031-9422(00)00094-7] [PMID: 10872202]

[91]   Semalty, M.; Semalty, A.; Badola, A.; Joshi, G.P.; Rawat, M.S.M. *Semecarpus anacardium* Linn.: A review. *Pharmacogn. Rev.,* **2010**, *4*(7), 88-94.
        [http://dx.doi.org/10.4103/0973-7847.65328] [PMID: 22228947]

[92]   Nadkarni, K.M.; Nadkarni, A.K. *Indian Materia Medica,* 3rd ed; M/S Popular Prakasan Pvt. Ltd.: Mumbai, **1976**, Vol. 1, .

[93]   Khosa, R.L.; Prasad, S.J. Pharmacognostical studies on Guduchi Tinospora cordifolia (Miers). *Res. Ind. Med,* **1971**, *6*, 261-269.

[94]   Chopra, R.N.; Nayar, S.L.; Chopra, I.C. *Glossary of Indian Medicinal Plants*; Council for Scientific and Industrial Research: New Delhi, **1956**, p. 21.

[95]   Zhao, T.F.; Wang, X.K.; Rimando, A.M.; Che, C.T. Folkloric medicinal plants: Tinospora sagittata var. cravaniana and Mahonia bealei. *Planta Med.,* **1991**, *57*(5), 505.
        [http://dx.doi.org/10.1055/s-2006-960188] [PMID: 1798808]

[96]   Chauhan, K. Successful treatment of throat cancer with Ayurvedic drugs. *Suchitra Ayurved.,* **1995**, *47*, 840-842.

[97]   Thippeswamy, G.; Salimath, B.P. Induction of caspase-3 activated DNase mediated apoptosis by hexane fraction of Tinospora cordifolia in EAT cells. *Environ. Toxicol. Pharmacol.,* **2007**, *23*(2), 212-220.
        [http://dx.doi.org/10.1016/j.etap.2006.10.004] [PMID: 21783760]

[98]   Jagetia, G.C.; Rao, S.K. Evaluation of the antineoplastic activity of guduchi (Tinospora cordifolia) in Ehrlich ascites carcinoma bearing mice. *Biol. Pharm. Bull.,* **2006**, *29*(3), 460-466.

[http://dx.doi.org/10.1248/bpb.29.460] [PMID: 16508146]

[99]   Singh, N.; Singh, S.M.; Prakash, ; Singh, G. Restoration of thymic homeostasis in a tumor-bearing host by *in vivo* administration of medicinal herb Tinospora cordifolia. *Immunopharmacol. Immunotoxicol.*, **2005**, *27*(4), 585-599.
[http://dx.doi.org/10.1080/08923970500416764] [PMID: 16435578]

[100]   Singh, N.; Singh, S.M.; Shrivastava, P. Effect of Tinospora cordifolia on the antitumor activity of tumor-associated macrophages-derived dendritic cells. *Immunopharmacol. Immunotoxicol.*, **2005**, *27*(1), 1-14.
[PMID: 15803856]

[101]   Singh, N.; Singh, S.M.; Shrivastava, P. Immunomodulatory and antitumor actions of medicinal plant Tinospora cordifolia are mediated through activation of tumor-associated macrophages. *Immunopharmacol. Immunotoxicol.*, **2004**, *26*(1), 145-162.
[http://dx.doi.org/10.1081/IPH-120029952] [PMID: 15106739]

[102]   Leyon, P.V.; Kuttan, G. Inhibitory effect of a polysaccharide from Tinospora cordifolia on experimental metastasis. *J. Ethnopharmacol.*, **2004**, *90*(2-3), 233-237.
[http://dx.doi.org/10.1016/j.jep.2003.09.046] [PMID: 15013186]

[103]   Thippeswamy, G.; Sheela, M.L.; Salimath, B.P. Octacosanol isolated from Tinospora cordifolia downregulates VEGF gene expression by inhibiting nuclear translocation of NF-<kappa>B and its DNA binding activity. *Eur. J. Pharmacol.*, **2008**, *588*(2-3), 141-150.
[http://dx.doi.org/10.1016/j.ejphar.2008.04.027] [PMID: 18513715]

[104]   Kapil, A.; Sharma, S. Immunopotentiating compounds from Tinospora cordifolia. *J. Ethnopharmacol.*, **1997**, *58*(2), 89-95.
[http://dx.doi.org/10.1016/S0378-8741(97)00086-X] [PMID: 9406896]

[105]   Bombardelli, E.; Morazzonni, P. Vitis vinifera L. *Fitoterapia,* **1995**, *66*, 291-317.

[106]   Paul, B.; Masih, I.; Deopujari, J.; Charpentier, C. Occurrence of resveratrol and pterostilbene in age-old darakchasava, an ayurvedic medicine from India. *J. Ethnopharmacol.,* **1999**, *68*(1-3), 71-76.
[http://dx.doi.org/10.1016/S0378-8741(99)00044-6] [PMID: 10624864]

[107]   Jang, M.; Cai, L.; Udeani, G.O.; Slowing, K.V.; Thomas, C.F.; Beecher, C.W.W.; Fong, H.H.; Farnsworth, N.R.; Kinghorn, A.D.; Mehta, R.G.; Moon, R.C.; Pezzuto, J.M. Cancer chemopreventive activity of resveratrol, a natural product derived from grapes. *Science,* **1997**, *275*(5297), 218-220.
[http://dx.doi.org/10.1126/science.275.5297.218] [PMID: 8985016]

[108]   Kapoor, L., Ed. *Handbook of Ayurvedic Medicinal Plants*; CRC Press: Boca Raton, **1990**.

[109]   Waffo-Téguo, P.; Hawthorne, M.E.; Cuendet, M.; Mérillon, J.M.; Kinghorn, A.D.; Pezzuto, J.M.; Mehta, R.G. Potential cancer-chemopreventive activities of wine stilbenoids and flavans extracted from grape (Vitis vinifera) cell cultures. *Nutr. Cancer,* **2001**, *40*(2), 173-179.
[http://dx.doi.org/10.1207/S15327914NC402_14] [PMID: 11962253]

[110]   Wadhwa, R.; Singh, R.; Gao, R.; Shah, N.; Widodo, N.; Nakamoto, T.; Ishida, Y.; Terao, K.; Kaul, S.C. Water extract of Ashwagandha leaves has anticancer activity: identification of an active component and its mechanism of action. *PLoS One,* **2013**, *8*(10), 1-11. :e77189.

[111]   Rai, M.; Jogee, P.S.; Agarkar, G.; dos Santos, C.A. Anticancer activities of Withania somnifera: Current research, formulations, and future perspectives. *Pharm. Biol.,* **2016**, *54*(2), 189-197.
[http://dx.doi.org/10.3109/13880209.2015.1027778] [PMID: 25845640]

[112]   Baliga, M.S.; Meera, S.; Vaishnav, L.K.; Rao, S.; Palatty, P.L. Rasayana drugs from the Ayurvedic system of medicine as possible radioprotective agents in cancer treatment. *Integr. Cancer Ther.,* **2013**, *12*(6), 455-463.
[http://dx.doi.org/10.1177/1534735413490233] [PMID: 23737641]

[113]   Nafiujjaman, M.; Nurunnabi, M.; Saha, S.K.; Jahan, R.; Lee, Y.K.; Rahmatullah, M. Anticancer activity of Arkeshwara Rasa - A herbo-metallic preparation. *Ayu,* **2015**, *36*(3), 346-350.

[http://dx.doi.org/10.4103/0974-8520.182757] [PMID: 27313425]

[114]   George, S.K.; Rajesh, R.; Kumar S, S.; Sulekha, B.; Balaram, P. A polyherbal ayurvedic drug-
-Indukantha Ghritha as an adjuvant to cancer chemotherapy via immunomodulation. *Immunobiology,*
2008, *213*(8), 641-649.
[http://dx.doi.org/10.1016/j.imbio.2008.02.004] [PMID: 18765169]

[115]   Penza, M.; Montani, C.; Jeremic, M.; Mazzoleni, G.; Hsiao, W.L.; Marra, M.; Sharma, H.; Di
Lorenzo, D. MAK-4 and -5 supplemented diet inhibits liver carcinogenesis in mice. *BMC
Complement. Altern. Med.,* **2007**, *7*(19), 19.
[http://dx.doi.org/10.1186/1472-6882-7-19] [PMID: 17559639]

[116]   Prasad, M.L.; Parry, P.; Chan, C. Ayurvedic agents produce differential effects on murine and human
melanoma cells *in vitro. Nutr. Cancer,* **1993**, *20*(1), 79-86.
[http://dx.doi.org/10.1080/01635589309514273] [PMID: 8415133]

[117]   Prasad, K.N.; Edwards-Prasad, J.; Kentroti, S.; Brodie, C.; Vernadakis, A. Ayurvedic (science of life)
agents induce differentiation in murine neuroblastoma cells in culture. *Neuropharmacology,* **1992**,
31(6), 599-607.
[http://dx.doi.org/10.1016/0028-3908(92)90193-S] [PMID: 1357573]

[118]   Inaba, R.; Sugiura, H.; Iwata, H. Immunomodulatory effects of Maharishi Amrit Kalash 4 and 5 in
mice. *Nippon Eiseigaku Zasshi,* **1995**, *50*(4), 901-905.
[http://dx.doi.org/10.1265/jjh.50.901] [PMID: 8538064]

[119]   Dileepan, K.N.; Varghese, S.T.; Page, J.C.; Stechschulte, D.J. Enhanced lymphoproliferative response,
macrophage mediated tumor cell killing and nitric oxide production after ingestion of an Ayurvedic
drug. *Biochem. Arch.,* **1993**, *9*, 365-374.

[120]   Patel, V.K.; Wang, J.; Shen, R.N.; Sharma, M.D.H.M.; Brahmi, Z. Reduction of metastases of Lewis
lung carcinoma by an Ayurvedic food supplement in mice. *Nutr. Res.,* **1992**, *12*, 667-676.
[http://dx.doi.org/10.1016/S0271-5317(05)80036-3]

[121]   Sharma, H.M.; Dwivedi, C.; Satter, B.C.; Abou-Issa, H. Antineoplastic properties of Maharishi Amrit
Kalash, an Ayurvedic food supplement, against 7,12-dimethylbenz(a)anthracene-induced mammary
tumors in rats. *J. Res. Educ. Indian Med.,* **1991**, *10*(3), 1-8.

[122]   Sharma, H.M.; Dwivedi, C.; Satter, B.C.; Gudehithlu, K.P.; Abou-Issa, H.; Malarkey, W.; Tejwani,
G.A. Antineoplastic properties of Maharishi-4 against DMBA-induced mammary tumors in rats.
Pharmacol. Biochem. Behav., **1990**, *35*(4), 767-773.
[http://dx.doi.org/10.1016/0091-3057(90)90356-M] [PMID: 2140606]

[123]   Saxena, A.; Dixit, S.; Aggarwal, S.; Seenu, V.; Prashad, R.; Bhushan, S.M.; Tranikanti, V.; Misra,
M.C.; Srivastava, A. An ayurvedic herbal compound to reduce toxicity to cancer chemotherapy: A
randomized controlled trial. *Indian J. Med. Paediatr. Oncol.,* **2008**, *29*, 11-18.
[http://dx.doi.org/10.4103/0971-5851.51426]

[124]   Baliga, M.S.; Meera, S.; Vaishnav, L.K.; Rao, S.; Palatty, P.L. Rasayana drugs from the Ayurvedic
system of medicine as possible radioprotective agents in cancer treatment. *Integr. Cancer Ther.,* **2013**,
12(6), 455-463.
[http://dx.doi.org/10.1177/1534735413490233] [PMID: 23737641]

[125]   Shamsi, T.N.; Parveen, R.; Fatima, S. Panchakola Reduces Oxidative Stress in MCF-7 Breast Cancer
and HEK293 Cells. *J. Diet. Suppl.,* **2017**, *1*, 11.
[PMID: 29144788]

[126]   Sandhya, T.; Mishra, K.P. Cytotoxic response of breast cancer cell lines, MCF 7 and T 47 D to triphala
and its modification by antioxidants. *Cancer Lett.,* **2006**, *238*(2), 304-313.
[http://dx.doi.org/10.1016/j.canlet.2005.07.013] [PMID: 16135398]

CHAPTER 7

Plant Based Bioactive Compounds as an Alternative for Cancer Therapy

Nikita Sharma[1], R. Mankamna Kumari[1], Nidhi Gupta[2] and **Surendra Nimesh[1,*]**

[1] *Department of Biotechnology, School of Life Sciences, Central University of Rajasthan, Ajmer 305817, Rajasthan, India*

[2] *Department of Biotechnology, The IIS University, Jaipur 302020, Rajasthan, India*

Abstract: Medicinal Plants have been known to be one of the oldest and most consistent sources for the production of novel drugs. Utilization of plant extracts as drugs can be attributed to their chemical and structural diversity along with their ability to interact with different biological targets in the cell. Moreover, they act as huge reservoirs for the phytochemicals which provide defense against a number of diseases. Cost effectiveness along with lesser adverse effects, allowed natural plants to be used as an alternative to conventional strategies for cancer treatment. Extracts from different natural plants have also been explored in the treatment of infectious diseases. The present chapter emphasizes on the use of plant extracts and their purified compound as cancer therapeutics. Cancer is one of the major causes of mortality worldwide. Owing to several limitations of current treatment regimens of cancer, the attention of researchers has been drawn towards exploration of natural sources. Herein, we will focus majorly on bioactive compounds as therapeutic agents for cancer treatment with emphasis on their other possible beneficiary roles.

Keywords: Anticancer Mechanism, Apoptosis, Cancer, Chemotherapy, Flavonoids, Medicinal Plants, Phytochemicals, Plant Extracts, Polyphenols, Saponins, Secondary Metabolites, Therapeutic Agents, Terpenes, Vinca Alkaloids.

INTRODUCTION

Cancer is the major growing health problem among both developed and developing countries. According to the recent report by American Cancer Society in "Cancer Facts and Figures 2017" it has been estimated that 1,688,780 number of new cases will be diagnosed and 600,920 cancer deaths in US in year 2017 [1].

---

[*] **Corresponding author Surendra Nimesh:** Department of Biotechnology, School of Life Sciences, Central University of Rajasthan, Ajmer 305817, Rajasthan, India; Tel: +91-1463-238734; Fax: +91-1463-238722; E-mails: surendranimesh@gmail.com, surendranimesh@curaj.ac.in

Currently, the available treatments of cancer include chemotherapy, radiation therapy, hormonal therapy, immunotherapy and surgical removal of the affected tissue. The commonly used chemotherapeutic drugs are DNA- interacting agents (Doxorubicin), antimetabolites (5 Fluorouracil, methotrexate), anti-tubulin agents (taxanes), hormones, antibodies, molecular targeting agents. It has been observed that combinatorial therapies work more effectively as compared to the classical therapies for an effective response in the patients. In spite of intensive interventions, these approaches are accompanied with certain side effects such as bone marrow suppression, loss of hair, gastrointestinal lesions, leukopenia and the development of resistance against drugs. These further results in low response rates, poor prognosis and reduces patient compliance. Therefore, there arises a need to search for effective methods with lower toxicities and higher efficiency.

Since ancient times, natural compounds have been used as remedies against several diseases. Traditional herbs and plants are well-known for their medicinal properties for *e.g.*, turmeric, cloves, ginger, cardamom, garlic and many more. Several bioactive compounds and phytochemicals including polyphenols, terpenoids, flavonoids and other organosulfur compounds have been reported for their anticancer and antimutagenic activity [2]. Many studies have shown that these compounds have enormous potential to reduce cell proliferation, decrease metastasis, enhance apoptosis and retard angiogenesis [3]. Currently, 60% of the clinically used anticancer agents have their origin from plants [4]. Some of them include Podophyllotoxin from *Podophyllumpeltatum*, Vincristine, Vinblastine, Camptothecin, Taxol and their analogs are found to be effective against different types of cancer [5]. In a study, it was revealed that atleast half of the cancer patients in US rely on herbal medicines. Generally, these bioactive compounds are given in combination with radiation therapy or other chemotherapy, and are proven to be much more effective as compared to be given alone [6]. The potential of the herbal system to be used as anticancer agents owes to the medicinal properties of not only reducing toxicity, but also boosting the immune system by decreasing level of oxidative stress. In order to identify novel pharmacophores from natural extracts for suppressing cancer, specific analytical markers are needed to be taken care of.

The present chapter highlights the alternative medicines derived from plants that show anticancer activity against several types of cancer. Natural bioactive compounds such as flavonoids, alkaloids, terpenoids, polyphenols possessing antitumor, anti-angiogenic, anti-oxidative activities have been discussed in the subsequent chapter that will further aid in understanding the approaches of chemoprevention.

1. POLYPHENOLS

These are secondary metabolites and are involved in defense mechanism against ultraviolet radiation and pathogen in the plants. Structurally, polyphenols are class of natural, semi synthetic and synthetic chemical compounds having multiple phenolic units. These can further be classified depending on the number of phenolic units in the compound. Studies have shown a great therapeutic potential against cancer, diabetes, neurodegenerative diseases, cardiovascular diseases [7]. Previous studies have reported that it inhibits the cell proliferation and angiogenesis, induce cell apoptosis, cell cycle arrest in the cancer cells. EGCG, resveratrol, curcumin, withaferin-A have been suggested as a potential adjuvants in chemotherapy [8]. Some of them are discussed in the following section:

1.1. Allicin

Allium sativum commonly known as garlic is well known for its several medicinal properties such as antidiabetic, antimicrobial, anti-hyperlipidemic and anticancer activity. It is one of the richest source of phenolic compounds among the daily consumed vegetables and is a major contributor of phenolic compounds in human diet [9]. It has been shown that phytochemical compounds and other organosulfur components of this plant possess anticancer properties and has the ability to suppress the progression of cancer. In an epidemiological study, colorectal adenomas patients were given garlic extract for a 6 month and 12 month period. It was observed that there was a decrease in size and number of colon adenomas lesions in the patient groups. The results suggested that the garlic extract and its sulfur components such as *S*-allylcysteine and *S*- allylmercaptocysteine has multiple role in the suppression of cancer [10]. In another molecular docking study, S-allyl-l-cysteine sulfoxide (component of garlic) showed higher affinity towards EGFR (Epidermal Growth factor Receptor, a transmembrane receptor which is highly expressed in cancerous cells). *In vitro* studies further confirmed the anticancer potential of S-allyl-l- cysteine sulfoxide [11]. It was observed that with the increase in the administration of garlic dose, the number and activity of natural killer cells also increased in the patients having advanced stages of digestive cancer [12].

1.2. Curcumin

Curcumin (diferuloylmethane) is an active polyphenol obtained from the rhizome of *Curcuma longa.* It helps in the prevention of oxidative and inflammatory environment, metabolic disorders, hyperlipidemia, pain and arthritis [13]. Studies have revealed the potential of curcumin against different types of cancer such as breast cancer, brain tumor, colorectal cancer, lung cancer without any adverse effects [14]. In addition, many researchers have proved the effect of curcumin at several stages of cancer including the initiation, promotion and progression level. It affects cell cycle regulators, mutagenesis, apoptosis, metastasis, invasion and oncogene expression through modulating many molecular targets and signaling pathways [15]. In a study, GO-Y030 curcumin analogue was used for targeting colorectal cancer stem cells. It was found that it inhibited the phosphorylation of STAT3, thus blocking the STAT pathway. A reduction in tumor size was also observed effectively in both *in vitro* and *in vivo* case [16]. One of the Nuclear factor, NF-kB, is very well known to control the transcription of DNA and cell survival. Curcumin have been found to block the NF-kB signaling pathway by various stimuli as TNF-α, hydrogen peroxide, phorbol esters. Aggarwal *et al.* demonstrated that curcumin interferes with the signaling pathway of NF-kB by inhibiting certain molecules involved in its activation [17]. In another study, HT29 human colon cancer cell lines were transfected with NF-kB luciferase construct and were challenged with lipopolysaccharide (LPS) stimulator. Results suggested that curcumin strongly inhibited LPS induced NF-kB activation and phosphorylation. Further it also promoted Caspase 3 activity [18]. In addition, it was also found to induce apoptosis through the generation of superoxide anions. Thus, it was evident that the anticancer activity of curcumin is independent of p53 levels in colon cancer cells [19]. Moreover, curcumin also affected Activator protein 1 (AP1); another transcription factor known to activate antiapoptotic, mitogenic and proangiogenic signals in cancer related cells. Some studies concluded that curcumin downregulates the activity of AP1, Matrix metallopeptidase 9 (MMP9) and inhibited Protein kinase-C (PKC) activity in astroglioma cells. It also modulates the activation of PKC by interfering with the release of Ca^{+2} from endoplasmic reticulum in HCT-116 human colon cancer cells [20].

The use of commercially available anticancer drugs is limited due to lack of specificity, toxicity and low bioavailability. A combinational therapy may reduce the non-specificity and increase the efficacy of these drugs. In a recent study, different drugs like docetaxel, 5-fluorouracil, doxorubicin, cisplatin were combined with curcumin and their combinational effect was studied on head and neck squamous cell carcinoma (HNSCC) NT8e cell lines. It was evident from the results that curcumin combined with 5-fluorouracil or doxorubicin showed considerable decrease in growth and increased apoptosis. An enhanced expression level of Bax, caspase 3, poly-ADP ribose polymerase (PARP) were observed with decrease in Bcl2 level in NT8e cells with the treatment of combined formulation. It was also shown that the formulation exhibited G1/S phase arrest, further conferred by the downregulation of CDK2, cyclins (D1, E2, B1, A2) and an enhanced p21 levels. Also, it was demonstrated that the combination interferes with the EGFR-ERK1/2 signaling by downregulation of certain molecules which are involved in the pathway [21]. Another study with curcumin showed an interventional anticancer effect on lung cancer stem cells in A549 and H1299 cells. The decrease in expression level of CSC lung markers (CD133, CD44, Nanog, Oct4) and a reduction in tumor size and number of CD133 positive cells were observed after the administration of curcumin in the cells. It was demonstrated that curcumin inhibits the lung cancer stem cells through altering the Wnt/β-catenin and sonic hedgehog pathways [22]. In order to enhance the bioavailability of curcumin in the body, various nanoformulations have been developed. This includes nanoparticles, liposomal encapsulation, micelles, emulsions, capsules and others. In a study, poly(lactic- co-glycolic) acid (PLGA) encapsulated curcumin nanospheres were designed against PC3, LNCaP, DU145 prostate cancer cell lines. The results showed that IC_{50} values of the nano-formulated particles were much lower than the curcumin alone [23]. Curcumin has undergone several human clinical trials for the evaluation of safety, tolerable dose, non-toxicity and efficiency of the anticancer activity [24]. In one of the phase I/II study, 8g/day oral curcumin with gemcitabine were given to 21 patients of gemcitabine resistance with prostate cancer. Both the phases reached their end points and no patients were withdrawn from the study due to toxicity. The combined gemcitabine-curcumin based chemotherapy was found to be safe and feasible in patients having pancreatic cancer and this could be further investigated regarding its anticancer efficacy [25].

1.3. Resveratrol

Resveratrol (3,5,4'-trihydroxy-*trans*-stilbene) is a phytoalexin and is produced during pathogenic attack or any injury in the plant. These are generally present in the skin of grapes, different types of berries, and some other fruits. It is known to exhibit anticancer, anti-inflammatory, anti-oxidant and antibacterial activity. It inhibits the proliferation of variety of cancer cells by altering the expression of certain transcription factors, signaling pathways, decrease in the levels of survivin, Bcl-2, cyclins and upregulation of p53, Bax, caspases and other apoptotic genes [26]. It has been reported that resveratrol affects the cancer at almost all the stages including initiation, promotion and progression of tumor [27]. In a study, it was shown that resveratrol possess anticancer property against colon cancer in animal models and in human by inhibiting Wnt signaling pathway. It suppresses the Wnt expression in normal colonic mucosa patients suffering from colon cancer. Thus, it affects the initiation, progression, metastasis, cell death stages of the carcinoma [28]. In another study, combinational approach was used on HT29 human colon cancer cell lines. Resveratrol and Quercetin (RQ) were given in a mixed ratio of 1:1 in HT29 to determine the anticancer activity. It reduced the production of reactive oxygen species (ROS) by 2.25 times and enhanced the cleavage activity of caspase 3 and PARP by 2 folds. Some transcription factors such as specificity proteins (Sp) are overexpressed in colon and other type of cancers which are required for cell survival and angiogenesis processes. However, it was observed that RQ treated cells showed a significant decrease in Sp1, Sp3, Sp4 mRNA and protein expression. Also, it showed lower expression level of oncogenic microRNA- 27a, proving the efficiency of anticancer activity of resveratrol against cancer [29].

In a clinical study, the concentration of resveratrol and their metabolites was determined after the administration of the drug in colorectal tissue of humans. Twenty patients with confirmed colorectal cancer report were allowed for 8 daily doses at 0.5 or 1.0 g before surgery. Resveratrol and its metabolites such as resveratrol-3-*O*-glucuronide, resveratrol-3-*O*-sulfate, resveratrol sulfate glucuronide and others were determined through high performance liquid chromatography (HPLC) or mass spectrometric analysis in colorectal section tissue. It was found that the maximum mean concentration of resveratrol and resveratrol-3-*O*-glucuronide recovered from the tissue were 674 nmol/g and 86.0 nmol/g respectively. Also, the tumor cell proliferation was reduced upto 5% after the consumption of the bioactive compound. Results suggest that resveratrol have a great potential to elicit anticancer effect [30]. In addition, resveratrol shows antioxidant, anti-inflammatory, anti-aging activity, modulatory effects of immune system, oxidative stress [31]. It can also act as a blocking agent by inhibiting the conversion of procarcinogen to carcinogen, as it stops the expression of monooxygenase cytochrome P450 isozyme CYP1 A1 which is responsible for liver metabolism of xenobiotics [32].

Extranodal NK/T cell lymphoma (NKTCL) is a rare type of non-Hodgkin lymphoma with poor identification. It was evident from the results that resveratrol shows anticancer activity by inducing DNA damage response pathway and inhibiting phosphorylation of AKT, Stat3 molecule. It also induces cell apoptosis through upregulating Bax, Bad, Caspase3, Caspase9 and suppressing MCl-1 and survivin expression. It was revealed that resveratrol inhibits NKTCL based cell lines (SNT-8, SNK-10, SNT-16) in a dose and time dependent manner [33]. Further to enhance the *in vivo* efficiency of the phytochemical compound, certain analogs possessing high anticarcinogenic and pharmacokinetic activity are studied. Resveratrol derivatives–imine analogs (IRA) showed a significant decrease in growth of colorectal carcinoma cell lines HCT-116wt, carrying p53 wild type gene [34]. Other modification includes the hydroxylic or methoxylic moiety on the phenolic rings of resveratrol, addition of 2,3-thiazolidin-4-one and 3-chloro-azetidin-2-one between the aromatic rings that displayed higher cytotoxicity and higher ability to suppress the growth of breast cancer cells. It was demonstrated that the inhibitory activity in *in vitro* breast cancer cells was enhanced several times as compared with the parent drug resveratrol [35]. Another resveratrol analogue, HS-1793 showed higher anticancer effect in many aspects as compared to the original resveratrol on MCF-7 and MDA-MB-231 cells. It altered and suppressed signaling pathways such as p53/p21WAF1/CIP1 dependent apoptosis in MCF-7 and p53 independent apoptosis in MDA-MB-231. The results suggested that HS-1793 could be used as a potential chemotherapeutic candidate against human breast cancer [36].

In order to overcome the limitations of multi drug resistance, poor bioavailability, solubility associated with resveratrol, combinatorial therapy can be implemented. Some of the researchers showed that the combination of drugs in a carrier inhibits the cancer growth and induces apoptosis in the cell. In a recent research, resveratrol was co-encapsulated with paclitaxel in a liposome based nanocarrier of 50 nm size and encapsulation efficiency of 50%. The results revealed that the nanoformulation showed an increased cytotoxicity against MCF-7/ADR drug resistant tumor cells and enhanced the retention time of drug in the body. *In vivo* administration of the formulation showed increased cell death and apoptosis with negligible signs of toxicity in the drug resistant tumor induced mice models [37].

1.4. Epigallocatechin Gallate

Tea has become one of the popular beverage worldwide in the form of black tea, green tea and oolong tea. All the varieties are generally derived from the plant *Camellia sinensis* that possess number of assorted compounds such as polyphenols [38]. Amongst the tea varieties, applications related to green tea is the widely explored field owing to their health benefits along with chemopreventive efficiency. Majority of its beneficial effects (such as anticancer, antidiabetic, antioxidant activity with potential role in obesity, stroke, Alzheimer and Parkinson's disease) are contributed by the polyphenolic compounds such as catechins that includes EGCG, (-)-epicatechin-3-gallate,(-)-epigallocatechin, and (-)-epicatechin. Amongst the available catechins EGCG accounts for more than 50-80% representing 200-300 mg/brewed cup of green tea [39]. It is proposed that this compound suppresses the inflammatory process that causes transformation, hyperproliferation, and initiation of carcinogenesis. This is mainly attributed by its radical scavenging activity, antioxidant activity and ability to regulate the signaling molecules related to mitosis, survival and cellular death modulating the cellular process involved in carcinogenesis: initiation, promotion and progression. Also, EGCG plays a vital role in cancer therapy by suppressing tumor suppressor p53 and nuclear factor kappa-light- chain, enhancer of activated B-cells (NF-kB) causing death of cancer cells [40]. Several studies have been conducted for the treatment of different types of cancer. Tissue factor pathway inhibitor 2 (TFPI-2) is predominantly downregulated due to its hypermethylation in bladder cancer cells. This activity was reversed in the presence of EGCG by restoring TFPI-2 expression and reducing the viability, invasion and apoptosis in bladder cancer cells (T24 cells) [41]. Similarly, recent studies have shown the effect of EGCG on breast cancer cells. The compound readily reduced the expression of ERα protein levels with 56% reduction using 60 μM EGCG in T-47D cells. Also, it showed potent activity when used in combination with siRNA against p53 in MCF-7 cells. The expression of p53 was higher in the EGCG-combined si-p53 treated group. Whereas, the expression level was lower in si-p53 group. The compound also exhibits its anticancer property by reducing cyclin-dependent protein activity, inhibition of β-catenin signalling and downregulating the expression of VEGF and MMP9 inhibiting growth and metastasis of breast cancer [42]. In addition, research on esophageal cancer using EGCG showed reduced Bcl2 protein expression and increased Bax and caspase3 protein expression with increased rate of apoptosis in the cancer cells. Interestingly, it was also shown that EGCG had enough potential in reversing multi-drug resistance by reducing ABCG2 expression [43]. Also, the effect of EGCG has been found to be positive in case of colon cancer and hepatocellular carcinoma. Moreover, the compound has more potential than SU11274 (specific Met tyrosine kinase inhibitor) to protect against chemotherapy side effects [44]. Studies suggest that EGCG with other chemotherapeutic molecule such as cisplatin, doxorubicin, 5-fluorouracil showed synergistic effect in suppressing cell proliferation, induce apoptosis and inhibit tumor angiogenesis and growth [45]. Thus, EGCG could be used for improving the overall health condition of patients.

Table 1. Represents few bioactive molecules and its anticancer potential studied *in-vitro*.Rosmarinic acid.

Plant Name and Part Used	Bioactive Compound	Cancer Treatment	References
Peganum harmala (Roots)	Harmine	Breast cancer	[46]
Curcuma longa (Rhizomes)	Curcumin and ascorbic acid	Leukaemia, glioblastoma and colon cancer	[47]
Allium wallichi (whole plant)	Steroids, terpenoids, flavonoids,*etc.*	Prostate cancer, breast cancer, cervical cancer	[48]
Debregeasia saeneb (Stem)	Tannins	Internal tumours	[49]
Ocimum sanctum (Leaves)	Eugenol, Orientin, vicenin	Breast, liver, fibrosarcoma cancer	[50]
Solanum nigrum (Leaves)	Solamargine, solasanine	Breast, liver, Lung and skin cancer	[51]
Aegle marmelos (Bark and root)	Lupeol	Lymphoma, melanoma and leukaemia	[52]
Zingiber officinale (Ginger)	Gingerol	Ovary, cervix, colon and urinary cancer	[53]
Panax ginseng (Roots)	Panaxadiol	Human colon cancer	[54]

Plant Name and Part Used	Bioactive Compound	Cancer Treatment	References
Broussonetia papyrifera (fruits, leaf and bark)	2S-abyssinone II, Verubulin	Glioblastoma and brain cancer	[55]
Glycyrrhiza uralensis (Roots)	Isoliquiritigenin	Human lung cancer	[56]
Boerhavia diffusa (Roots)	Punarnavine	Malignant melanoma cancer	[57]
Croton macrobothrys (Leaves)	Corydine, salutaridine	Leukaemia and lung cancer	[58]
Clausena lansium (seeds)	Clausenalansamid A and B	Gastric, liver cancer	[59]
Linum usitatissimum (Leaves and Flowers)	Cyanogenic glycosides	Breast cancer	[60]
Calvatia caelata (Fruiting bodies)	Laccases	Liver and breast cancer	[61]
Aloe vera (whole plant)	Aloesin, emodin	Anti-angiogenic activity	[62]
Emblica officinalis	Polyphenols, tannins	Lymphoma and melanoma	[62]
Momordica charantia (Leaves and Roots)	Charantin, cucurbitane-type triterpene	Colon cancer and breast cancer	[63]
Lavatera cashmeriana (Seeds)	Lavatera cashmeriana protease inhibitors	Leukemia, lung, colon cancer	[64]

1.5. Rosmarinic Acid

Rosmarinic acid (RA) and carnosic acid are the two main polyphenols that are predominantly found in the rosemary extract of the plant, *Rosmarinus officinalis L.* The two polyphenols have been widely explored in the field of cancer and are found to be beneficial in suppressing several cancers such as colon, liver, breast and stomach cancer [65]. Alterations in the COX-2 pathway and increase in the prostaglandin E2 (PGE2) are common in the development and progression of colorectal cancer, that is stimulated by the activation of ERK-signaling pathway [66]. This activity is reversed in the presence of RA through its anti-inflammatory properties. At a dose level of 5-20 μmol/L, the COX-2 promoter activity was significantly reduced along with reduction in binding of AP-1 factors, c-Jun and c-Fos to the COX-2 promoter. In addition, RA also antagonized the activation of signal-regulated protein kinase-1/2 (ERK1/2). However, the alterations in the signaling pathway mediated by RA can vary from one cell line to another [67]. At a concentration of 55-832 μM, ROS levels significantly decreased along with reduction in the migration and adhesion rates in the Ls174-T colon cells. Further, RA can protect against BCNU-induced DNA damage in CO115 cells, suggesting a possible role in chemopreventive effects at a dose level of 50 μM [68]. Besides the role of COX-2, several other cancer markers such as intercellular adhesion molecule-1 (ICAM-1) and vascular cell adhesion molecule-1 (VCAM-1) are known to play pivotal role in the progression of cancers. It is reported that ICAM-1 and VCAM-1 circulating levels are higher in nasopharyngeal carcinoma and are associated with poor prognosis in pancreatic cancer and breast cancer leading to tumour growth and metastasis [69]. Also, RA is known to play an effective role in melanoma, which is considered to be the most dangerous form of skin cancer. In a study, the polyphenolic compound act as radiosensitizer and increased cellular death by 42% in B16F10 melanoma cells. This shows the dual capability of RA in protecting the normal, while sensitizing the cancer cells. In human leukemic cell lines U937, RA suppressed the activation of NF-kappa B and inhibited the nuclear translocation of p50 and p65 along with activation of caspases for induction of apoptosis [70]. RA has also found its application in breast cancer by inhibiting the activity of methyltransferase in MCF-7 cancer cells. Also, it has shown to inhibit migration of MDA-MB-231BO human bone- homing breast cancer cells suggesting that RA can inhibit the breast cancer metastasis [71]. RA, in combination with cisplatin also showed noteworthy effect on human ovarian cancer cells by inducing apoptosis [72]. Moreover, the compound also displayed antiangiogenic activity by inhibiting proliferation, migration, adhesion, and tube formation of human umbilical vein endothelial cells, that can predominantly decrease tumour growth and metastasis [73]. In addition to this, effect of orally administered RA in 7,12- dimethylbenz(a)anthracene (DMBA) induced skin carcinogenesis in Swiss albino mice effectively reduced the tumor formation and modulated antioxidant status and apoptosis markers [74]. RA also showed 50% inhibition in the proliferation of A549 lung carcinoma cells by inhibiting COX-2 activity. Similar results were observed in case of oral cancer induced in golden Syrian hamsters by DMBA, that improved the antioxidant status and downregulated the expressions of p53 and Bcl2 [75]. Moreover, it was found to suppress the inflammatory related cytokines such as IL6, IL-1β, IL-22, level of COX-2 protein and inducible nitric oxide synthase (iNOS) in mice with dextran sulphate sodium induced colitis. In addition, it inhibited NF-kappaB and STAT3 pleiotropically, ensuring the reduction in pro-survival genes [76]. Thus, the polyphenolic compound RA can prove to be a promising drug for chemoprevention and treatment of cancer.

2. ALKALOIDS

These are one of the most diverse groups possessing both anti-proliferative and anti-metastatic activity against various cancers. Chemically, these are heterocyclic ring compounds containing nitrogen atom. Several alkaloids exhibit medicinal properties such as analgesic effect of morphine, ephedrine in asthma, and anticancer activity of vincristine [77]. These are one of the most bioactive compounds and have been successfully used as chemotherapeutic agents against various diseases.

Vinca alkaloids

These are a class of organic compounds that are extracted from *Catharanthus roseus* of apocyanaceae family. These are found widely all over the world and it has been used for centuries as a medicinal source for high blood pressure, diabetes, scurvy and ulcer. These are among the oldest group of plant alkaloids that are being used to treat cancer. Clinically, the four major vinca alkaloids that are used includes vincristine, vinorelbine, vinblastine and vindesine [78]. The main mechanism of action is by cell cycle arrest at metaphase stage due to the interaction of tubulin and disruption of microtubule function and inhibiting spindle formation [79]. Vinblastine interferes with proliferation of endothelium thereby blocking the angiogenesis by binding to the microtubule. It is used in the treatment of both Hodgkins and non-hodgkins lymphoma, small lung cell carcinoma, breast cancer and other tumors. Vincristine binds with the tubulin and blocks the polymerization, thereby arresting the cell cycle. Vinrelbine and vindesine inhibits cell proliferation and showed effective anticancer activity against breast and small cell lung cancer. Vinorelbine has been approved in USA in 1994 for the treatment of small cell lung cancer [80]. In a study it was evident that vincristine activity was enhanced with crocetin in HeLa, SKOV3 and A549 cells. Results showed p53 dependent and independent induced cancer death which was analysed through the release of lactate dehydrogenase (LDH). Vinca alkaloids can be used in combination to enhance their anticancer activity against different cancers. Currently, vincristine and vinblastine with other chemotherapeutic agents such as bryostatin I, nilotinib, bevacizumab and doxorubicin are under clinical trials against acute lymphoblastic leukemia (ALL), lymphoma [81].

Camptothecin

Camptothecin, a quinoline alkaloid obtained from bark and stem of *Camptotheca acuminata*, a Chinese tree have been used for a long time as a traditional medicine against cancer. This bioactive compound selectively inhibits topoisomerase I, which is involved in the relaxation of DNA helix. Various derivatives of camptothecin have been synthesised and have undergone clinical trials at different phases. In clinical phase I study, 25 patients were administered with liposomal 9-nitro-20(s)-camptothecin analogue to analyse the safety of the therapy in cancer patients. 6.7-26.6 µg/kg/day dose was given gradually in a stepwise manner for 8 weeks to the patients having primary and metastatic lung cancer. Aerosolized administration showed a positive result with no significant toxic effect among the patients [82]. Additionally, it has been found that it is a potent inhibitor of nuclear factor erythroid 2-related factor 2 (NRF-2) which plays an important role in developing chemotherapeutic drug resistance in patients. The expression of NRF-

2 in human hepatocellular carcinoma biopsies was determined through immunostaining, western blotting, reverse transcriptase quantitative real time PCR (RT-qPCR) and luciferase reporter assay. Camptothecin treatment markedly decreased the gene expression and transcriptional activity of NRF-2 in various cell lines such as HepG2, A549 [83]. Also, camptothecin decreased the Nitric oxide(NO) production, mRNA expression level of inducible nitric oxide synthase (iNOS) in SW480, human colon cancer cell lines. The results proved the inhibitory activity of camptothecin on lipopolysaccharide alongwith interlukin (IL) 1β stimulation of NO generation through the suppression of transcription of iNOS gene [84]. The results suggest the efficiency of camptothecin as an anti-carcinogenic drug where certain modifications can further enhance the bioavailability, targeted delivery of the drug to particular tissues, thereby reducing the chances of toxicity.

3. SAPONINS AND TERPENOIDS

Terpenes are aromatic organic compounds commonly produced by plants, mainly conifers. These compounds are reported to possess therapeutic potential owing to their anti-inflammatory, anti-tumorigenic and neurodegenerative properties for treating various diseases. Oxidized product of terpenes is known as terpenoids. One of the class, sesquiterpenoids are known to target the mediators involved in inflammation and cancer and are under clinical trials [85]. Saponins are triterpenoid glycosides that are known to possess cytotoxicity against different human cancer cell lines. Also, these are being used as adjuvant in vaccines due to their cell penetrating mechanisms.

3.1. Diosgenin

Diosgenin is a steroidal saponin extracted from Dioscorea plants including *Trigonella foenum graecum, Costus speciosus,* Yam and others. It belongs to the family of triterpene which has a great importance in the field of pharmacy. The antioxidant property of diosgenin is known to affect the inflammatory cytokine levels. Therefore, this approach can be used for the treatment of cancer. Plethora of work has been done to show the anti-tumorogenic effect of diosgenin on cancer cells including breast cancer [86], colon cancer [87], hepatocellular carcinoma [88], lung cancer [89] and others. In one of the study, it was analysed that diosgenin exhibits anticancer activity through the reduction of peroxidation reaction and marker enzymes and in turn enhances the antioxidant defense system. N-Methyl-N-Nitrosourea (NMU) is a specific carcinogen of mammary gland, which mimics the breast cancer tissue in many aspects. During investigation, Sprague Dawley rats were induced with breast cancer through intraperitoneal injection of NMU (in concentration of 50mg/kg body weight) in a single dose. Diosgenin was given orally with a dose of 20 mg/kg body weight to these cancer induced rats for a period of 45 days. A significant decrease in the level of lipid peroxidation reaction and marker enzymes was observed, which further enhanced the antioxidant defense system [90].

Cancer cells possess activated telomerase property, while such activity is not easily identified in healthy cells. In of the studies, researchers showed the efficiency of fenugreek extract and pure isolated diosgenin to suppress the human telomerase reverse transcriptase (hTERT) gene expression in lung cancer A549 cell lines. A markedly decreased level of hTERT gene expression was observed when the cancer cells were treated with the extract and diosgenin for a period of 24, 48, 72 hrs respectively. The cytotoxicity effects were analysed through qPCR, MTT assays in A549 cells. IC50 values calculated were 47, 44, 43 μM and 49, 48, 47μM for pure diosgenin and extract respectively. The results revealed that pure diosgenin is highly effective against cancer as compared to the fenugreek extract [89, 91]. Diosgenin also induces apoptosis in cancer cell lines through multiple signalling pathways. One of the group analysed the effect of diosgenin in colorectal cancer cell lines HCT-116 and HT-29. It was observed that diosgenin sensitizes HT-29 cells through the activation of p38 MAPK pathway and further increased the expression of DR5. Subsequently, there was an increase in the level of -2 expression which can further be reduced through the use of COX-2 inhibitor, in turn enhanced the apoptosis induction [87]. It was observed that on treatment with diosgenin, the growth of Bel-7402, SMMC-7721 and HepG2 hepatocellular carcinoma cell lines (HCC) was inhibited. It inhibited the Akt phosphorylation, upregulated p21, p27, caspase -3,-8,-9 expression with induction in G2/M phase arrest and apoptosis in HCC [88]. In case of myeloid leukemia cells, diosgenin induces the production of ROS, and results in the generation of cytotoxic effect. Thus, induces autophagy in the cells [92]. Novel diosgenin (Dgn) analogs were designed and investigated for their antiproliferative activity against various cancer cell lines such as breast (HBL-100), lung (A549), colon (HT-29, HCT-116) by [3-(4,5-dimethylthiazolyl-2)-2,5-diphenyltetrazoliumbromide] MTT assay. Dgn1 (simple phenyl R moiety bonded with the original molecule through triazole) showed the highest antiproliferative activity in A549 cells with an IC50 value of 5.54μM followed by Dgn 2(with o-nitrophenyl) and Dgn 5(o- cyanophenyl) with an IC50 in the range of 5.77-9.44μM. The study revealed the potential of diosgenin analogues as antiproliferative agent against human cancer cell lines and this can be used for further studies [93].

3.2. Punicic Acid

It is a bioactive compound generated from pomegranate seed oil. Chemically, it is trichosanic acid consisting of omega-5 polyunsaturated fatty acid long chains.

Pomegranate extract has been used as anticancer therapy and includes a variety of phytochemicals and active biological compounds. Punicic acid inhibited proliferation of cells by 92 and 96% for estrogen insensitive breast cancer cell lines (MDA-MB-231) and estrogen sensitive breast cancer cell lines generated from MDA-MB-231 (MDA-ERalpha7) when treated with 40µM punicic acid. It also induced apoptosis in MDA-MB-231 and MDA-ERalpha7 by 86 and 91%, respectively as compared with the untreated control through disruption of mitochondrial membrane potential of cell. The results suggested the potential ability of punicic acid to inhibit proliferation of breast cancer to be dependent on lipid peroxidation and PKC pathway [94]. Clinical studies have shown the carcinogenic activity of pomegranate juice in prostate cancer cell lines. The major components include luteolin (L), ellagic acid (E) and punicic acid (P) which act synergistically to inhibit the growth of Prostate cancer (PCa) in either hormone dependent or independent cells. It also inhibited the migration and chemotaxis towards a chemokine CXCL12 required for PC metastasis. For *in vivo* study, immunodeficient mouse models were injected with luciferase expressing human PCa cells subcutaneously to prostate to investigate the effect of punicic acid on tumor growth. Weekly administration of tumor growth was monitored with the help of bioluminescence imaging technique. Results revealed that L, E and P in combination suppressed the PC-3M-luc tumor growth, inhibited CXCL12/CXCR4 involved in metastasis. Moreover, it was found that L+E+P inhibited *in vivo* angiogenesis by suppressing angiogenic factors, such as interleukin 8 and other vascular endothelial factors involved in various signaling. Thus, it inhibits the invasion, progression and metastasis of the prostate cancer [95]. In a study, punicic acid was shown to inhibit the estrogen receptors selectively. It was determined to inhibit the estrogen receptor (ER) alpha, beta with an IC50 value of 7.2µM and 8.8µM, respectively. Also, it induced mRNA expression of ERalpha and ERbeta in MCF-7 but not MDA- MB-231 cell lines. So, these are selective estrogen receptor modulators (SERM) for their concentration dependent modulation of estrogen receptor activity in different cell lines [96].

3.3. Thymol

Thymol also known as 2-isopropyl-5-methylphenol, is a natural monoterpene phenol derivative, extracted from *Thymus vulgaris* (common thyme), *Trachyspermum ammi* and other similar plants. Plethora of studies have demonstrated its antiseptic, antibacterial, antifungal, antioxidant, antimicrobial and anti-inflammatory properties. As per the regulations of Environmental Protection agencies, thymol has been regarded as safe and no adverse effects were found when administered on both the animals and humans [97]. Despite many potential uses, its anticancer mechanism in the cells has not yet been elucidated.

In a study, it was demonstrated that thymol affects the AGS Human gastric carcinoma cells through an intrinsic mitochondrial pathway. Results showed that thymol inhibited the cellular growth and induced the expression of pro-apoptotic mitochondrial proteins, such as Bax, Caspase, poly ADP ribose polymerase in human gastric AGS cancer cell lines [98]. Additionally, it was found to induce cell cycle arrest at G1/G0 phase in HL-60, acute promyelotic leukemia cells. There was a considerable increase in the ROS, production of mitochondrial H_2O_2 and Bax protein level. Further, Western blot analysis showed a significant decrease in the Bcl2 protein expression level. It was also found that the expression of caspase 9, 8 and PARP cleavage was also altered. Thymol induced apoptosis showed the involvement of both caspase dependent and independent pathways [99]. It was also shown to exhibit a protective effect against DNA damage caused by the oxidants present in the cell. Any antioxidant or bioactive compound protects the DNA break by quenching the free radicals and thereby decreasing the chances of cancer. Similarly, in *in vitro* study on HepG2 and Caco2, thymol shielded the DNA from hydrogen peroxide induced cytotoxicity. The protection ability of thymol, carvacrol (one of the components of essential plant oils) was demonstrated and showed to be a potent antioxidant and inhibitor against cancer [100]. Recently, it was observed that thymol also regulated the motility of tumor cell in a dose dependent manner. The effect of signaling proteins involved in the migration of C6 glioma cells on treatment with thymol including extracellular signal regulated kinases (ERK)1/2, matrix metallopeptidase (MMP)2 and MMP9, protein kinase Cα (PKCα) were investigated. The results revealed that thymol (30μM) altered the glioma cell migration by affecting the PKCα, ERK1/2 signaling proteins and suppression of MMP synthesis [101].

Mechanism Associated with Cancer Chemoprevention and its Treatment

There are several factors that gets altered during the tumor formation including transcription factors, growth factors, various kinases and their associated receptors and cell survival proteins (Fig. **1**). Some of the key features have been discussed below:

Phytochemical Induced Apoptosis

Apoptosis is characterised by programmed cell death that takes place in multicellular organisms. Different stages of apoptosis includes blebbing, cell shrinkage followed by nuclear fragmentation. Various phytochemicals are shown to involve in apoptosis mediated signaling. There are a number of signal transduction pathways that regulate the apoptosis process. Any alteration in the signaling pathways results in an uncontrolled cell proliferation. The apoptotic proteins may either function by increasing the permeability of the membrane,

Camptothecin
Curcumin
Resveratrol
Thymol
Diosgenin
Punicic acid
EGCG
Rosmarinic acid
Vincristine

Fig. (1). Represents chemical structures of different Bioactive compounds.

creating the membrane pores and causing swelling in mitochondria, thereby leaking out apoptotic effectors [108]. Caspases, a member of the protease family plays an important role in cell degradation during the apoptosis process. These are suppressed by the activity of inhibitor of apoptotic proteins (IAPs). Small mitochondrial-derived activators of caspases (SMAC) are released from mitochondria and binds with IAPs, deactivates it and stimulates the apoptotic pathway. On the other side, cytochrome c is released from mitochondria through mitochondrial apoptosis-induced channel (MAC) formed in the outer membrane of mitochondria. Cytochrome c binds with apoptotic protease activating factor 1 (Apaf-1) and ATP, which then attaches with pro-caspase9 to form protein apoptosome complex. This further converts into caspase9 and activates the effector caspase3 which is required for the apoptosis pathway to proceed [109]. A proper balance is maintained and established between the pro-apoptotic protein (Bax, Bak, Bad) and anti-apoptotic proteins (Bcl-Xl, Bcl2) of Bcl2 family to regulate the various processes within the cell. Bcl2 proteins control mitochondrial outer membrane permeabilization pore (MOMPP) and MAC either to form pores through pro-apoptotic Bax/Bak or inhibit the formation of pore through anti-apoptotic Bcl2, Bcl-Xl. Thus regulating the apoptotic signaling pathway [110]. In support to this, epidemiological studies have shown an inverse interrelation between the intake of fruits and vegetables and risk of cancer. The cranberry phytochemical extracts showed significant decrease in cell proliferation levels of MCF-7 breast cancer cell lines, at doses of 5- 30mg/mL. It was observed that at 50mg/mL dose of phytochemical extract, ratio of apoptotic cells to total cells increased to 25% as compared to the control groups [111]. In another study, Curcumin also showed similar results. There was a considerable decrease in the levels of Bcl2 protein and increase in Bax, apoptotic protein, thus increasing the Bax/Bcl2 ratio. MDA-MB-231 xenograft tumor mice showed significant decrease in tumor size and mass on administration of curcumin compared with the control [112].

Table 2. Represents bioactive molecules with its clinical relevance.

Bioactive Compound	Plant Source	Formulation (Trade Name)	Cancer Treatment	Clinical Status	Reference
Vincristine	*Catharanthus roseus*	Sphingomyelin/cholesterol (SM/Chol) liposomal vincristine (Marqibo)	Relapsed acute lymphoblastic leukaemia	FDA approved (2012)	NDA*:202497
Vinorelbine		Vinorelbine	Non-small cell lung cancer	Single and combination; Phase I and III trials	[102]
Vinflunine		Vinflunine	solid tumors	Phase III clinical trials	[102, 103]
Paclitaxel	*Taxus brevifolia*	Paclitaxel lecithin/cholesterol liposome (Lipusu)	ovarian, breast, non-SCLC, gastric and head and neck cancers	Approved in chinese market	[104]
		Injectable nanoparticle albumin-bound paclitaxel (Abraxane)	improvement in neuropathy side effects after the therapy discontinuation	FDA approved (2005)	NDA 21-660/S-031
		Docetaxel (Paclitaxel mimics)- (Taxotere)	Breast, ovarian, prostate cancer	Approved (1995)	NDA-022234Orig1s000
Homoharri-ngtonine	*Cephalotaxus fortunei*	Synribo	chronic myeloid leukaemia	FDA approved (2012)	NDA-3208987
Ingenol mebutate	*Euphorbia peplus*	PEP005	Human non-melanoma skin cancer	Clinical phase I/II	[105]
		Picato	Cutaneous treatment of non-hyperkeratotic actinic keratosis	FDA approved (2012)	NDA-3829544
Combretastatin A4	*Combretum caffrum*	Combretastatin A4 (CA4P)	anaplastic thyroid carcinoma	Clinical phase II	[106]
Resveratrol	*Vitis vinifera L.*	Resveratrol	colon cancer	Clinical phase I/II	NCT00256334
Roscovitine	Derived from olomucine; *Raphanus sativus L.*	Roscovitine	Inhibition of cell cycle progression	Phase II clinical trials in Europe	[103, 107]

(Table 2) cont.....

Bioactive Compound	Plant Source	Formulation (Trade Name)	Cancer Treatment	Clinical Status	Reference
Flavopirido-l	Rohitukine based structure; *Dysoxylum binectariferumHook.f.* (Meliaceae)	Flavopiridol	Solid tumors, lymphomas	Phase I and Phase II clinical trials	[103, 107]

*NDA: New Drug Application.

Epigenetics-DNA Methylation and Histone Modifications

DNA methylation and histone modifications can be used as a platform for epigenetics targeting against the cancer therapy. DNA methylation involves the covalent addition of methyl group at 5' position of cytosine or 6' position of adenine ring. It generally occurs at CpG sites, where the cytosine and guanine are separated by phosphate moiety in the somatic cells. In a study it was found that more than 98% of DNA methylation occurs at CpG sites in somatic cells and around a quarter of methylation appears in non CpG sites in embryonic stem cells [113]. Under cancerous state, these CpG islands undergoes abnormal hypermethylation resulting in transcriptional silencing of certain genes which is further inherited in daughter cells during cell division process. On the contrary, hypomethylation of CpG sites within the gene promoter leads to the overexpression of oncogenes within the cell [114]. Additionally, methyl-CpG-binding domain proteins (MBDs) bind to the methylated DNA to form condensed inactive heterochromatin and cause gene silencing. In a study, it was revealed that hypermethylated genes in cancer contribute to methyl-CpG- binding domain protein 2 mediated transcriptional silencing [115].

Another epigenetic factor that contributes is histone modifications. Histones are highly alkaline proteins that are arranged in an octamer form. DNA gets wrapped onto these histone proteins in an intricate manner to form structural units called chromosomes. These are packaged in a compact form so that it gets fit inside the cell nuclei. Some of the modifications of histone proteins include acetylation, methylation, phosphorylation, ubiquitylation of different tails *etc* [116]. Through the various histone modifications, an alteration in the gene expression can occur i.e, either silencing or overexpression of specific genes which are involved in the histone packaging. For instance, methylated DNA when gets attached to MBD proteins, it initiates the association of histone deacetylase and other chromatin related proteins that in turn modify to form heterochromatin. In a recent study, gallic acid showed the inhibitory effect on DNA methyltransferase(DNMT) activity and proved to be an effective strategy against tobacco-associated cancer. It was revealed that EGCG modulate the gene expression through gallic acid mediated targeting of DNMT. It also reactivates the GADD45 signaling pathway through demethylation of CCNE2 and CCNB1 in H1299 cells [117].

Cyclooxygenases-2 (COX-2)

Cyclooxygenase also known as prostaglandins-endoperoxide synthase (PTGS), are bifunctional membrane bound enzymes required for the formation of prostanoids [118]. These are of 3 different types namely COX-1, COX-2 and COX-3. Generally, COX-1 gene is constitutively expressed in cells of tissues and contributes to housekeeping functions, while COX-3 is specifically expressed in tissues such as brain and spinal cord. Expression of COX-2 is normally low in most of the cells but is found relatively higher in 80-90% colorectal and other cancers. It is transiently expressed in response to the inflammatory stimuli in the cancer cells [119]. One of the reason for such a difference in the expression levels can be the cross-talk between various mediators including interleukins and cytokines (IL-1, IL-6 and TNF-α) [120]. Another reason behind this could be the increased production of prostaglandins, which then binds with the cell surface receptors and alters the cellular growth [119]. Moreover, it was found that COX-2 expression was also related to the large tumor size and poor survival rate in colorectal cancer [121]. Thus, COX-2 expression can be the potential target for colon cancer prevention. Studies have revealed the ability of natural extracts to inhibit the expression of COX. Cerella *et al.* have shown the inhibition of COX expression through different natural compounds at various stages including transcriptional, post transcriptional, post translational and other modifications [122]. Also, curcumin was found to inhibit the metabolites of cyclooxygenase, and provide a chemopreventive measure through the induction of apoptosis pathway [123]. In a recent study it was shown that resveratrol inhibited the expression of COX-2 protein in human colorectal cancer HCT116 cells. Results revealed a significant decrease in the cell proliferation activity and quantitative real time PCR analysis, western blot further conferred the decreased mRNA expression of COX-2 in treated group as compared with the control group [124].

Angiogenesis Inhibition

Angiogenesis is a physiological process of formation of new blood vessels from pre-existing vessels. This mainly includes the migration, differentiation and development of endothelial cells which line the inner wall of the blood vessels. The angiogenesis process is regulated from the chemical signals of the body. Tumor stimulates the growth of blood vessels by releasing different endogenous signal molecules, such as vascular endothelial growth factor (VEGF), fibroblast growth factor (FGF), transforming growth factor-α (TGF-α), angiogenin which in turn activates the capillary growth. Therefore, angiogenic inhibitors can be used as a therapeutic strategy to reduce the formation of blood vessels and thereby tumor proliferation [125].

In a study, it was observed that grape seed extract (GSE) inhibited angiogenesis through the suppression of vascular endothelial growth signaling pathway. It was shown that the extract could directly inhibit the kinase activity of VEGF receptor/mitogen activated protein kinase in endothelial cells. The results were further corroborated in tumor bearing mice models. *In vivo* assays revealed the decrease in the density of blood vessels and phosphorylation of mitogen activated protein kinase in GSE administered mice [126]. Similarly, *Nelumbo nucifera* leaf extract showed the anti-angiogenic effect in human umbilical vein endothelial cells (HUVECs). Results showed the potency of *N. nucifera* extract as an antioxidant and anti-angiogenic agent on VEGF induced proliferation, tube formation and *in vivo* chick chorioallantoic membrane (CAM) formation [127]. In a study, anti-tumor effect of RA was evaluated against hepatocellular carcinoma. RA at concentration of 75, 150, 300mg/kg were intragastrically administered in H22 tumor bearing mice daily for 10 days. The effect on the levels of cytokines including IL-1β, IL-6, TNF-α, VEGF, TGF-β was analysed through ELISA. Results showed a significant decrease in the elevation of all cytokines as compared with the control group. qPCR and Western blot studies revealed a decrease in mRNA and protein expression levels of NF-κB p65 [128].

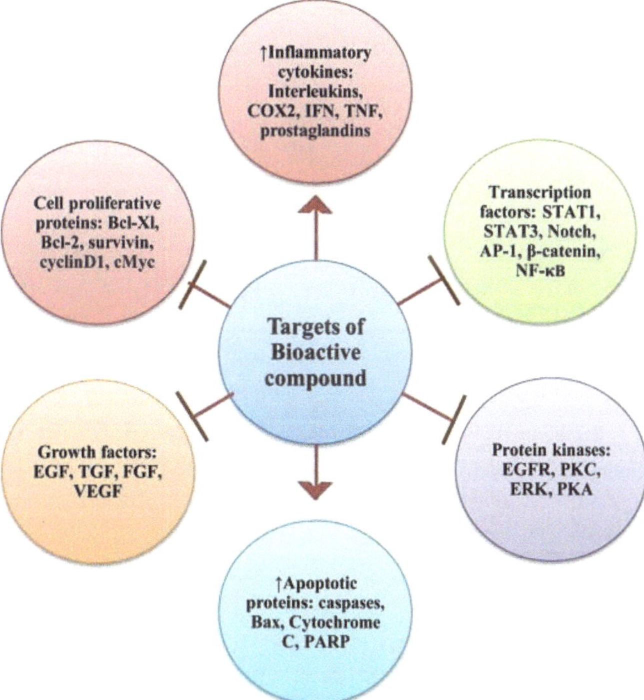

Fig. (2). Represents some possible mechanisms of action of bioactive compound relevant to block cancer cell growth.

Other Mechanisms

Apart from the above mentioned mechanisms, several other pathways contribute for the cancer proliferation and migration. These include hedgehog signaling, NF-κB pathway, PI-3 kinase pathway, STAT-3, Wnt pathway, and Nrf-2 signaling. Recent studies have shown that several plant derived phytochemicals possess anticancer activity through altering cell signaling cascades at different stages as in transcriptional level, post transcriptional level, protein activation [129]. Therefore, specific natural compounds can be investigated that reduce further proliferation of tumor cells within the tissue.

Limitations of Natural Compounds

It is evident from the chapter that bioactive compounds have potential benefits as a preventive as well as therapeutic agent [130]. Although, with its long history of application as diet and traditional medicines, they are known to carry deleterious effects even at pharmacological concentrations in some population [131]. There are reports that signify the antioxidant property of compounds *in vitro,* but non-effective *in vivo.* The pro-oxidative effect was best demonstrated with the use of tea catechins such as (-)-epigallocatechin-3-gallate (EGCG). It was observed that EGCG was unstable *in vitro* conditions and underwent oxidative polymerization and generation of H_2O_2 [132]. The oxidative stress generated during this condition actually aided in the inhibition of cancer cell proliferation. It is also reported that high concentration of green tea derived preparations induced toxicity of liver, kidney and intestine in dogs [133]. Another major challenge in the field of development of natural compounds as drugs is bioavailability. A well-known compound, curcumin is reported to show low bioavailability. Thus, in order to increase its bioavailability, nanoformulations such as micelles, liposomes can be designed to deliver the compound [134]. In one of the study, Genistein was complexed with high- amylose corn starch that increased the genistein plasma concentration twice as high when genistein was given alone [135]. In addition, it is discerned that phytochemical crystal structures, salt selection, excipient comparability should be taken into account to develop a competent drug. The physical form of the compounds can affect solubility, absorption and pharmacokinetic properties of the drug. A detailed description of importance and characterization of crystal form of the drug has been reviewed by *Clas.* The phytochemicals, when taken orally showed low bioavailability due to metabolism by Phase I and Phase II drug metabolising enzymes (DMEs). Phase I enzymes are mainly composed of cytochrome P450 that are involved in oxidation, reduction and hydrolysis to increase its polarity. Phase II DME makes use of glucuronidation, sulfation to increase water solubility and excretability of a drug. Herein, excessive metabolism shows drugs poor availability [136].

CONCLUSION

It is clearly evident from the present chapter that phytochemicals of most of the commonly available plant species and not only can those of medicinal plant species serve as promising and effective compounds for the treatment of cancer. Chemically derived drugs developed for the treatment have proved to be effective; however, carry several limitations such as toxicity and high cost. Under this scenario, an alternative approach, incorporating the use of phytochemicals can revolutionize the treatment of cancer. This comprehensive chapter highlights the essential bioactive compounds possessing a potential role in cancer treatment including its *in vitro* and clinical studies. The major advantage of implementing natural compounds for cancer therapy is their multitargeting ability, blocking more than one signaling pathway. Further, most of the studied compounds are required to be taken clinical research to evaluate their actual applications and toxicity. Also, as a chemopreventive approach, these natural phytochemicals can be used for the treatment and various efforts should be made to understand their potencies, pharmacokinetics and pharmacodynamics, drug-drug interaction, stabilities, metabolism and dosage period. These herbal compounds with medicinal properties have tremendous potential to be used as an alternative against chemotherapeutic drugs and continue to be an attractive research topic in the upcoming future.

CONSENT FOR PUBLICATION

Not applicable.

CONFLICT OF INTEREST

The authors declare that they do not have any conflict of interest regarding the present work.

ACKNOWLEDGMENTS

Declared none.

REFERENCES

[1]   *Cancer Facts and Figures,* **2017**.*American Cancer Society https://www.cancer.org/research/cancer-facts-statistics/all-cancer-facts- figures/cancer-facts-figures-2017.html (accessed 1st January, 2018),*

[2]   Iqbal, J.; Abbasi, B.A.; Mahmood, T.; Kanwal, S.; Ali, B.; Khalil, A.T. Plant- derived anticancer agents: A green anticancer approach. *Asian Pac. J. Trop. Biomed.,* **2017**, *7*(12), 1129-1150.
[http://dx.doi.org/10.1016/j.apjtb.2017.10.016]

[3]   Mazumder, A.; Cerella, C.; Diederich, M. Natural scaffolds in anticancer therapy and precision medicine. *Biotechnol. Adv.,* **2018**, *36*(6), 1563-1585.
[http://dx.doi.org/10.1016/j.biotechadv.2018.04.009] [PMID: 29729870]

[4]   Seelinger, M.; Popescu, R.; Giessrigl, B.; Jarukamjorn, K.; Unger, C.; Wallnöfer, B.; Fritzer-Szekeres, M.; Szekeres, T.; Diaz, R.; Jäger, W.; Frisch, R.; Kopp, B.; Krupitza, G. Methanol extract of the ethnopharmaceutical remedy Smilax spinosa exhibits anti-neoplastic activity. *Int. J. Oncol.,* **2012**, *41*(3), 1164-1172.
[http://dx.doi.org/10.3892/ijo.2012.1538] [PMID: 22752086]

[5]   Merina, N.; Chandra, K.J.; Jibon, K. Medicinal plants with potential anticancer activities: a review. *Int. Res. J. Pharm.,* **2012**, *3*(6), 26-30.

[6]   Goyal, S.; Gupta, N.; Chatterjee, S.; Nimesh, S. Natural plant extracts as potential therapeutic agents for the treatment of cancer. *Curr. Top. Med. Chem.,* **2017**, *17*(2), 96-106.
[http://dx.doi.org/10.2174/1568026616666160530154407] [PMID: 27237328]

[7]   Pandey, K.B.; Rizvi, S.I. Plant polyphenols as dietary antioxidants in human health and disease. *Oxid. Med. Cell. Longev.,* **2009**, *2*(5), 270-278.
[http://dx.doi.org/10.4161/oxim.2.5.9498] [PMID: 20716914]

[8]   Pistollato, F.; Calderón Iglesias, R.; Ruiz, R.; Aparicio, S.; Crespo, J.; Dzul Lopez, L.; Giampieri, F.; Battino, M. The use of natural compounds for the targeting and chemoprevention of ovarian cancer. *Cancer Lett.,* **2017**, *411*, 191-200.
[http://dx.doi.org/10.1016/j.canlet.2017.09.050] [PMID: 29017913]

[9]   Martins, N.; Petropoulos, S.; Ferreira, I.C. Chemical composition and bioactive compounds of garlic (Allium sativum L.) as affected by pre- and post-harvest conditions: A review. *Food Chem.,* **2016**, *211*, 41-50.
[http://dx.doi.org/10.1016/j.foodchem.2016.05.029] [PMID: 27283605]

[10]   Tanaka, S.; Haruma, K.; Yoshihara, M.; Kajiyama, G.; Kira, K.; Amagase, H.; Chayama, K. Aged garlic extract has potential suppressive effect on colorectal adenomas in humans. *J. Nutr.,* **2006**, *136*(3) Suppl., 821S-826S.
[http://dx.doi.org/10.1093/jn/136.3.821S] [PMID: 16484573]

[11]   Roy, N.; Nazeem, P.A.; Babu, T.D.; Abida, P.S.; Narayanankutty, A.; Valsalan, R.; Valsala, P.A.; Raghavamenon, A.C. EGFR gene regulation in colorectal cancer cells by garlic phytocompounds with special emphasis on S-Allyl-L-Cysteine Sulfoxide. *Interdiscip. Sci.,* **2018**, *10*(4), 686-693.
[http://dx.doi.org/10.1007/s12539-017-0227-6] [PMID: 28349439]

[12]   Ishikawa, H.; Saeki, T.; Otani, T.; Suzuki, T.; Shimozuma, K.; Nishino, H.; Fukuda, S.; Morimoto, K. Aged garlic extract prevents a decline of NK cell number and activity in patients with advanced cancer. *J. Nutr.,* **2006**, *136*(3) Suppl., 816S-820S.
[http://dx.doi.org/10.1093/jn/136.3.816S] [PMID: 16484572]

[13]   Hewlings, S.J.; Kalman, D.S. Curcumin: A Review of Its' Effects on Human Health. *Foods,* **2017**, *6*(10), 92.
[http://dx.doi.org/10.3390/foods6100092] [PMID: 29065496]

[14]   Senft, C.; Polacin, M.; Priester, M.; Seifert, V.; Kögel, D.; Weissenberger, J. The nontoxic natural compound Curcumin exerts anti-proliferative, anti-migratory, and anti-invasive properties against malignant gliomas. *BMC Cancer,* **2010**, *10*(1), 491.
[http://dx.doi.org/10.1186/1471-2407-10-491] [PMID: 20840775]

[15]   Wilken, R.; Veena, M.S.; Wang, M.B.; Srivatsan, E.S. Curcumin: A review of anti-cancer properties and therapeutic activity in head and neck squamous cell carcinoma. *Mol. Cancer,* **2011**, *10*(1), 12.
[http://dx.doi.org/10.1186/1476-4598-10-12] [PMID: 21299897]

[16]   Lin, L.; Liu, Y.; Li, H.; Li, P.K.; Fuchs, J.; Shibata, H.; Iwabuchi, Y.; Lin, J. Targeting colon cancer stem cells using a new curcumin analogue, GO-Y030. *Br. J. Cancer,* **2011**, *105*(2), 212-220.
[http://dx.doi.org/10.1038/bjc.2011.200] [PMID: 21694723]

[17]   Aggarwal, B.B.; Ichikawa, H.; Garodia, P.; Weerasinghe, P.; Sethi, G.; Bhatt, I.D.; Pandey, M.K.; Shishodia, S.; Nair, M.G. From traditional Ayurvedic medicine to modern medicine: identification of

therapeutic targets for suppression of inflammation and cancer. *Expert Opin. Ther. Targets,* **2006**, *10*(1), 87-118.
[http://dx.doi.org/10.1517/14728222.10.1.87] [PMID: 16441231]

[18]   Jeong, W-S.; Kim, I-W.; Hu, R.; Kong, A-N.T. Modulatory properties of various natural chemopreventive agents on the activation of NF-kappaB signaling pathway. *Pharm. Res.,* **2004**, *21*(4), 661-670.
[http://dx.doi.org/10.1023/B:PHAM.0000022413.43212.cf] [PMID: 15139523]

[19]   Kasi, P.D.; Tamilselvam, R.; Skalicka-Woźniak, K.; Nabavi, S.F.; Daglia, M.; Bishayee, A.; Pazoki-Toroudi, H.; Nabavi, S.M. Molecular targets of curcumin for cancer therapy: an updated review. *Tumour Biol.,* **2016**, *37*(10), 13017-13028.
[http://dx.doi.org/10.1007/s13277-016-5183-y] [PMID: 27468716]

[20]   Dyer, J.L.; Khan, S.Z.; Bilmen, J.G.; Hawtin, S.R.; Wheatley, M.; Javed, M.U.; Michelangeli, F. Curcumin: a new cell-permeant inhibitor of the inositol 1,4,5-trisphosphate receptor. *Cell Calcium,* **2002**, *31*(1), 45-52.
[http://dx.doi.org/10.1054/ceca.2001.0259] [PMID: 11990299]

[21]   Sivanantham, B.; Sethuraman, S.; Krishnan, U.M. Combinatorial effects of curcumin with an anti-neoplastic agent on head and neck squamous cell carcinoma through the regulation of EGFR-ERK1/2 and apoptotic signaling pathways. *ACS Comb. Sci.,* **2016**, *18*(1), 22-35.
[http://dx.doi.org/10.1021/acscombsci.5b00043] [PMID: 26505786]

[22]   Zhu, J.Y.; Yang, X.; Chen, Y.; Jiang, Y.; Wang, S.J.; Li, Y.; Wang, X.Q.; Meng, Y.; Zhu, M.M.; Ma, X.; Huang, C.; Wu, R.; Xie, C.F.; Li, X.T.; Geng, S.S.; Wu, J.S.; Zhong, C.Y.; Han, H.Y. Curcumin Suppresses Lung Cancer Stem Cells *via* Inhibiting Wnt/β-catenin and Sonic Hedgehog Pathways. *Phytother. Res.,* **2017**, *31*(4), 680-688.
[http://dx.doi.org/10.1002/ptr.5791] [PMID: 28198062]

[23]   Gera, M.; Sharma, N.; Ghosh, M.; Huynh, D.L.; Lee, S.J.; Min, T.; Kwon, T.; Jeong, D.K. Nanoformulations of curcumin: an emerging paradigm for improved remedial application. *Oncotarget,* **2017**, *8*(39), 66680-66698.
[http://dx.doi.org/10.18632/oncotarget.19164] [PMID: 29029547]

[24]   Gupta, S.C.; Patchva, S.; Aggarwal, B.B. Therapeutic roles of curcumin: lessons learned from clinical trials. *AAPS J.,* **2013**, *15*(1), 195-218.
[http://dx.doi.org/10.1208/s12248-012-9432-8] [PMID: 23143785]

[25]   Kanai, M.; Yoshimura, K.; Asada, M.; Imaizumi, A.; Suzuki, C.; Matsumoto, S.; Nishimura, T.; Mori, Y.; Masui, T.; Kawaguchi, Y.; Yanagihara, K.; Yazumi, S.; Chiba, T.; Guha, S.; Aggarwal, B.B. A phase I/II study of gemcitabine-based chemotherapy plus curcumin for patients with gemcitabine-resistant pancreatic cancer. *Cancer Chemother. Pharmacol.,* **2011**, *68*(1), 157-164.
[http://dx.doi.org/10.1007/s00280-010-1470-2] [PMID: 20859741]

[26]   Aggarwal, B.B.; Bhardwaj, A.; Aggarwal, R.S.; Seeram, N.P.; Shishodia, S.; Takada, Y. Role of resveratrol in prevention and therapy of cancer: preclinical and clinical studies. *Anticancer Res.,* **2004**, *24*(5A), 2783-2840.
[PMID: 15517885]

[27]   Smoliga, J.M.; Baur, J.A.; Hausenblas, H.A. Resveratrol and health--a comprehensive review of human clinical trials. *Mol. Nutr. Food Res.,* **2011**, *55*(8), 1129-1141.
[http://dx.doi.org/10.1002/mnfr.201100143] [PMID: 21688389]

[28]   Nguyen, A.V.; Martinez, M.; Stamos, M.J.; Moyer, M.P.; Planutis, K.; Hope, C.; Holcombe, R.F. Results of a phase I pilot clinical trial examining the effect of plant-derived resveratrol and grape powder on Wnt pathway target gene expression in colonic mucosa and colon cancer. *Cancer Manag. Res.,* **2009**, *1*, 25-37.
[http://dx.doi.org/10.2147/CMAR.S4544] [PMID: 21188121]

[29]   Del Follo-Martinez, A.; Banerjee, N.; Li, X.; Safe, S.; Mertens-Talcott, S. Resveratrol and quercetin in

combination have anticancer activity in colon cancer cells and repress oncogenic microRNA-27a. *Nutr. Cancer,* **2013**, *65*(3), 494-504.
[http://dx.doi.org/10.1080/01635581.2012.725194] [PMID: 23530649]

[30]   Patel, K.R.; Brown, V.A.; Jones, D.J.; Britton, R.G.; Hemingway, D.; Miller, A.S.; West, K.P.; Booth, T.D.; Perloff, M.; Crowell, J.A.; Brenner, D.E.; Steward, W.P.; Gescher, A.J.; Brown, K. Clinical pharmacology of resveratrol and its metabolites in colorectal cancer patients. *Cancer Res.,* **2010**, *70*(19), 7392-7399.
[http://dx.doi.org/10.1158/0008-5472.CAN-10-2027] [PMID: 20841478]

[31]   Varoni, E.M.; Lo Faro, A.F.; Sharifi-Rad, J.; Iriti, M. Anticancer molecular mechanisms of resveratrol. *Front. Nutr.,* **2016**, *3*, 8.
[http://dx.doi.org/10.3389/fnut.2016.00008] [PMID: 27148534]

[32]   Diaz-Gerevini, G.T.; Repossi, G.; Dain, A.; Tarres, M.C.; Das, U.N.; Eynard, A.R. Beneficial action of resveratrol: How and why? *Nutrition,* **2016**, *32*(2), 174-178.
[http://dx.doi.org/10.1016/j.nut.2015.08.017] [PMID: 26706021]

[33]   Sui, X.; Zhang, C.; Zhou, J.; Cao, S.; Xu, C.; Tang, F.; Zhi, X.; Chen, B.; Wang, S.; Yin, L. Resveratrol inhibits Extranodal NK/T cell lymphoma through activation of DNA damage response pathway. *J. Exp. Clin. Cancer Res.,* **2017**, *36*(1), 133.
[http://dx.doi.org/10.1186/s13046-017-0601-6] [PMID: 28950914]

[34]   Wang, S.; Willenberg, I.; Krohn, M.; Hecker, T.; Meckelmann, S.; Li, C.; Pan, Y.; Schebb, N.H.; Steinberg, P.; Empl, M.T. Growth-Inhibiting Activity of Resveratrol Imine Analogs on Tumor Cells *In Vitro. PLoS One,* **2017**, *12*(1), e0170502.
[http://dx.doi.org/10.1371/journal.pone.0170502] [PMID: 28114318]

[35]   Chimento, A.; Sirianni, R.; Saturnino, C.; Caruso, A.; Sinicropi, M.S.; Pezzi, V. Resveratrol and its analogs as antitumoral agents for breast cancer treatment. *Mini Rev. Med. Chem.,* **2016**, *16*(9), 699-709.
[http://dx.doi.org/10.2174/1389557516666160321113255] [PMID: 26996623]

[36]   Kim, J-A.; Kim, D.H.; Hossain, M.A.; Kim, M.Y.; Sung, B.; Yoon, J-H.; Suh, H.; Jeong, T.C.; Chung, H.Y.; Kim, N.D. HS-1793, a resveratrol analogue, induces cell cycle arrest and apoptotic cell death in human breast cancer cells. *Int. J. Oncol.,* **2014**, *44*(2), 473-480.
[http://dx.doi.org/10.3892/ijo.2013.2207] [PMID: 24316714]

[37]   Meng, J.; Guo, F.; Xu, H.; Liang, W.; Wang, C.; Yang, X-D. Combination therapy using co-encapsulated resveratrol and paclitaxel in liposomes for drug resistance reversal in breast cancer cells *in vivo. Sci. Rep.,* **2016**, *6*, 22390.
[http://dx.doi.org/10.1038/srep22390] [PMID: 26947928]

[38]   Siddiqui, I.A.; Asim, M.; Hafeez, B.B.; Adhami, V.M.; Tarapore, R.S.; Mukhtar, H. Green tea polyphenol EGCG blunts androgen receptor function in prostate cancer. *FASEB J.,* **2011**, *25*(4), 1198-1207.
[http://dx.doi.org/10.1096/fj.10-167924] [PMID: 21177307]

[39]   Khan, N.; Afaq, F.; Saleem, M.; Ahmad, N.; Mukhtar, H. Targeting multiple signaling pathways by green tea polyphenol (-)-epigallocatechin-3-gallate. *Cancer Res.,* **2006**, *66*(5), 2500-2505.
[http://dx.doi.org/10.1158/0008-5472.CAN-05-3636] [PMID: 16510563]

[40]   Farhan, M.; Khan, H.Y.; Oves, M.; Al-Harrasi, A.; Rehmani, N.; Arif, H.; Hadi, S.M.; Ahmad, A. Cancer therapy by catechins involves redox cycling of copper ions and generation of reactive oxygen species. *Toxins (Basel),* **2016**, *8*(2), 37.
[http://dx.doi.org/10.3390/toxins8020037] [PMID: 26861392]

[41]   Feng, C.; Ho, Y.; Sun, C.; Xia, G.; Ding, Q.; Gu, B. Epigallocatechin gallate inhibits the growth and promotes the apoptosis of bladder cancer cells. *Exp. Ther. Med.,* **2017**, *14*(4), 3513-3518.
[http://dx.doi.org/10.3892/etm.2017.4981] [PMID: 29042941]

[42]   Huang, C-Y.; Han, Z.; Li, X.; Xie, H-H.; Zhu, S-S. Mechanism of EGCG promoting apoptosis of

MCF-7 cell line in human breast cancer. *Oncol. Lett.,* **2017**, *14*(3), 3623-3627.
[http://dx.doi.org/10.3892/ol.2017.6641] [PMID: 28927122]

[43]   Liu, L.; Ju, Y.; Wang, J.; Zhou, R. Epigallocatechin-3-gallate promotes apoptosis and reversal of multidrug resistance in esophageal cancer cells. *Pathol. Res. Pract.,* **2017**, *213*(10), 1242-1250.
[http://dx.doi.org/10.1016/j.prp.2017.09.006] [PMID: 28964574]

[44]   Wen, Y.; Zhao, R-Q.; Zhang, Y-K.; Gupta, P.; Fu, L-X.; Tang, A-Z.; Liu, B-M.; Chen, Z-S.; Yang, D-H.; Liang, G. Effect of Y6, an epigallocatechin gallate derivative, on reversing doxorubicin drug resistance in human hepatocellular carcinoma cells. *Oncotarget,* **2017**, *8*(18), 29760-29770.
[http://dx.doi.org/10.18632/oncotarget.15964] [PMID: 28423656]

[45]   Rady, I.; Mohamed, H.; Rady, M.; Siddiqui, I.A.; Mukhtar, H. Cancer preventive and therapeutic effects of egcg, the major polyphenol in green tea. *Egypt. J. Basic Appl. Sci.,* **2017**.

[46]   Ayoob, I.; Hazari, Y.M.; Lone, S.H.; Khuroo, M.A.; Fazili, K.M.; Bhat, K.A. Phytochemical and cytotoxic evaluation of Peganum Harmala: Structure activity relationship studies of harmine. *ChemistrySelect,* **2017**, *2*(10), 2965-2968.
[http://dx.doi.org/10.1002/slct.201700232]

[47]   Ooko, E.; Kadioglu, O.; Greten, H.J.; Efferth, T. Pharmacogenomic Characterization and Isobologram Analysis of the Combination of Ascorbic Acid and Curcumin-Two Main Metabolites of *Curcuma longa*-in Cancer Cells. *Front. Pharmacol.,* **2017**, *8*, 38.
[http://dx.doi.org/10.3389/fphar.2017.00038] [PMID: 28210221]

[48]   Bhandari, J.; Muhammad, B.; Thapa, P.; Shrestha, B.G. Study of phytochemical, anti-microbial, anti-oxidant, and anti-cancer properties of Allium wallichii. *BMC Complement. Altern. Med.,* **2017**, *17*(1), 102.
[http://dx.doi.org/10.1186/s12906-017-1622-6] [PMID: 28178952]

[49]   Tariq, A.; Sadia, S.; Pan, K.; Ullah, I.; Mussarat, S.; Sun, F.; Abiodun, O.O.; Batbaatar, A.; Li, Z.; Song, D.; Xiong, Q.; Ullah, R.; Khan, S.; Basnet, B.B.; Kumar, B.; Islam, R.; Adnan, M. A systematic review on ethnomedicines of anti-cancer plants. *Phytother. Res.,* **2017**, *31*(2), 202-264.
[http://dx.doi.org/10.1002/ptr.5751] [PMID: 28093828]

[50]   Preethi, R.; Padma, P. Biosynthesis and bioactivity of silver nanobioconjugates from grape (vitis vinifera) seeds and its active component resveratrol. *Int. J. Pharm. Sci. Res.,* **2016**, *7*(10), 4253.

[51]   Al Sinani, S.S.; Eltayeb, E.A.; Coomber, B.L.; Adham, S.A. Solamargine triggers cellular necrosis selectively in different types of human melanoma cancer cells through extrinsic lysosomal mitochondrial death pathway. *Cancer Cell Int.,* **2016**, *16*(1), 11.
[http://dx.doi.org/10.1186/s12935-016-0287-4] [PMID: 26889092]

[52]   Wal, A.; Srivastava, R.; Wal, P.; Rai, A.; Sharma, S. Lupeol as a magical drug. *Pharmaceutical and Biological Evaluations,* **2015**, *2*(5), 142-151.

[53]   Rastogi, N.; Duggal, S.; Singh, S.K.; Porwal, K.; Srivastava, V.K.; Maurya, R.; Bhatt, M.L.; Mishra, D.P. Proteasome inhibition mediates p53 reactivation and anti-cancer activity of 6-gingerol in cervical cancer cells. *Oncotarget,* **2015**, *6*(41), 43310-43325.
[http://dx.doi.org/10.18632/oncotarget.6383] [PMID: 26621832]

[54]   Wang, C-Z.; Zhang, Z.; Wan, J-Y.; Zhang, C-F.; Anderson, S.; He, X.; Yu, C.; He, T-C.; Qi, L-W.; Yuan, C-S. Protopanaxadiol, an active ginseng metabolite, significantly enhances the effects of fluorouracil on colon cancer. *Nutrients,* **2015**, *7*(2), 799-814.
[http://dx.doi.org/10.3390/nu7020799] [PMID: 25625815]

[55]   Pang, S-Q.; Wang, G-Q.; Lin, J.S.; Diao, Y.; Xu, R.A. Cytotoxic activity of the alkaloids from Broussonetia papyrifera fruits. *Pharm. Biol.,* **2014**, *52*(10), 1315-1319.
[http://dx.doi.org/10.3109/13880209.2014.891139] [PMID: 24992202]

[56]   Jung, S.K.; Lee, M-H.; Lim, D.Y.; Kim, J.E.; Singh, P.; Lee, S.Y.; Jeong, C.H.; Lim, T.G.; Chen, H.; Chi, Y.I.; Kundu, J.K.; Lee, N.H.; Lee, C.C.; Cho, Y.Y.; Bode, A.M.; Lee, K.W.; Dong, Z.

Isoliquiritigenin induces apoptosis and inhibits xenograft tumor growth of human lung cancer cells by targeting both wild type and L858R/T790M mutant EGFR. *J. Biol. Chem.*, **2014**, *289*(52), 35839-35848.
[http://dx.doi.org/10.1074/jbc.M114.585513] [PMID: 25368326]

[57]   Mishra, S.; Aeri, V.; Gaur, P. K.; Jachak, S. M. Phytochemical, therapeutic, and ethnopharmacological overview for a traditionally important herb: Boerhavia diffusa Linn *BioMed Res. Int,* **2014**.

[58]   Motta, L.B.; Furlan, C.M.; Santos, D.Y.; Salatino, M.L.; Duarte-Almeida, J.M.; Negri, G.; Carvalho, J.E.d.; Ruiz, A.L.T.; Cordeiro, I.; Salatino, A. Constituents and antiproliferative activity of extracts from leaves of Croton macrobothrys. *Rev. Bras. Farmacogn.*, **2011**, *21*(6), 972-977.
[http://dx.doi.org/10.1590/S0102-695X2011005000174]

[59]   Maneerat, W.; Tha-In, S.; Cheenpracha, S.; Prawat, U.; Laphookhieo, S. New amides from the seeds of Clausana lansium. *J. Med. Plants Res.*, **2011**, *5*(13), 2812-2815.

[60]   Sakarkar, D.; Deshmukh, V. Ethnopharmacological review of traditional medicinal plants for anticancer activity. *Int. J. Pharm. Tech. Res.*, **2011**, *3*(1), 298-308.

[61]   Xu, L.N.; Lu, B.N.; Hu, M.M.; Xu, Y.W.; Han, X.; Qi, Y.; Peng, J.Y. Mechanisms involved in the cytotoxic effects of berberine on human colon cancer HCT-8 cells. *Biocell,* **2012**, *36*(3), 113-120.
[PMID: 23682426]

[62]   Rahman, S.; Carter, P.; Bhattarai, N. Aloe vera for tissue engineering applications. *J. Funct. Biomater.*, **2017**, *8*(1), 6.
[http://dx.doi.org/10.3390/jfb8010006] [PMID: 28216559]

[63]   Weng, J.-R.; Bai, L.-Y.; Chiu, C.-F.; Hu, J.-L.; Chiu, S.-J.; Wu, C.-Y. Cucurbitane triterpenoid from Momordica charantia induces apoptosis and autophagy in breast cancer cells, in part, through peroxisome proliferator-activated receptor γ activation *Evid-Based Complementary Altern. Med,* **2013**.

[64]   Rakashanda, S.; Mubashir, S.; Qurishi, Y.; Hamid, A.; Masood, A.; Amin, S. Trypsin inhibitors from Lavatera cashmeriana Camb. seeds: isolation, characterization and in-vitro cytotoxicity activity. *Int. J. Pharm. Sci. Inven.*, **2013**, *2*(5), 55-65.

[65]   Ngo, S.N.; Williams, D.B.; Head, R.J. Rosemary and cancer prevention: preclinical perspectives. *Crit. Rev. Food Sci. Nutr.*, **2011**, *51*(10), 946-954.
[http://dx.doi.org/10.1080/10408398.2010.490883] [PMID: 21955093]

[66]   Greenhough, A.; Smartt, H.J.; Moore, A.E.; Roberts, H.R.; Williams, A.C.; Paraskeva, C.; Kaidi, A. The COX-2/PGE2 pathway: key roles in the hallmarks of cancer and adaptation to the tumour microenvironment. *Carcinogenesis,* **2009**, *30*(3), 377-386.
[http://dx.doi.org/10.1093/carcin/bgp014] [PMID: 19136477]

[67]   Ramos, A.A.; Pedro, D.; Collins, A.R.; Pereira-Wilson, C. Protection by Salvia extracts against oxidative and alkylation damage to DNA in human HCT15 and CO115 cells. *J. Toxicol. Environ. Health A,* **2012**, *75*(13-15), 765-775.
[http://dx.doi.org/10.1080/15287394.2012.689804] [PMID: 22788364]

[68]   Roland, C.L.; Dineen, S.P.; Toombs, J.E.; Carbon, J.G.; Smith, C.W.; Brekken, R.A.; Barnett, C.C., Jr Tumor-derived intercellular adhesion molecule-1 mediates tumor-associated leukocyte infiltration in orthotopic pancreatic xenografts. *Exp. Biol. Med. (Maywood),* **2010**, *235*(2), 263-270.
[http://dx.doi.org/10.1258/ebm.2009.009215] [PMID: 20404043]

[69]   Moon, D-O.; Kim, M-O.; Lee, J-D.; Choi, Y.H.; Kim, G-Y. Rosmarinic acid sensitizes cell death through suppression of TNF-α-induced NF-kappaB activation and ROS generation in human leukemia U937 cells. *Cancer Lett.*, **2010**, *288*(2), 183-191.
[http://dx.doi.org/10.1016/j.canlet.2009.06.033] [PMID: 19619938]

[70]   Xu, Y.; Jiang, Z.; Ji, G.; Liu, J. Inhibition of bone metastasis from breast carcinoma by rosmarinic acid. *Planta Med.*, **2010**, *76*(10), 956-962.
[http://dx.doi.org/10.1055/s-0029-1240893] [PMID: 20157877]

[71]   Moore, J.; Megaly, M.; MacNeil, A.J.; Klentrou, P.; Tsiani, E. Rosemary extract reduces Akt/mTOR/p70S6K activation and inhibits proliferation and survival of A549 human lung cancer cells. *Biomed. Pharmacother.,* **2016**, *83*, 725-732.
[http://dx.doi.org/10.1016/j.biopha.2016.07.043] [PMID: 27470574]

[72]   Visanji, J.M.; Thompson, D.G.; Padfield, P.J. Induction of G2/M phase cell cycle arrest by carnosol and carnosic acid is associated with alteration of cyclin A and cyclin B1 levels. *Cancer Lett.,* **2006**, *237*(1), 130-136.
[http://dx.doi.org/10.1016/j.canlet.2005.05.045] [PMID: 16019137]

[73]   Kontogianni, V.G.; Tomic, G.; Nikolic, I.; Nerantzaki, A.A.; Sayyad, N.; Stosic-Grujicic, S.; Stojanovic, I.; Gerothanassis, I.P.; Tzakos, A.G. Phytochemical profile of Rosmarinus officinalis and Salvia officinalis extracts and correlation to their antioxidant and anti-proliferative activity. *Food Chem.,* **2013**, *136*(1), 120-129.
[http://dx.doi.org/10.1016/j.foodchem.2012.07.091] [PMID: 23017402]

[74]   Tao, L.; Wang, S.; Zhao, Y.; Sheng, X.; Wang, A.; Zheng, S.; Lu, Y. Phenolcarboxylic acids from medicinal herbs exert anticancer effects through disruption of COX-2 activity. *Phytomedicine,* **2014**, *21*(11), 1473-1482.
[http://dx.doi.org/10.1016/j.phymed.2014.05.001] [PMID: 24916702]

[75]   Jin, B-R.; Chung, K-S.; Cheon, S-Y.; Lee, M.; Hwang, S.; Noh Hwang, S.; Rhee, K-J.; An, H-J. Rosmarinic acid suppresses colonic inflammation in dextran sulphate sodium (DSS)-induced mice *via* dual inhibition of NF-κB and STAT3 activation. *Sci. Rep.,* **2017**, *7*, 46252.
[http://dx.doi.org/10.1038/srep46252] [PMID: 28383063]

[76]   Lu, J.-J.; Bao, J.-L.; Chen, X.-P.; Huang, M.; Wang, Y.-T. Alkaloids isolated from natural herbs as the anticancer agents *Evid. Based Complementary Altern. Med,* **2012**.

[77]   Anitha, S. Pharmacological activity of vinca alkaloids. *Res Rev J Pharmacognosy Phytochem,* **2016**, *4*(3), 27-34.

[78]   Moudi, M.; Go, R.; Yien, C.Y.S.; Nazre, M. Vinca alkaloids. *Int. J. Prev. Med.,* **2013**, *4*(11), 1231-1235.
[PMID: 24404355]

[79]   Schutz, F.A.; Bellmunt, J.; Rosenberg, J.E.; Choueiri, T.K. Vinflunine: drug safety evaluation of this novel synthetic vinca alkaloid. *Expert Opin. Drug Saf.,* **2011**, *10*(4), 645-653.
[http://dx.doi.org/10.1517/14740338.2011.581660] [PMID: 21524237]

[80]   Zhong, Y.J.; Shi, F.; Zheng, X.L.; Wang, Q.; Yang, L.; Sun, H.; He, F.; Zhang, L.; Lin, Y.; Qin, Y.; Liao, L.C.; Wang, X. Crocetin induces cytotoxicity and enhances vincristine-induced cancer cell death *via* p53-dependent and -independent mechanisms. *Acta Pharmacol. Sin.,* **2011**, *32*(12), 1529-1536.
[http://dx.doi.org/10.1038/aps.2011.109] [PMID: 21986580]

[81]   Verschraegen, C.F.; Gilbert, B.E.; Loyer, E.; Huaringa, A.; Walsh, G.; Newman, R.A.; Knight, V. Clinical evaluation of the delivery and safety of aerosolized liposomal 9-nitro-20(s)-camptothecin in patients with advanced pulmonary malignancies. *Clin. Cancer Res.,* **2004**, *10*(7), 2319-2326.
[http://dx.doi.org/10.1158/1078-0432.CCR-0929-3] [PMID: 15073107]

[82]   Chen, F.; Wang, H.; Zhu, J.; Zhao, R.; Xue, P.; Zhang, Q.; Bud Nelson, M.; Qu, W.; Feng, B.; Pi, J. Camptothecin suppresses NRF2-ARE activity and sensitises hepatocellular carcinoma cells to anticancer drugs. *Br. J. Cancer,* **2017**, *117*(10), 1495-1506.
[http://dx.doi.org/10.1038/bjc.2017.317] [PMID: 28910823]

[83]   Shen, X.; Chen, J.; Qiu, R.; Fan, X.; Xin, Y. Effect of camptothecin on inducible nitric oxide synthase expression in the colon cancer SW480 cell line. *Oncol. Lett.,* **2015**, *10*(5), 3157-3160.
[http://dx.doi.org/10.3892/ol.2015.3658] [PMID: 26722304]

[84]   Qin, J.; Wang, W.; Zhang, R. Novel natural product therapeutics targeting both inflammation and cancer. *Chin. J. Nat. Med.,* **2017**, *15*(6), 401-416.

[http://dx.doi.org/10.1016/S1875-5364(17)30062-6] [PMID: 28629530]

[85]   Bhuvanalakshmi, G.; Basappa, K.S.R.; Rangappa, K.S.; Dharmarajan, A.; Sethi, G.; Kumar, A.P.; Warrier, S. Breast Cancer Stem-Like Cells Are Inhibited by Diosgenin, a Steroidal Saponin, by the Attenuation of the Wnt β-Catenin Signaling *via* the Wnt Antagonist Secreted Frizzled Related Protein-4. *Front. Pharmacol.,* **2017**, *8*, 124.
[http://dx.doi.org/10.3389/fphar.2017.00124] [PMID: 28373842]

[86]   Lepage, C.; Léger, D.Y.; Bertrand, J.; Martin, F.; Beneytout, J.L.; Liagre, B. Diosgenin induces death receptor-5 through activation of p38 pathway and promotes TRAIL-induced apoptosis in colon cancer cells. *Cancer Lett.,* **2011**, *301*(2), 193-202.
[http://dx.doi.org/10.1016/j.canlet.2010.12.003] [PMID: 21195543]

[87]   Li, Y.; Wang, X.; Cheng, S.; Du, J.; Deng, Z.; Zhang, Y.; Liu, Q.; Gao, J.; Cheng, B.; Ling, C. Diosgenin induces G2/M cell cycle arrest and apoptosis in human hepatocellular carcinoma cells. *Oncol. Rep.,* **2015**, *33*(2), 693-698.
[http://dx.doi.org/10.3892/or.2014.3629] [PMID: 25434486]

[88]   Rahmati-Yamchi, M.; Ghareghomi, S.; Haddadchi, G.; Milani, M.; Aghazadeh, M.; Daroushnejad, H. Fenugreek extract diosgenin and pure diosgenin inhibit the hTERT gene expression in A549 lung cancer cell line. *Mol. Biol. Rep.,* **2014**, *41*(9), 6247-6252.
[http://dx.doi.org/10.1007/s11033-014-3505-y] [PMID: 24973886]

[89]   Jagadeesan, J.; Nandakumar, N.; Rengarajan, T.; Balasubramanian, M.P. Diosgenin, a steroidal saponin, exhibits anticancer activity by attenuating lipid peroxidation *via* enhancing antioxidant defense system during NMU-induced breast carcinoma. *J. Environ. Pathol. Toxicol. Oncol.,* **2012**, *31*(2), 121-129.
[http://dx.doi.org/10.1615/JEnvironPatholToxicolOncol.v31.i2.40] [PMID: 23216637]

[90]   Mohammad, R.Y.; Somayyeh, G.; Gholamreza, H.; Majid, M.; Yousef, R. Diosgenin inhibits hTERT gene expression in the A549 lung cancer cell line. *Asian Pac. J. Cancer Prev.,* **2013**, *14*(11), 6945-6948.
[http://dx.doi.org/10.7314/APJCP.2013.14.11.6945] [PMID: 24377630]

[91]   Jiang, S.; Fan, J.; Wang, Q.; Ju, D.; Feng, M.; Li, J.; Guan, Z.B.; An, D.; Wang, X.; Ye, L. Diosgenin induces ROS-dependent autophagy and cytotoxicity *via* mTOR signaling pathway in chronic myeloid leukemia cells. *Phytomedicine,* **2016**, *23*(3), 243-252.
[http://dx.doi.org/10.1016/j.phymed.2016.01.010] [PMID: 26969378]

[92]   Masood-Ur-Rahman, ; Mohammad, Y.; Fazili, K.M.; Bhat, K.A.; Ara, T. Synthesis and biological evaluation of novel 3-O-tethered triazoles of diosgenin as potent antiproliferative agents. *Steroids,* **2017**, *118*, 1-8.
[http://dx.doi.org/10.1016/j.steroids.2016.11.003] [PMID: 27864018]

[93]   Grossmann, M.E.; Mizuno, N.K.; Schuster, T.; Cleary, M.P. Punicic acid is an ω-5 fatty acid capable of inhibiting breast cancer proliferation. *Int. J. Oncol.,* **2010**, *36*(2), 421-426.
[PMID: 20043077]

[94]   Wang, L.; Li, W.; Lin, M.; Garcia, M.; Mulholland, D.; Lilly, M.; Martins-Green, M. Luteolin, ellagic acid and punicic acid are natural products that inhibit prostate cancer metastasis. *Carcinogenesis,* **2014**, *35*(10), 2321-2330.
[http://dx.doi.org/10.1093/carcin/bgu145] [PMID: 25023990]

[95]   Tran, H.N.A.; Bae, S-Y.; Song, B-H.; Lee, B-H.; Bae, Y-S.; Kim, Y-H.; Lansky, E.P.; Newman, R.A. Pomegranate (Punica granatum) seed linolenic acid isomers: concentration-dependent modulation of estrogen receptor activity. *Endocr. Res.,* **2010**, *35*(1), 1-16.
[http://dx.doi.org/10.3109/07435800903524161] [PMID: 20136514]

[96]   Nagoor Meeran, M.F.; Javed, H.; Al Taee, H.; Azimullah, S.; Ojha, S.K.; Ojha, S.K. Pharmacological properties and molecular mechanisms of thymol: prospects for its therapeutic potential and pharmaceutical development. *Front. Pharmacol.,* **2017**, *8*, 380.

[http://dx.doi.org/10.3389/fphar.2017.00380] [PMID: 28694777]

[97]   Kang, S-H.; Kim, Y-S.; Kim, E-K.; Hwang, J-W.; Jeong, J-H.; Dong, X.; Lee, J-W.; Moon, S-H.; Jeon, B-T.; Park, P-J. Anticancer effect of thymol on AGS human gastric carcinoma cells. *J. Microbiol. Biotechnol.,* **2016**, *26*(1), 28-37.
[http://dx.doi.org/10.4014/jmb.1506.06073] [PMID: 26437948]

[98]   Deb, D.D.; Parimala, G.; Saravana Devi, S.; Chakraborty, T. Effect of thymol on peripheral blood mononuclear cell PBMC and acute promyelotic cancer cell line HL-60. *Chem. Biol. Interact.,* **2011**, *193*(1), 97-106.
[http://dx.doi.org/10.1016/j.cbi.2011.05.009] [PMID: 21640085]

[99]   Slamenová, D.; Horváthová, E.; Sramková, M.; Marsálková, L. DNA-protective effects of two components of essential plant oils carvacrol and thymol on mammalian cells cultured *in vitro*. *Neoplasma,* **2007**, *54*(2), 108-112.
[PMID: 17319782]

[100] Lee, K.P.; Kim, J.E.; Park, W.H.; Hong, H. Regulation of C6 glioma cell migration by thymol. *Oncol. Lett.,* **2016**, *11*(4), 2619-2624.
[http://dx.doi.org/10.3892/ol.2016.4237] [PMID: 27073528]

[101] Amin, A.; Gali-Muhtasib, H.; Ocker, M.; Schneider-Stock, R. Overview of major classes of plant-derived anticancer drugs. *Int. J. Biomed. Sci.,* **2009**, *5*(1), 1-11.
[PMID: 23675107]

[102] Jordan, M.A.; Wilson, L. Microtubules as a target for anticancer drugs. *Nat. Rev. Cancer,* **2004**, *4*(4), 253-265.
[http://dx.doi.org/10.1038/nrc1317] [PMID: 15057285]

[103] Shah, U.; Shah, R.; Acharya, S.; Acharya, N. Novel anticancer agents from plant sources. *Chin. J. Nat. Med.,* **2013**, *11*(1), 16-23.
[http://dx.doi.org/10.3724/SP.J.1009.2013.00016]

[104] Bernabeu, E.; Cagel, M.; Lagomarsino, E.; Moretton, M.; Chiappetta, D.A. Paclitaxel: What has been done and the challenges remain ahead. *Int. J. Pharm.,* **2017**, *526*(1-2), 474-495.
[http://dx.doi.org/10.1016/j.ijpharm.2017.05.016] [PMID: 28501439]

[105] Ogbourne, S.M.; Parsons, P.G. The value of nature's natural product library for the discovery of New Chemical Entities: the discovery of ingenol mebutate. *Fitoterapia,* **2014**, *98*, 36-44.
[http://dx.doi.org/10.1016/j.fitote.2014.07.002] [PMID: 25016953]

[106] West, C.M.; Price, P. Combretastatin A4 phosphate. *Anticancer Drugs,* **2004**, *15*(3), 179-187.
[http://dx.doi.org/10.1097/00001813-200403000-00001] [PMID: 15014350]

[107] Cragg, G.M.; Newman, D.J. Plants as a source of anti-cancer agents. *J. Ethnopharmacol.,* **2005**, *100*(1-2), 72-79.
[http://dx.doi.org/10.1016/j.jep.2005.05.011] [PMID: 16009521]

[108] Lemasters, J.J.; Theruvath, T.P.; Zhong, Z.; Nieminen, A-L. Mitochondrial calcium and the permeability transition in cell death. *Biochim. Biophys. Acta,* **2009**, *1787*(11), 1395-1401.
[http://dx.doi.org/10.1016/j.bbabio.2009.06.009] [PMID: 19576166]

[109] Dejean, L.M.; Martinez-Caballero, S.; Kinnally, K.W. Is MAC the knife that cuts cytochrome c from mitochondria during apoptosis? *Cell Death Differ.,* **2006**, *13*(8), 1387-1395.
[http://dx.doi.org/10.1038/sj.cdd.4401949] [PMID: 16676005]

[110] Dejean, L.M.; Martinez-Caballero, S.; Manon, S.; Kinnally, K.W. Regulation of the mitochondrial apoptosis-induced channel, MAC, by BCL-2 family proteins. *Biochim. Biophys. Acta,* **2006**, *1762*(2), 191-201.
[http://dx.doi.org/10.1016/j.bbadis.2005.07.002] [PMID: 16055309]

[111] Sun, J.; Hai Liu, R. Cranberry phytochemical extracts induce cell cycle arrest and apoptosis in human MCF-7 breast cancer cells. *Cancer Lett.,* **2006**, *241*(1), 124-134.

[http://dx.doi.org/10.1016/j.canlet.2005.10.027] [PMID: 16377076]

[112] Lv, Z-D.; Liu, X-P.; Zhao, W-J.; Dong, Q.; Li, F-N.; Wang, H-B.; Kong, B. Curcumin induces apoptosis in breast cancer cells and inhibits tumor growth *in vitro* and *in vivo*. *Int. J. Clin. Exp. Pathol.,* **2014**, *7*(6), 2818-2824.
[PMID: 25031701]

[113] Jin, B.; Li, Y.; Robertson, K.D. DNA methylation: superior or subordinate in the epigenetic hierarchy? *Genes Cancer,* **2011**, *2*(6), 607-617.
[http://dx.doi.org/10.1177/1947601910393957] [PMID: 21941617]

[114] Daura-Oller, E.; Cabre, M.; Montero, M.A.; Paternain, J.L.; Romeu, A. Specific gene hypomethylation and cancer: new insights into coding region feature trends. *Bioinformation,* **2009**, *3*(8), 340-343.
[http://dx.doi.org/10.6026/97320630003340] [PMID: 19707296]

[115] Wang, H.; Khor, T.O.; Shu, L.; Su, Z-Y.; Fuentes, F.; Lee, J-H.; Kong, A.N. Plants *vs.* cancer: a review on natural phytochemicals in preventing and treating cancers and their druggability. *Anticancer. Agents Med. Chem.,* **2012**, *12*(10), 1281-1305.
[http://dx.doi.org/10.2174/187152012803833026] [PMID: 22583408]

[116] Luijsterburg, M.S.; van Attikum, H. Chromatin and the DNA damage response: the cancer connection. *Mol. Oncol.,* **2011**, *5*(4), 349-367.
[http://dx.doi.org/10.1016/j.molonc.2011.06.001] [PMID: 21782533]

[117] Weng, Y.P.; Hung, P.F.; Ku, W.Y.; Chang, C.Y.; Wu, B.H.; Wu, M.H.; Yao, J.Y.; Yang, J.R.; Lee, C.H. The inhibitory activity of gallic acid against DNA methylation: application of gallic acid on epigenetic therapy of human cancers. *Oncotarget,* **2017**, *9*(1), 361-374.
[PMID: 29416619]

[118] Garavito, R.M.; Mulichak, A.M. The structure of mammalian cyclooxygenases. *Annu. Rev. Biophys. Biomol. Struct.,* **2003**, *32*(1), 183-206.
[http://dx.doi.org/10.1146/annurev.biophys.32.110601.141906] [PMID: 12574066]

[119] Tober, K.L.; Thomas-Ahner, J.M.; Kusewitt, D.F.; Oberyszyn, T.M. Effects of UVB on E prostanoid receptor expression in murine skin. *J. Invest. Dermatol.,* **2007**, *127*(1), 214-221.
[http://dx.doi.org/10.1038/sj.jid.5700502] [PMID: 16917495]

[120] Wang, D.; Dubois, R.N. The role of COX-2 in intestinal inflammation and colorectal cancer. *Oncogene,* **2010**, *29*(6), 781-788.
[http://dx.doi.org/10.1038/onc.2009.421] [PMID: 19946329]

[121] Sheehan, K.M.; Sheahan, K.; O'Donoghue, D.P.; MacSweeney, F.; Conroy, R.M.; Fitzgerald, D.J.; Murray, F.E. The relationship between cyclooxygenase-2 expression and colorectal cancer. *JAMA,* **1999**, *282*(13), 1254-1257.
[http://dx.doi.org/10.1001/jama.282.13.1254] [PMID: 10517428]

[122] Cerella, C.; Sobolewski, C.; Dicato, M.; Diederich, M. Targeting COX-2 expression by natural compounds: a promising alternative strategy to synthetic COX-2 inhibitors for cancer chemoprevention and therapy. *Biochem. Pharmacol.,* **2010**, *80*(12), 1801-1815.
[http://dx.doi.org/10.1016/j.bcp.2010.06.050] [PMID: 20615394]

[123] Rao, C.V.; Desai, D.; Rivenson, A.; Simi, B.; Amin, S.; Reddy, B.S. Chemoprevention of colon carcinogenesis by phenylethyl-3-methylcaffeate. *Cancer Res.,* **1995**, *55*(11), 2310-2315.
[PMID: 7757981]

[124] Gong, W.H.; Zhao, N.; Zhang, Z.M.; Zhang, Y.X.; Yan, L.; Li, J.B. The inhibitory effect of resveratrol on COX-2 expression in human colorectal cancer: a promising therapeutic strategy. *Eur. Rev. Med. Pharmacol. Sci.,* **2017**, *21*(5), 1136-1143.
[PMID: 28338176]

[125] Nishida, N.; Yano, H.; Nishida, T.; Kamura, T.; Kojiro, M. Angiogenesis in cancer. *Vasc. Health Risk Manag.,* **2006**, *2*(3), 213-219.

[http://dx.doi.org/10.2147/vhrm.2006.2.3.213] [PMID: 17326328]

[126]   Wen, W.; Lu, J.; Zhang, K.; Chen, S. Grape seed extract inhibits angiogenesis *via* suppression of the vascular endothelial growth factor receptor signaling pathway. *Cancer Prev. Res. (Phila.),* **2008**, *1*(7), 554-561.
[http://dx.doi.org/10.1158/1940-6207.CAPR-08-0040] [PMID: 19139005]

[127]   Lee, J.S.; Shukla, S.; Kim, J-A.; Kim, M. Anti-angiogenic effect of Nelumbo nucifera leaf extracts in human umbilical vein endothelial cells with antioxidant potential. *PLoS One,* **2015**, *10*(2), e0118552.
[http://dx.doi.org/10.1371/journal.pone.0118552] [PMID: 25714482]

[128]   Cao, W.; Hu, C.; Wu, L.; Xu, L.; Jiang, W. Rosmarinic acid inhibits inflammation and angiogenesis of hepatocellular carcinoma by suppression of NF-κB signaling in H22 tumor-bearing mice. *J. Pharmacol. Sci.,* **2016**, *132*(2), 131-137.
[http://dx.doi.org/10.1016/j.jphs.2016.09.003] [PMID: 27707649]

[129]   Chen, H.; Liu, R.H. Potential Mechanisms of Action of Dietary Phytochemicals for Cancer Prevention by Targeting Cellular Signaling Transduction Pathways. *J. Agric. Food Chem.,* **2018**, *66*(13), 3260-3276.
[http://dx.doi.org/10.1021/acs.jafc.7b04975] [PMID: 29498272]

[130]   Lambert, J.D.; Hong, J.; Yang, G.Y.; Liao, J.; Yang, C.S. Inhibition of carcinogenesis by polyphenols: evidence from laboratory investigations. *Am. J. Clin. Nutr.,* **2005**, *81*(1) Suppl., 284S-291S.
[http://dx.doi.org/10.1093/ajcn/81.1.284S] [PMID: 15640492]

[131]   Schilter, B.; Andersson, C.; Anton, R.; Constable, A.; Kleiner, J.; O'Brien, J.; Renwick, A.G.; Korver, O.; Smit, F.; Walker, R. Guidance for the safety assessment of botanicals and botanical preparations for use in food and food supplements. *Food Chem. Toxicol.,* **2003**, *41*(12), 1625-1649.
[http://dx.doi.org/10.1016/S0278-6915(03)00221-7] [PMID: 14563389]

[132]   Weisburg, J.H.; Weissman, D.B.; Sedaghat, T.; Babich, H. *In vitro* cytotoxicity of epigallocatechin gallate and tea extracts to cancerous and normal cells from the human oral cavity. *Basic Clin. Pharmacol. Toxicol.,* **2004**, *95*(4), 191-200.
[http://dx.doi.org/10.1111/j.1742-7843.2004.pto_950407.x] [PMID: 15504155]

[133]   Isbrucker, R.A.; Edwards, J.A.; Wolz, E.; Davidovich, A.; Bausch, J. Safety studies on epigallocatechin gallate (EGCG) preparations. Part 2: dermal, acute and short-term toxicity studies. *Food Chem. Toxicol.,* **2006**, *44*(5), 636-650.
[http://dx.doi.org/10.1016/j.fct.2005.11.003] [PMID: 16387402]

[134]   Eisenstein, S.A.; Clapper, J.R.; Holmes, P.V.; Piomelli, D.; Hohmann, A.G. A role for 2-arachidonoylglycerol and endocannabinoid signaling in the locomotor response to novelty induced by olfactory bulbectomy. *Pharmacol. Res.,* **2010**, *61*(5), 419-429.
[http://dx.doi.org/10.1016/j.phrs.2009.12.013] [PMID: 20044005]

[135]   Cohen, R.; Schwartz, B.; Peri, I.; Shimoni, E. Improving bioavailability and stability of genistein by complexation with high-amylose corn starch. *J. Agric. Food Chem.,* **2011**, *59*(14), 7932-7938.
[http://dx.doi.org/10.1021/jf2013277] [PMID: 21688810]

[136]   Bailey, D.G.; Dresser, G.K. Interactions between grapefruit juice and cardiovascular drugs. *Am. J. Cardiovasc. Drugs,* **2004**, *4*(5), 281-297.
[http://dx.doi.org/10.2165/00129784-200404050-00002] [PMID: 15449971]

CHAPTER 8

Promoting Melanocyte Regeneration Using Different Plants and Their Constituents

Sharique A. Ali[*]**, Naima Parveen** and **Ayesha S. Ali**

Postgraduate Department of Biotechnology and Zoology, Saifia College of Science, Bhopal-462001, India

Abstract: Earth's landform is highly rich in biodiversity holding thousands of flora exhibiting tremendous therapeutic potential which has been extensively used in traditional systems of medicine including Ayurveda, Unani, Siddha, Homeopathy and Tibb. However, due to the advancement in allopathic medicines, the use of herbs becomes shaded. Vitiligo is a skin depigmentation disease in which the loss of melanocytes results in the appearance of irreversible white patches on the body. As it is one of the most conspicuous traits, variation in skin color or spotted skin has led some societies to attach labels and fabricate myths about people having pigmented macules on their face and body. Therefore, several treatment modes have been unleashed. But the current treatments of vitiligo including phototherapy, surgery, use of topical corticosteroid and immune modulators come under increasing scrutiny due to their aftereffects, underscoring the requirement of such treatment strategies which have low or no side effects. Hence, the use of plants and their constituents for preparation of dermatological formulation for the treatment of vitiligo is highly recommended. In the present chapter, we have discussed the types and pathogenesis of vitiligo and the modern treatment modalities with the problems associated with them, with reference to the validated clinical use of herbal products. Furthermore, the results of our own studies and controlled clinical trials by other investigators enlighten the varying efficacies of different plants and their active components for melanocyte proliferation and regeneration which might be clinically used for the treatment of vitiligo, thus opening a platform for further research and development.

Keywords: Depigmentation, Melanocytes, Keratinocytes, UV, Vitiligo.

INTRODUCTION

There is a myriad of diverse flora existing on our land which has incredible medicinal values and can be employed to prevent, improve or cure various human diseases, which otherwise are almost incurable [1, 2]. There has been a long

[*] **Corresponding Author Sharique A. Ali:** Department of Biotechnology, Saifia College of Science, Bhopal-462001, India; Tel: +91-9893015818; E-mail: drshariqali@yahoo.com

history of the use of plants and their allied products against human and other livestock ailments [3]. But with the remarkable advances made in allopathic medicine, the use of plants has been ignored for various reasons. Synthetic drugs and chemicals in spite of accurately treating diseases show severe side effects, making us re-think for returning to nature for a better and scientifically validated use of herbal medicines. Recent phytochemical and pharmacological studies support that these natural botanicals have better ethnobotanical efficacies for the treatment of various life threatening diseases including cancer [3 - 6].

Vitiligo, a skin disease has shown to have unsatisfactory results with allopathic medicines, allowing us to focus on the use of herbs for therapeutic intervention of this dreadful social stigma, where the loss of functioning melanocytes causes the appearance of irreversible white patches on skin. Several triggers have been found to be involved with vitiligo, ranging from sunburn to mechanical trauma and chemical exposures that ultimately cause an autoimmune response, which targets melanocytes, consequently resulting in progressive skin depigmentation [7]. Vitiligo affects about 1-2% of the world population and can develop at any age, but several studies report that it makes its debut often in childhood and adolescence. It can significantly impact quality of life and has potential systemic complications; often represents a therapeutic challenge to clinicians and researchers alike [8, 9].

There are multiple research papers measuring the clinical efficacy of narrow band ultraviolet light B exposure (UVB), psoralen with ultraviolet light A exposure (PUVA), excimer laser, topical corticosteroid, topical immunomodulator, calcipotriol, 1-phenylalanine, stem cell therapy, and surgical therapy in the management of symptoms associated with vitiligo. The papers conclude that there is some evidence that these treatment modalities are of benefit, but concerns are raised about their after effects including phototoxic reactions, blistering, and long term risk of skin cancer [10, 11].

Thus, in recent years treatment strategies have focussed on the development of novel therapeutic options which may provide higher efficacy with a good safety profile. As plants are one of the richest sources of bioactive chemicals that are mostly free from harmful side-effects [12], therefore there is an increased interest in identifying natural melanogenic agents from plants. Although in Ayurveda and Unani, there is a significant use of herbs for the treatment of vitiligo, but there is no proper scientific validation of the mechanism of action of the plants and their constituents. Here in this chapter, we have discussed the results of our own studies as well as controlled clinical trials by others investigating the efficacy of herbal extracts of certain plants like *Psoralea corylifolia, Withania somnifera, Ficus carica, Piper nigrum, Nigella sativa, Berberis vulgaris, Ammi majus etc.* in the treatment of vitiligo. The treatment strategies using these plants not only halt disease progression but also promote repigmentation through melanocyte regeneration, proliferation and migration.

SKIN PIGMENTATION AT A GLANCE

Skin coloration of all human beings is due to the unique distribution of melanin pigment throughout the body. Melanin is a biopolymer produced inside the special pigment cells called melanocytes through a process of melanogenesis. Development of melanocytes and the process of pigmentation is explained here:

Melanocyte Development

Melanocytes are the pigment producing cells populated in skin, eyes and inner ears of vertebrates. They arise from the pluripotent neural crest cells after undergoing various complex developmental processes. Neural crest cells (NCC) are the multipotent cells originated from the ectoderm. They are grouped into four regionally distributed populations-cranial, vagal, trunk and sacral [13, 14]. Origin of melanocytes present in skin of head region is from cranial NCCs whereas melanocytes of remaining body are originated from trunk NCC. The trunk NCC is divided into dorsally and ventrally migrating cells. Dorso-laterally migrating cells are the chief source of melanocytes while the ventrally migrating cells are supposed to form peripheral nervous system and adrenal medulla [15]. But, there is evidence in support of the fact that melanocytes arise from the cells migrating ventrally first and then along the nerve. Cells of nerve sheath called Schwann cells are able to produce melanocytes. Therefore, the cells migrating ventrally either differentiate into neurons or melanocytes [16, 17].

Melanoblasts, precursors to melanocytes travel through the dermis and proliferate. While travelling, melanoblasts express several melanogenic genes, most of them are regulated by micropthalmia associated transcription factor (MITF). Melanocyte proliferation involves several signalling pathways such as MAPK-kinase signalling, α-MSH/cAMP/PKA, endothelin/PKA/PKC pathways. Different growth factors and hormones as potent mitogens are also evolved including hepatocyte growth factor, stem cell factor, endothelins, α- MSH, ACTH [18]. After specification and proliferation, they spread to their final destination in the epidermis and hair follicles where they differentiate. Maturation of melanocytes is recognized by the appearance of enzyme tyrosinase. Finally the matured melanocytes populate in the skin, hair follicles, choroid and iris of the eye and the inner ear. Microscopic analysis of melanocytes indicates that they are oval, fusiform, dendritic cells smaller than keratinocytes [19].

Melanogenesis

Melanogenesis is a complex biochemical pathway responsible for melanin production. It takes place in special organelles called melanosomes of melanocytes. Melanin has various functions such as protection from UV light, absorption of free radicals, storage of ions and coupled oxidation reduction reaction [20, 21]. Based on the availability of substrate and functioning of melanogenic enzymes, two types of melanin are produced: Pheomelanin and eumelanin. Tyrosinase, a copper containing enzyme catalyzes the hydroxylation of tyrosine into 3, 4 dihydroxyphenylalanine (DOPA) which is then oxidized to DOPA quinone [22]. In the presence of cystein, 3 or 5 cysteinyl DOPAs are formed, which get oxidized and polymerize to form yellow red melanin-pheomelanin. But in the absence of cystein or other thiols, DOPA quinone undergoes cyclization and forms DOPA chrome. DOPA chrome spontaneously loses carboxylic acid and forms DHI, which further gets oxidized to form dark brown black, DHI melanin. However, if tyrosinase related protein 2 (TRP2) is present, DOPA chrome is converted to DHI 2 carboxylic acid (DHICA). Tyrosinase related protein 1 (TRP1) further catalyzes the conversion of DHICA into DHICA melanin and finally brown black melanin-eumelanin is produced. Human skin is composed of all types of melanin in a particular ratio, and this ratio determines visible pigmentation. Eumelanin is found to be more efficient in terms of photo protection than pheomelanin [23 - 25].

MelaninTransfer to Keratinocytes

Special membrane bound organelles present in the cytoplasm of melanocytes produce melanin. This melanin when transferred to neighbouring keratinocytes through the dendritic processes of melanocytes imparts color to the skin. In the basal layer of epidermis, melanocytes form epidermal melanin unit as a result of the association between 30-40 keratinocytes within each melanocyte. Hence, the ratio of melanocytes to keratinocytes is 1:10 in the epidermal layer. Melanocytes and keratinocytes communicate with each other by cell to cell contact through cell adhesion molecules like E- and P-catherine. This contact between melanocytes and keratinocytes is necessary for melanin transfer to keratinocytes which then determines the color of the skin [26 - 29].

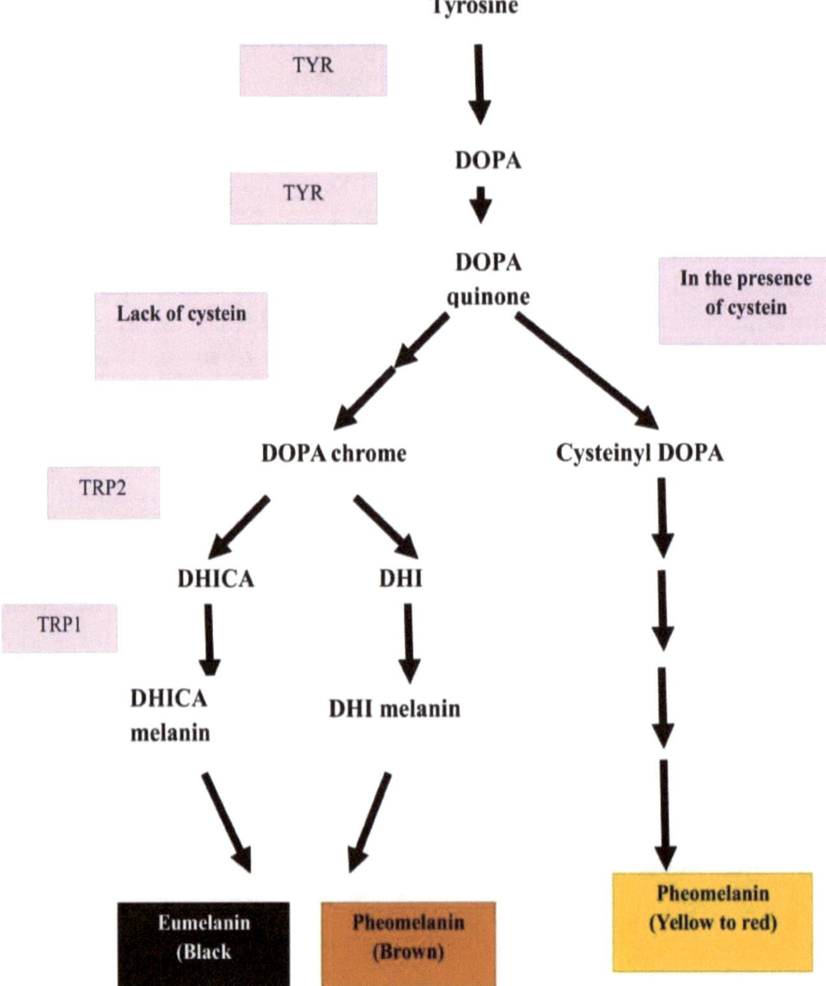

Fig. (1). Production of different types of melanin.

PIGMENTARY DISORDERS

Color of the skin is due to the melanin produced by melanocytes. Normal structure and function of melanocytes results in normal pigmentation. But if there is even a minor change in the complex process of pigmentation, it may lead to serious aesthetic problems in the form of hyperpigmentation and hypopig-mentation. Accumulation of excess melanin and its distribution results in hyperpigmentation. Hyperpigmentary diseases include melasma, post inflam-matory hyperpigmentation, senile lentigos, ephelides *etc.* On the contrary, hypopigmenation is the condition when there is less or lack of melanin produced by melanocytes. It may be congenital or acquired, generalized or localized. Commonly occurring hypopigmentary conditions are albinism, idiopathic guttate hypomelanosis, vitiligo *etc.* Most widespread causes of skin hypo and hyperpigmentation are inflammation caused by sunlight, skin damage, allergic reactions, certain medications and several other genetic and climatic factors. Treatments of these disorders are diverse and somehow depend on the cause of the disease [30, 31].

VITILIGO

Vitiligo is an acquired, idiopathic disease characterized by destroyed melanocytes, which results in patchy depigmentation.Vitiligo affects almost 0.2-2% of the world population. Aulus Cornelius Celsus used the term 'vitiligo' for the first time in his medical treatise *De medicina* during the second century B.C [32, 33]. The name vitiligo comes from a latin word *vitium*, meaning defect or blemish [34]. Patients with vitiligo have one to many amelanotic, white or milk white macules. Generally the macules are round and oval in shape. Most essential characteristic of vitiligo is variation in melanocyte ratio of the dermal-epidermal region of the skin [35, 36]. Vitiligo is neither contagious nor it is life threatening but it can alter quality of life of an affected person. It is due to consequent social and psychological problems rather than clinical issues [37].

Epidemiology

Vitiligo is the most common skin pigmentary disorder. Various studies have been conducted around the world concerning epidemiology of vitiligo. The largest epidemiological survey for vitiligo was done by Howitz *et al.* [38], on the island of Bornholm in Denmark, where 0.38% of population was affected with vitiligo. The population prevalence of vitiligo often ranges from 0.2% to 2%, although the exact prevalence is not easy to estimate [39, 40]. The highest incidence of the disease has been reported in Indian citizens from the Indian subcontinents. Vitiligo is more frequently reported in females than in males. Girls and women are often more curious for treatment because of the greater social consequences for the women affected with vitiligo than for men. Children and adults of both the sexes are uniformly affected; but vitiligo is widely reported during the stages of active development. Findings from epidemiological studies showed that vitiligo occurs in any age but usually develops in young people between the ages of 10 to 30 years. Almost 50% of the patients develop vitiligo before 20 years and nearly 70-80% develop before 30 years [37].

Types of Vitiligo

Vitiligo is classified into two major forms: Segmental vitiligo and non segmental vitiligo. According to the review conducted between 2011-2012 by the *Vitiligo and Global Issues Consensus Conference*, vitiligo can be classified as:

1. Non segmental vitiligo

It is characterized by depigmented macules or patches that vary in size ranging from few to many centimetres in diameter. Most often, involving both side of the body and having tendency of symmetrical distribution. Non segmental vitiligo is considered as a broad group comprises the following types or forms:

  i. Acrofacial: It can preferably affect the perioral region. But also affects head, hands and feet
 ii. Mucosal: It affects the oral and genital mucosa
iii. Generalized or common: It can affect any part of tegument, generally face, hands, fingers and trauma exposed areas
 iv. Universal: It is the most common form, occurs in adulthood. It affects 80-90% of the body surface and corresponds to complete or usually complete depigmentation
  v. Mixed vitiligo: It is the concomitant involvement of segmental and non segmental vitiligo

2. Segmental Vitiligo

Koga first proposed that segmental vitiligo was different from non segmental [41]. Segmental vitiligo typically has a rapid progression, but depigmentation spreads within the segment. Extension of macule occurs over a period of 6-24 months and then stops. In addition to limited, segmental vitiligo has another distinguishable characteristic compared with non segmental vitiligo. Segmental vitiligo usually has earlier age of onset than non segmental vitiligo. It can be further divided into three forms: Unisegmental, when one segment is affected; Bisegmental, two segments are affected; Plurisegmental, more than two segments are affected.

3. Undetermined or Unclassifiable Forms of Vitiligo

  i. Focal: Focal vitiligo is acquired, small, isolated hypo pigmented macule. It does not fit to segmental distribution nor has it evolved into non segmental vitiligo.
 ii. Mucosal: When it occurs in context of non segmental vitiligo, it has been classified as non segmental. But, if mucosal vitiligo occurs in isolation then it is readily classified as undetermined vitiligo [40].

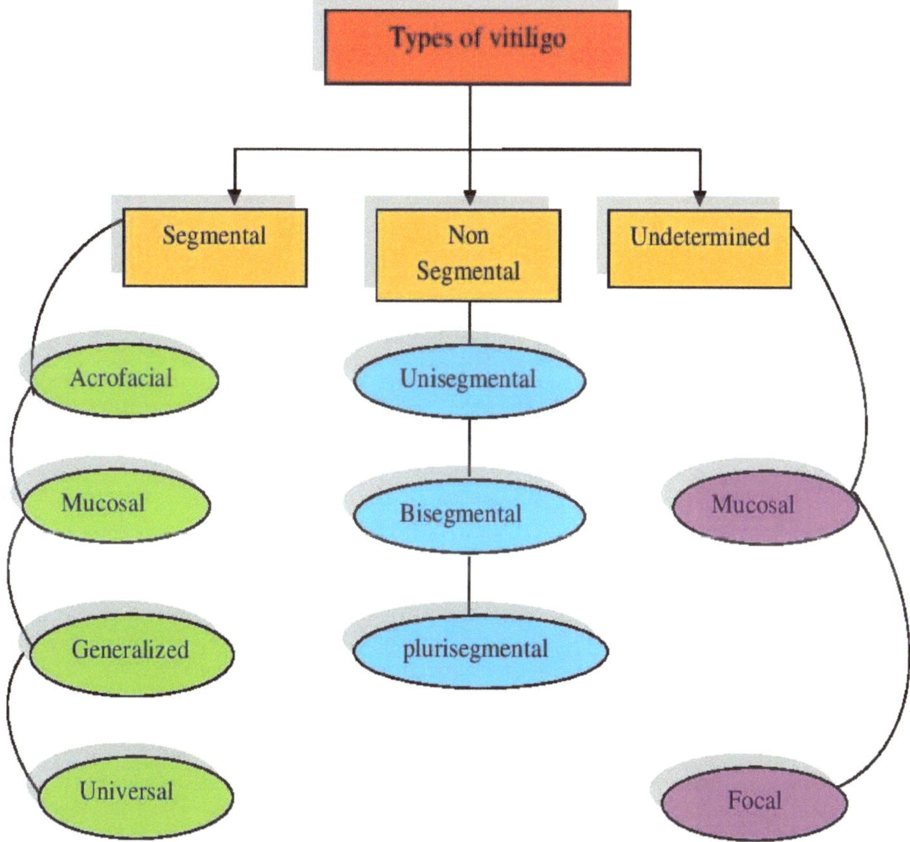

Fig. (2). Types of vitiligo.

Pathogenesis of Vitiligo

Several theories have been proposed for explaining the pathogenesis of vitiligo:

Genetic Hypothesis

Most human diseases result from an interaction between genetic variants and environmental factors, and to establish the actual contribution of genetic factors is the first step of genetic studies that evaluate complex diseases. Epidemiological studies based on genetics concluded that vitiligo can be considered as a genetic disease because: (i) the disease vary in symptom rigorousness and the age of onset, which hampers the definition of the appropriate phenotype and the selection of the most favourable study population; the onset of disease in the early age was associated with familial occurrence of generalized vitiligo [42, 43]. Early onset vitiigo is also associated with more severe disease; (ii) the etiological mechanisms of the disease can vary; vitiligo's etiopathogenesis has not yet been fully understood, and various theories have been proposed; (iii) More often, the complex genetic diseases are oligogenic or even polygenic and each gene takes part to a fraction of the overall relative risk.

The involvement of genetic factors in the susceptibility to vitiligo became evident in familial studies, which demonstrated that vitiligo segregates with a complex standard of multifactorial and polygenic inheritance. Ando *et al.* [44], during one of their experiments found that there was a significant interaction between HLA-B46 and familial non segmental vitiligo in 131 Japanese patients, whereas HLA-A31 and CW4 were found in nonfamilial patients.

Additionally, around 50 candidate genes have already been investigated in association studies for susceptibility to vitiligo. However, only a few genes present a clear association with vitiligo. On the one hand, there are non-HLA genes, including DDR1, XBP1, NLRP1, PTPN22 and COMT; on the other hand, there are HLA-associated genes, including HLA-A2, HLA-DR4 and HLA-DR7 alleles [8, 45]. Hence, genetic factors probably play an essential role in the pathogenesis of vitiligo, but the exact genetic defects remain to be identified.

Autoimmune Hypothesis

Autoimmune hypothesis is one of the most significant and popular hypotheses. This hypothesis suggests that abnormality of the immune system results in destruction of melanocytes. Substantial new data implicate immune mechanisms in the pathogenesis of vitiligo and indicate that vitiligo may share common linkages with other autoimmune diseases (thyroid disorders, juvenile diabetes mellitus, and Addison's disease, pernicious anaemia) [42, 46].

Vitiligo is accompanied by abnormal cellular and humoral immunity. Elevated levels of serum circulating autoantibodies particularly of the IgG class have been observed in 5-10% of vitiligo patients. However, the function of antimelanocyte antibodies in vitiligo pathogenesis remains unsure and it has been suggested that their presence may be secondary to melanocyte and keratinocyte damages [47, 48].

In the margins of lesional and normal pigmented skin of patients with active vitiligo or inflammatory vitiligo, a mild mononuclear cell infiltrate can be observed. Immuno histochemical studies indicated that it is T cells that are abundant in these infiltrates; T cells may therefore play a major role in the destruction of melanocytes. More recently, an *in vitro* study showed that cytotoxic T lymphocytes infiltrated in common vitiligo perilesional area destroyed neighbouring melanocytes [49, 50]. Different abnormalities in peripheral blood mononuclear cells have also been described. Levels of natural killer cells, CD4+ and CD8+ have been reported to be normal, increased or decreased. Various factors are known to influence these parameters and they are not standardized in any of the studies conducted [51].

Neural Hypothesis

The neural hypothesis was first suggested by Lerner [52]. It was reported that there is a presence of certain neurochemical mediators that are cytotoxic to melanocytes secreted from nearby nerve endings. This theory is supported by the following clinical interpretations:

1. The existence of the localized form of vitiligo that seems to be limited to one segment of the body. This 'segemental' vitiligo is approximately non dermatomal but normally affects portions of multiple dermatomes. It is also assumed that segmental vitiligo does not act in response to classical vitiligo therapies, such as PUVA, but to agents that modulate neural function.
2. The onset of vitiligo is reported after a severe emotional stress. The mechanism by which stress results into depigmentation is not clear.
3. It is also reported that vitiligo occurs in patients with neurological disorders, in a child with viral encephalitis, in multiple sclerosis and in a patient with peripheral nerve injury [53].

Autocytotoxic Hypothesis

This theory proposed that the precursors of melanogenesis are toxic to melanocytes. Melanocytes have an intracellular protective mechanism in order to eliminate toxic melanin precursors (*e.g.* dopa, dopachrome and 5,6-dihydroxyindole) and free radicals. In vitiligo, there may be some hindrance of this mechanism, resulting in an accumulation of indoles and free radicals that destruct melanocytes [54].

Growth Factor Defect Hypothesis

In 1987, Puri *et al.* [55], postulated that the defective growth of melanocyteoriginated from non lesional and perilesional skin. Surprisingly, the investigators observed that the defects were corrected partially by *in vitro* supplementation of fetal lung fibroblast derived growth factors. Their finding suggests that growth defects play an essential role in pathogenesis of vitiligo. Further studies are required to evaluate the use of growth factors, as a part of repigmentation therapy in vitiligo.

Adhesion Defect Theory

Gautier *et al.*, in 2003 [56] proposed that non segmental vitiligo might be caused by a chronic detachment of melanocytes stimulated by trauma, mainly a mechanical rubbing of healthy skin. This concept is called as "melanocytorrhagy theory". Furthermore, Gauthier *et al.* hypothesized that an autoimmune activation could be provoked by dendritic cells or memory T cells detecting auto-antigens during melanocytorrhagy through the epidermis basal layer [57].

Convergence Theory

It has been suggested that a combined theory rather than a separate theory is more suitable in the etiology. Furthermore, the studies that the patients' exhibit a variety of clinical forms and various histories of onset of disease make us believe that the etiology of vitiligo may vary among individual patients. This theory suggests that stress, genetic factors, autoimmunity, accumulation of toxic compounds, infections, mutation, varied cellular environment and impaired melanocyte migration and proliferation can all contribute to the phenomenon of vitiligo [58].

CURRENT TREATMENT MODALITIES FOR VITILIGO

The aim of the treatment is to control the damage of melanocytes and stimulates its migration and distribution to surrounding cells. Conventional treatment for vitiligo including topical treatment and physical or phototherapy remains the mainstay of current treatment. Overall treatment strategies are divided into physical, pharmacological and surgical:

(i). Physical Treatment

Physical treatment involves the utilization of light or radiation. Generally, ultraviolet (UV) radiation of both UVA and UVB spectrum has been used with varying efficacies.

a). Narrow Band UVB- NBUVB

Narrow band UV of wavelength 311-313 nm can be given to the whole body of vitiligo patient using lamps. Previously it was considered as an effective and safe treatment for vitiligo. But, longer exposure to UV radiation may cause skin ageing or skin cancer. A comparative study conducted by Westerhof and Nieuweboer-Krobotova in 1997 [59], comparing the effect of NBUV and PUVA, the authors reported 46% repigmentation with PUVA while 67% with NBUV. Due to the better results achieved by NBUV as compared to PUVA, it can be used more. Combination therapy of NBUV with topical compounds such as afamelanotide was also found effective to induce repigmentation in vitiligo patients [60]. Janus kinase (JAK) inhibitors are the promising class of targeted therapy to achieve repigmentation. They have been used in combination with low dose narrow UV-B phototherapy. Tofacitinib and ruxolitinib are the JAK inhibitors which can be taken orally, followed by treatment with narrow band UV-B [61].

b). PUVA Therapy

Oral PUVA therapy is considered as one of the most popular treatment introduced in 1968. It consists of UV radiation of wavelength 320-400 nm and the photosensitizing drugs usually psoralen in the form of 5- methoxypsoralen or 8-methoxypsoralen [62]. The drug can be administered orally 2 hours before light treatment. More frequent side effects associated with these treatment modalities are cutaneous phototoxicities, photo ageing, nausea and the risk of skin cancer [63].

c). Monochromatic Excimer Light

In this method, specific wavelength of 308 nm is delivered with xenon chloride gas. This light can be produced by two forms either through excimer laser that produces a coherent and monochromatic light or the excimer lamp that produces non-coherent light [64]. A double blind comparative study showed that lamps are time consuming to deliver a specific dose needed when compared with Laser, though there is no difference in response rate found. Additionally as opposed to NBUVB these forms of treatment may be applied in a more localized way in lesion [65, 66].

(ii). Pharmacological Treatment

a). Topical Corticosteroid

The use of topical corticosteroid in vitiligo treatment is considered as first line treatment due to its cost effectiveness and easy application [67]. The application of corticosteroid topically, is appropriate for the treatment of localized vitiligo and hence used on small affected areas particularly elbow, knees, and face [62]. A retrospective study showed that the efficacy of class 3 corticosteroid is higher than that of class 4 corticosteroid. The incidence of atrophy was also observed with class 4 corticosteroid [68].

However studies recommended the use of high power corticosteroid but its use is limited to 2-3 months only. So the use of low power corticosteroid is considered in order to minimize the adverse effects. It is also recommended that if there is no clinical response observed in patient of localized vitiligo after topical corticosteroid application, its use should be discontinued [69].

b). Immunomodulators

Topical immunomodulators are the potent therapeutic agents that work *via* immunological pathway. It can either suppress or enhance immune and inflammatory response in skin. Generally tacrolimus and pimecrolimus are used as immunomodulators for the treatment of vitiligo. The mechanism of action of these drugs involves calcineurin inhibition which results in down regulation of T-cell reactivity and disturbance in transcription of proinflammatory cytokine genes which is essential in the pathophysiology of the early immune response [70]. Similarly, prostaglandin E has immunomodulatory effect on melanocytes and controls their proliferation. It has been used for the treatment of vitiligo and there was significant improvement in vitiligo conditions observed during treatment with the use of topical prostaglandin E [71].

(iii). Surgical Treatment

Vitiligo patient who failed to respond to classical therapies having stable vitiligo are treated with surgical therapy. These methods are generally used for the areas not easy to treat such as elbows, eyelids, knees, and lips. Tissue grafting and cell suspension grafting are the two broad techniques of surgical treatment which consist of following types:

Tissue Grafting

Punch Grafting

Punch grafting is performed by making multiple punches of different size on affected areas and then transplanting it with 1-2 mm thickness punch biopsies from the donar area. Better repigmentation with good cosmetic results is observed with punch grafting. Malakar and Dharin [72] observed 90-100% repigmentation rates in around 75% patients treated with punch graft. There are certain adverse effects found with larger grafts such as cobblestoning which has been corrected with electro fulguration. Studies also proved that punch graft combined with NBUV or topical corticosteroid gives much better results [73, 74].

Suction Blister Epidermal Grafting

In this technique, dermoepidermal separation from the donor site is done by applying constant suction in order to obtain thin graft and the recipient area is prepared by laser therapy and dermabrasion. A retrospective study showed that more than 75% repigmentation has achieved in 89% patients under study [75]. This method offers good therapeutic results but is time consuming.

Split Thickness Grafting

Like suction blister grafting, this technique also involves the preparation of recipient area by dermabrasion followed by split thickness graft of donor area. To obtain thin skin graft, a dermatone is needed and hence this procedure requires skill and experience person to handle dermatone. Although it gives good results with 90-100% repigmentation rates as proved by Agrawal and Agrawal [76], there are some side effects associated with this technique like scarring at normally pigmented donor area and incompatibility of color at recipient area [76, 77].

Epidermal Cell Suspension Grafting

Cultured Epidermal Cell Suspension Grafting

This method is definitely beneficial as it increases the number of cells by using tissue culture technique. Using less donor tissue it is able to treat larger recipient areas. But this method is costly and require sophisticated tissue culture laboratory, also the use of certain mitogens in culture medium raised question about safety [78]. Non cultured method on the other hand is much better than cultured method as it is faster and gives better results [79].

Non- cultured Epidermal Cell Suspension Grafting

In this method, skin fragment is extracted as biopsy from the donor area. Epidermis is separated from the dermis by treating the skin fragment with trypsin. After consequent steps, suspension of keratinocytes and melanocytes are obtained which is then transplanted to recipient area. It offers good results with excellent color compatibility at recipient site [79 - 81].

Despite the fact that vitiligo is a well characterized autoimmune disease, it is considered as 'cosmetic' by health insurance companies in many countries of the world. The management of vitiligo is associated with direct and indirect cost paid by the patient. Most of the patients with vitiligo experience greater financial burden as they cannot afford the treatment of their disease, which is very expensive. They often face difficulties in receiving financial support for their treatment from third party payers including insurance companies, government agencies *etc.* Due to this reason and also the adverse effects found associated with these treatment modalities, people have started looking back towards ancient treatment systems like Unani and Ayurveda, where they have used herbal remedies to cure various diseases including leucoderma or vitiligo. Although the ancient system of treatment uses plant and its products which is no doubt safe and free from any side effects but the mechanism of action of those plants are not described. This provide an impetus to the researchers to carry out studies on efficacies of plants used in Unani and Ayurveda for the treatment of vitiligo and several other plants with proper mechanisms of their action.

PROMOTING MELANOCYTE REGENERATION USING DIFFERENT PLANTS AND THEIR CONSTITUENTS

As plants are one of the richest sources of bioactive compounds which are free from any adverse effects, there is an increased interest to identify natural melanogenesis stimulator from plants. Several studies have been conducted using different plants in order to promote melanocytes regeneration with varying efficacies. Some of them are briefly described:

Psoralea Corylifolia

Psoralea corylifolia is a plant of Fabaceae family and has been extensively used in Ayurveda and Siddha system of Indian medicine. Extract of this plant contains a variety of chemical compounds including coumarins, flavonoids and meroterpenes. It has been experimentally proved that psoralen, a type of furocoumarin found in seeds of *Psoralea corylifolia* has potential of inducing repigmentation [82]. A clinical study on 10 patients with the onset of disease between 6 months to two years has been carried out using *Psoralea corylifolia* seed powder in combination with some other plants. 60-70% of the patients show positive response [83]. Ethanolic extract of *Psoralea corylifolia* has an effect on enzyme tyrosinase and enhances melanin production by improving tyrosinase activity [84, 85].

A study conducted by our team on isolated fish melanophores showed melanin granules dispersion when treated with lyophilized extract of *Psoralea corylifolia*. It is indicated from the results that the melanin dispersion leading to skin darkening is mediated by cholino-muscarinic or cholino-psoralen like receptors found on melanophores [86]. Recently, Hussain *et al.* [87], formulated anti vitiligo cream using *Psoralea corylifolia* seed extract and tested on different vitiligo patients. Patients were advised to apply ointment on white patches once in a day and exposed the area to sun rays. After application of ointment to few days, white patches became reddish and vascularised and finally the whole patches were disappeared [87].

Nigella Sativa

Nigella sativa is the small elegant annual herb, popularly known as black seeds or *kalaunji*. It is most widely used medicinal plant in traditional system of medicines like Ayurveda, Sidha, Unani and Tibb. In Islam, it is considered as one of the greatest forms of medicine available to cure various ailments [88]. Thymoquinone is the major component of *Nigella sativa* seeds. It has several therapeutic properties including anti inflammation, antitumour, antibacterial, antioxidant and immune boosting. Skin darkening effect of lyophilized seed extract of *Nigella sativa* and its active ingredient thymoquinone on wall lizard melanophores was observed by our team. Results of our findings showed that thymoquionone extracted from *Nigella sativa* impersonate the action of acetylcholine in melanin dispersion leading to skin darkening *via* stimulation of cholinergic receptors of muscarinic nature. The study suggested that *Nigella sativa* and its active principle can be used as novel melanogen for the treatment of vitiligo [89].

A retrospective study conducted on 52 vitiligo patients divided into two groups having 26 patients in each group. Vitiligo lesions of one group of patients were treated with *Nigella sativa* oil and other with fish oil. During the treatment, lesions of patients were evaluated by observers using vitiligo area scoring index (VASI). After six months improvement was observed in most of the patients of both the group, but *Nigella sativa* oil was found more effective in comparison to fish oil. Hence the authors suggested the use of *Nigella sativa* along with the major drug for the treatment of vitiligo [90].

Withania Somnifera

Withania somnifera, commonly known as Ashwagandha or Indian ginseng is a plant of Solanaceae family native to India, Nepal, China and Yemen. It is used as the main ingredient in plenty of medicines. Various studies indicated that *Withania somnifera* possesses antioxidant, anti-inflammatory, anti tumor, immunomodulatory properties [91, 92]. So in recent years, several *in vitro* and *in vivo* studies have been conducted in order to validate more therapeutic potentials of *Withania somnifera* including repigmentation.

Two individual studies were carried out by our team using isolated melanophores of Indian Frog *Rana tigerina* and wall lizard *Hemidactylus flaviviridis* to determine the effect of *Withania somnifera* and its active principle withaferin A on melanophores of skin. Dispersion of melanin was observed in isolated melanophores of both Indian Frog *Rana tigerina* as well as wall lizard *H. flaviviridis* after treatment with lyophilized root extract of *Withania somnifera* and pure withaferin A. Melanin dispersion effect was antagonised by atropine and hyoscine. These studies suggested that *Withania somnifera* and pure withaferin A mimic the melanin dispersal effect of acetylcholine *via* stimulation of cholinergic receptor leading to skin darkening. It also appears that phylogenetic development of *Rana tigerina* melanophores is homologous to more evolved *H. flaviviridis*-melanophore receptor system [93, 94].

Piper Nigrum

Piper nigrum is a flowering climbing vine, popularly known as black pepper and belongs to Piperaceae family. It is grown in many tropical regions of India, Indonesia and Brazil. It contains a variety of phytochemicals including alkaloids, amides, phenolics, flavonoids, terpenes *etc.* An alkaloid- piperine is the major active component isolated from black pepper having wide range of pharmacological activities like anti-inflammatory, anti-cancer, anti-asthmatic, anti-oxidant, melanogenic etc [95 - 98].

Effects of lyophilized extract of *Piper nigrum* and its active principle piperine were studied by our team on isolated tail melanophores of tadpoles of *Rana tigerina*. Dispersion of melanin occurred leading to skin darkening which was mediated by cholinergic-piperine like receptors [96]. The results of the study was similar to the work of Lin *et al.* [99], who have observed the stimulatory effect of *Piper nigrum* and its main alkaloid- piperine on cultured mouse melanocytes proliferation. They have found nearly 300% stimulation of the growth of cultured melanocyte cell line by the action of aqueous extract of *Piper nigrum*. In continuation to this work Lin *et al.* [100], also studied the comparative effect of certain amides extracted from *Piper nigrum*. They observed that along with piperine, *Piper nigrum* also contains several amides with the ability to stimulate melanocyte proliferation. Piperine isolated from *Piper nigrum* was formulated into cream and topically tested on goat skin. It was found that melanocyte proliferate at around 69% after application of piperine cream. It was also observed that piperine cream has no side effects as confirmed by irritancy test [101].

Ficus Carica

Ficus carica is an important member of the family Moraceae, native to Southwest Asia and the Eastern Mediterranean and commonly referred as 'fig'. It has been used for its medicinal benefits as anti-inflammatory, cardiovascular, respiratory, metabolic remedies. Edible part of the fig plant is fruit and has been dried and freshly consumed which contains vitamins, minerals, sugars, phenolic compounds and organic acids. It can be eaten raw, dried, canned, or in other preserved forms [102, 103]. The fruits bark and leaves have been used in ancient medicines in order to treat various ailments such as respiratory, gastrointestinal, diabetes, ulcers *etc* [104]. Inspite of its various therapeutic potentials, no work has been done to evaluate the effect of *Ficus carica* on skin melanophores leading to darkening. In this regard, we have studied the effect of leaf extract of *Ficus carica* and its active ingredient psoralen on isolated melanophores of *Hemidactylus flaviviridis*. This was the first report of its kind where the leaf extract of *Ficus carica* has been found to cause skin darkening *via* activation of muscarinic cholinergic receptors [105].

Berberis Vulgaris

Berberis vulgaris is a shrub of Berberidaceae family and native of moderate and semitropical regions of Asia, Europe, Africa, South America, and North America. *Berberis vulgaris* is widely used as food, medicine, and also as decorative plant. In traditional system of medicines, *Berberis vulgaris* is used to treat various diseases such as fever, cough, liver disease, hyperglycemia, hyperlipidemia etc [106, 107]. A variety of pharmacologically active ingredients are found in *Berberis vulgaris* including alkaloids, flavonoids, phenolics *etc.* but berberine is the major alkaloid isolated from *Berberis vulgaris.* Berberine was found to exhibit many therapeutic properties such as antioxidation, anti-inflammation, hypotension, hypoglycaemic *etc* [108].

The potential of *Berberis vulgaris* to induce skin darkening was evaluated by our team through testing the effect of *Berberis vulgaris* root extract and its active compound berberine on isolated skin melanophores of toad *Bufo melanostictus.* Melanin dispersion was observed leading to skin darkening in response to *Berberis vulgaris* root extract and pure berberine mediated by beta-adrenergic receptors [109]. This was the first study of its kind where *Berberis vulgaris* and its active ingredient berberine was found to cause skin darkening *via* melanin displacement within the melanophores of *Bufo melanostictus.* Therefore, further assessment and controlled clinical trials are needed to produce skin darkening agent from *Berberis vulgaris.*

Nelumbo Nucifera

Nelumbo nucifera is an aquatic perennial plant of Nelumbonaceae family native to Tropical Asia, and Australia. It is commonly grown in water gardens and known as Indian lotus, bean of India, sacred lotus. It has been extensively used for nutritional and medicinal purpose by people all over the World. Studies suggested that lotus has antidiarheal, anti-inflammatory, antioxidant, hypoglycaemic and antimicrobial activities [110]. Effect of *Nelumbo nucifera* on melanogenesis was studied by Jeon *et al.* [111], on human melanocytes. In their study they have extracted essential oil from *Nelumbo nucifera* and assessed its effect on cultured human melanocyte. It was shown to stimulate melanin synthesis and induced the expression of tyrosinase and microphthalmia associated transcription factor (MITF). With the purpose of validate the effective component of *Nelumbo nucifera* essential oil, the authors had assessed its composition and essential oil found comprised of palmitic acid methyl ester, linoleic acid methyl ester, palmitoleic acid methyl ester, linolenic acid methyl ester. Among all components, palmitic acid methyl ester was noticeably induced melanogenesis [111].

Polygoni Multiflorum

Polygoni multiflorum also called as *Fallopia multiflori* and tuber fleece flower is a species of flowering plant belonging to the family Polygonaceae. It is most commonly used in traditional Chinese medicines. It has been evaluated for various biological activities such as antioxidation, lipid regulation, radical scavenging, melanogenesis stimulation *etc* [112 - 114]. It has been observed that 2, 3, 5, 4'-tetrahydroxystilbene-2-O-beta-D-glucoside (THSG), a main component of *Polygoni multiflorum* was able to induce melanogenesis [115].

Polygoni multiflorum root extract was examined for its effect on melanogenesis in zebra fish embryos and found to produce increased level of pigmentation. Elevated level of melanin biosynthesis or pigmentation was due to activation of tyrosinase. So, *Polygoni multiflorum* can be used as a potential agent for the treatment of vitiligo. But there are some negative effects observed with the root extract of *Polygoni multiflorum* hence it has not been recommended for women during pregnancy [116].

Angelica Sinensis

Angelica sinensis is a herb of Apiaceae family, commonly known as dong quai or female ginseng. Many studies have evaluated *Angelica sinensis* and its active ingredients as antioxidant, anti-inflammatory, anti-hypertensive agents [117]. Raman *et al.* [118], have investigated the effect of *Angelica sinensis* root extract on proliferation of cultured mouse melanocytes. At low concentration root extract was not able to propagate melanocytes but at high concentration it stimulates melanocyte cell division. In another study conducted by Deng and Yang [119], also considered *Angelica sinensis* as potent agent for its clinical use in the treatment of vitiligo. They concluded that *Angelica sinensis* not only promotes melanocyte regeneration but also increases melanin synthesis and tyrosinase activity [119].

Ammi Majus

Ammi majus commonly known as bishop's weed, bullwort, lady's lace etc is a white lace like flowering plant which belongs to the family Apiaceae. It is an effective medicinal plant with a long history of its use in Egyptian traditional medicine for the treatment of vitiligo. The crystalline extract of *Ammi majus* was proved to have remarkable effect on a patient with vitiligo. Several experiments with this plant showed that a high percentage of vitiligo cases promptly responded, improved or completely recovered within short period of time during treatment or after treatment [120 - 122]. An experiment conducted on a lady who was disappointed by the treatment of dermatologists showed positive and satisfactory results when treated with seed extract of *Ammi majus*. Through chromatographic and other biological techniques active components of plant were identified as furanocoumarins (5-methoxy psoralen, 8-methoxypsoralen) and oxypeucedanin [123].

Several other plants including *Azaridacta indica, Bituminaria bituminosa, Eclipta alba, Foeniculum vulgare, Ginkgo biloba, Helectoris isora, Ocimum sanctum, Polypodium leucotomos, Semecarpus anacardium, Silybum marianum* [124 - 132] *etc.* were also proved to have melanocyte proliferation and regeneration ability. The list of plants and their active ingredients studied for their stimulatory effect on melanogenesisis shown in Table **1**.

Table 1. Reported herbs that are claimed to regenerate and proliferate melanocytes and stimulate melanogenesis.

Plant (Botanical Name)	Common Name	Family	Active Compound	Reference
Psoralea corylifolia	Babchi	Fabaceae	Psoralen	[82, 84-86]
Nigella sativa	Black seeds, Kalaunji	Ranunculaceae	Thymoquionone	[89]
Withania somnifera	Indian ginseng	Solanaceae	Withaferin A	[93, 94]
Piper nigrum	Black pepper	Piperaceae	Piperine	[96, 101]
Ficus carica	Fig	Moraceae	Psoralen	[105]
Berberis vulgaris	Common barberry	Berberidaceae	Berberine	[109]
Nelumbo nucifera	Lotus	Nelumbonaceae	Palmitic acid methyl ester	[111]
Polygoni multiflorum	Tuber fleece flower	Polygonaceae.	Hydroxystilbene	[115, 116]
Angelica sinensis	Dong quai or female ginseng.	Apiaceae	Ferulic acid	[119]
Ammi majus	Bishop's weed, bullwort, lady's lace	Apiaceae	Furanocoumarins	[123]
Ginkgo biloba	Ginkgo	Ginkgoeceae	Furanocoumarins	[132]
Ocimum sanctum	Tulsi	Lamiaceae	Eugenol, oleanolic acid	[130]
Polypodium leucotomos	Golden polypody	Polypodiaceae	Furanocoumarins	[125]
Azadiracta indica	Neem	Meliaceae	Azadirachtinol, nimbosterol	[127]
Eclipta alba	Bhringraj	Asteraceae	Steroids, flavonoids	[126]

(Table 1) cont.....

Plant (Botanical Name)	Common Name	Family	Active Compound	Reference
Silybum marianum	Marian thistle, Milk thistle	Asteraceae	Triterpene glycoside, Flavanolignan	[131]
Semecarpus anacardium	Bhilwa	Anacardiaceae	Sterols, flavonoids, glycosides	[131]
Helectoris isora	Indian screw fruit	Sterculiaceae	Sitosterols, flavonoids	[129]
Bituminaria bituminosa	Arabian pea	Fabaceae	Furanocoumarins	[128]
Foeniculum vulgare	Fennel	Umbelliferae	Furanocoumarins	[124]

CONCLUSION

Vitiligo is more concisely considered as social stigma instead of disease, as physical appearance is the most important status characteristic for human beings. Hence various treatment strategies have been developed till date including phototherapy, surgical grafting, topical application of various chemicals *etc.* but none of them have been found to be entirely satisfactory. Vitiligo treatment with herbs was used in traditional system of Indian, Chinese and Egyptian medicines which have become less popular due to the availability of advance treatment options. Since these treatments impart long term side effects hence the use of herbs and its ingredients is now again becoming more popular due to its non-toxicity and having lesser side effects. However further advancements in treatments using different derivatives of these plants are required in order to get complete recovery of vitiligo patient with decreased possibility of side effects. Additionally, more data from the clinical trials on human subjects must be collected to achieve treatment with stable and reasonable solutions to the condition.

CONSENT FOR PUBLICATION

Not applicable.

CONFLICT OF INTEREST

The authors confirm that this chapter content has no conflict of interest.

ACKNOWLEDGEMENT

The authors extend gratitude to the Secretary and Principal of Saifia College of Science, Bhopal, India, for encouragement.

REFERENCES

[1]   Samuelsson, G.; Bohlin, L. *Drugs of natural origin: A textbook of pharmacognosy,* 5th ed; Taylor & Francis: Abingdon, **2004**, pp. 620-621.

[2]   Bouasla, A.; Bouasla, I. Ethnobotanical survey of medicinal plants in northeastern of Algeria. *Phytomedicine,* **2017**, *36*(36), 68-81.
[http://dx.doi.org/10.1016/j.phymed.2017.09.007] [PMID: 29157830]

[3]   Rathore, B.; Ali Mahdi, A.; Nath Paul, B.; Narayan Saxena, P.; Kumar Das, S. Indian herbal medicines: possible potent therapeutic agents for rheumatoid arthritis. *J. Clin. Biochem. Nutr.,* **2007**, *41*(1), 12-17.
[http://dx.doi.org/10.3164/jcbn.2007002] [PMID: 18392103]

[4]   Kandil, F.E.; Nassar, M.I. A tannin anti-cancer promotor from *Terminalia arjuna. Phytochemistry,* **1998**, *47*(8), 1567-1568.
[http://dx.doi.org/10.1016/S0031-9422(97)01078-9] [PMID: 9612958]

[5]   Chekole, G. Ethnobotanical study of medicinal plants used against human ailments in Gubalafto District, Northern Ethiopia. *J. Ethnobiol. Ethnomed.,* **2017**, *13*(1), 55.
[http://dx.doi.org/10.1186/s13002-017-0182-7] [PMID: 28978342]

[6]   Ali, S.A.; Naaz, I.; Zaidi, K.U.; Ali, A.S. Recent Updates in Melanocyte Function: The Use of Promising Bioactive Compounds for the Treatment of Hypopigmentary Disorders. *Mini Rev. Med. Chem.,* **2017**, *17*(9), 785-798.
[http://dx.doi.org/10.2174/1389557516666161223153953] [PMID: 28019642]

[7]   Arianayagam, S.; Ryan, T.J. Disorders of pigmentation of the skin hypothesisunderlying interventions by multiple systems of medicine: is there a role for integrated medicine? *Curr. Sci.,* **2016**, *111*(2), 325-336.
[http://dx.doi.org/10.18520/cs/v111/i2/325-336]

[8]   Spritz, R.A. Modern vitiligo genetics sheds new light on an ancient disease. *J. Dermatol.,* **2013**, *40*(5), 310-318.
[http://dx.doi.org/10.1111/1346-8138.12147] [PMID: 23668538]

[9]   Jang, H.J.; Seo, Y.K. Pigmentation Effect of Rice Bran Extracted Minerals Comprising Soluble Silicic Acids *Evid Based Complementary and Altern Med,* **2016**, 1-8.
[http://dx.doi.org/10.1155/2016/3137486]

[10]   Arca, E.; Taştan, H.B.; Erbil, A.H.; Sezer, E.; Koç, E.; Kurumlu, Z. Narrow-band ultraviolet B as monotherapy and in combination with topical calcipotriol in the treatment of vitiligo. *J. Dermatol.,* **2006**, *33*(5), 338-343.
[http://dx.doi.org/10.1111/j.1346-8138.2006.00079.x] [PMID: 16700666]

[11]   Borderé, A.C.; Lambert, J.; van Geel, N. Current and emerging therapy for the management of vitiligo. *Clin. Cosmet. Investig. Dermatol.,* **2009**, *2*, 15-25.
[PMID: 21436965]

[12]   Petrovska, B.B. Historical review of medicinal plants' usage. *Pharmacogn. Rev.,* **2012**, *6*(11), 1-5.
[http://dx.doi.org/10.4103/0973-7847.95849] [PMID: 22654398]

[13]   Le Douarin, N.M.; Creuzet, S.; Couly, G.; Dupin, E. Neural crest cell plasticity and its limits. *Development,* **2004**, *131*(19), 4637-4650.
[http://dx.doi.org/10.1242/dev.01350] [PMID: 15358668]

[14]   Sommer, L. Generation of melanocytes from neural crest cells. *Pigment Cell Melanoma Res.,* **2011**, *24*(3), 411-421.
[http://dx.doi.org/10.1111/j.1755-148X.2011.00834.x] [PMID: 21310010]

[15]   Zabierowski, S.E.; Fukunaga-Kalabis, M.; Li, L.; Herlyn, M. Dermis-derived stem cells: a source of epidermal melanocytes and melanoma? *Pigment Cell Melanoma Res.,* **2011**, *24*(3), 422-429.
[http://dx.doi.org/10.1111/j.1755-148X.2011.00847.x] [PMID: 21410654]

[16]   Cramer, S.F. The histogenesis of acquired melanocytic nevi. Based on a new concept of melanocytic differentiation. *Am. J. Dermatopathol.,* **1984**, *6* Suppl., 289-298.
[PMID: 6528932]

[17]   Adameyko, I.; Lallemend, F.; Aquino, J.B.; Pereira, J.A.; Topilko, P.; Müller, T.; Fritz, N.; Beljajeva, A.; Mochii, M.; Liste, I.; Usoskin, D.; Suter, U.; Birchmeier, C.; Ernfors, P. Schwann cell precursors from nerve innervation are a cellular origin of melanocytes in skin. *Cell,* **2009**, *139*(2), 366-379.
[http://dx.doi.org/10.1016/j.cell.2009.07.049] [PMID: 19837037]

[18]   Costin, G.E.; Hearing, V.J. Human skin pigmentation: melanocytes modulate skin color in response to stress. *FASEB J.,* **2007**, *21*(4), 976-994.
[http://dx.doi.org/10.1096/fj.06-6649rev] [PMID: 17242160]

[19]   Ernfors, P. Cellular origin and developmental mechanisms during the formation of skin melanocytes. *Exp. Cell Res.,* **2010**, *316*(8), 1397-1407.
[http://dx.doi.org/10.1016/j.yexcr.2010.02.042] [PMID: 20211169]

[20]   Riley, P.A. Melanin. *Int. J. Biochem. Cell Biol.,* **1997**, *29*(11), 1235-1239.
[http://dx.doi.org/10.1016/S1357-2725(97)00013-7] [PMID: 9451820]

[21]   Simon, J.D.; Peles, D.; Wakamatsu, K.; Ito, S. Current challenges in understanding melanogenesis: bridging chemistry, biological control, morphology, and function. *Pigment Cell Melanoma Res.,* **2009**, *22*(5), 563-579.
[http://dx.doi.org/10.1111/j.1755-148X.2009.00610.x] [PMID: 19627559]

[22]   Fitzpatrick, T.B.; Miyamoto, M.; Ishikawa, K. The evolution of concepts of melanin biology. *Arch. Dermatol.,* **1967**, *96*(3), 305-323.
[http://dx.doi.org/10.1001/archderm.1967.01610030083015] [PMID: 5341550]

[23]   Sugumaran, M. Molecular mechanisms for mammalian melanogenesis. Comparison with insect cuticular sclerotization. *FEBS Lett.,* **1991**, *295*(1-3), 233-239.
[http://dx.doi.org/10.1016/0014-5793(91)81431-7] [PMID: 1765160]

[24]   del Marmol, V.; Beermann, F. Tyrosinase and related proteins in mammalian pigmentation. *FEBS Lett.,* **1996**, *381*(3), 165-168.
[http://dx.doi.org/10.1016/0014-5793(96)00109-3] [PMID: 8601447]

[25]   Hearing, V.J. Determination of melanin synthetic pathway. *J. Invest. Dermatol.,* **2011**, *131*, 8-11.
[http://dx.doi.org/10.1038/skinbio.2011.4] [PMID: 21157421]

[26]   Fitzpatrick, T.B.; Breathnach, A.S. The epidermal melanin unit system. *Dermatol. Wochenschr.,* **1963**, *147*, 481-489.
[PMID: 14172128]

[27]   Haass, N.K.; Herlyn, M. Normal human melanocyte homeostasis as a paradigm for understanding melanoma. *J. Investig. Dermatol. Symp. Proc.,* **2005**, *10*(2), 153-163.
[http://dx.doi.org/10.1111/j.1087-0024.2005.200407.x] [PMID: 16358819]

[28]   Yamaguchi, Y.; Brenner, M.; Hearing, V.J. The regulations of skin pigmentation. *J. Biol. Chem.,* **2007**, *13*, 1-11.

[29]   Lee, A.Y. Role of keratinocytes in the development of vitiligo. *Ann. Dermatol.,* **2012**, *24*(2), 115-125.
[http://dx.doi.org/10.5021/ad.2012.24.2.115] [PMID: 22577260]

[30]   Ali, S.A.; Naaz, I. Current Challenges in Understanding the Story of Skin Pigmentation — Bridging the Morpho-Anatomical and Functional Aspects of Mammalian Melanocytes. *Muscles cells and Tissue. In tech Publications*; Europe, **2015**.
[http://dx.doi.org/10.5772/60714]

[31]   Pirrone, J.; Broyer, J.; Otte, N.; Reich, K.; Boer-Auer, A. Extensive hyperpigmentation of the face in a Filipina. *J. Dtsch. Dermatol. Ges.,* **2017**, *15*(11), 1167-1168.
[http://dx.doi.org/10.1111/ddg.13329] [PMID: 29024494]

[32]   Nair, B.K. Vitiligo--a retrospect. *Int. J. Dermatol.,* **1978**, *17*(9), 755-757.
        [http://dx.doi.org/10.1111/ijd.1978.17.9.755] [PMID: 365814]

[33]   Gauthier, Y.; Benzekri, L. Historical aspects.*Vitiligo*; Picardo, M.; Taïeb, A., Eds.; Springer Verlag: Heidelberg, **2010**, pp. 3-9.
        [http://dx.doi.org/10.1007/978-3-540-69361-1_1]

[34]   Koranne, R.V.; Sachdeva, K.G. Vitiligo. *Int. J. Dermatol.,* **1988**, *27*(10), 676-681.
        [http://dx.doi.org/10.1111/j.1365-4362.1988.tb01260.x] [PMID: 3069756]

[35]   Moellmann, G.; Klein-Angerer, S.; Scollay, D.A.; Nordlund, J.J.; Lerner, A.B. Extracellular granular material and degeneration of keratinocytes in the normally pigmented epidermis of patients with vitiligo. *J. Invest. Dermatol.,* **1982**, *79*(5), 321-330.
        [http://dx.doi.org/10.1111/1523-1747.ep12500086] [PMID: 7130745]

[36]   Allam, M.; Riad, H. Concise review of recent studies in vitiligo. *Qatar Med. J.,* **2013**, *2013*(2), 1-19.
        [http://dx.doi.org/10.5339/qmj.2013.10] [PMID: 25003059]

[37]   Sehgal, V.N.; Srivastava, G. Vitiligo: compendium of clinico-epidemiological features. *Indian J. Dermatol. Venereol. Leprol.,* **2007**, *73*(3), 149-156.
        [http://dx.doi.org/10.4103/0378-6323.32708] [PMID: 17558045]

[38]   Howitz, J.; Brodthagen, H.; Schwartz, M.; Thomsen, K. Prevalence of vitiligo. Epidemiological survey on the Isle of Bornholm, Denmark. *Arch. Dermatol.,* **1977**, *113*(1), 47-52.
        [http://dx.doi.org/10.1001/archderm.1977.01640010049006] [PMID: 831622]

[39]   Bolognia, J.L.; Nordlund, J.J.; Ortonne, J.P. Vitiligo vulgaris.*The pigmentary system*; Nordlund, J.J.; Boissy, R.E.; Hearing, V.J.; King, R.A.; Ortonne, J.P., Eds.; Oxford University Press: New York, **1998**, pp. 513-551.

[40]   Ezzedine, K.; Lim, H.W.; Suzuki, T.; Katayama, I.; Hamzavi, I.; Lan, C.C.; Goh, B.K.; Anbar, T.; Silva de Castro, C.; Lee, A.Y.; Parsad, D.; van Geel, N.; Le Poole, I.C.; Oiso, N.; Benzekri, L.; Spritz, R.; Gauthier, Y.; Hann, S.K.; Picardo, M.; Taieb, A. Revised classification/nomenclature of vitiligo and related issues: the Vitiligo Global Issues Consensus Conference. *Pigment Cell Melanoma Res.,* **2012**, *25*(3), E1-E13.
        [http://dx.doi.org/10.1111/j.1755-148X.2012.00997.x] [PMID: 22417114]

[41]   Koga, M.; Tango, T. Clinical features and course of type A and type B vitiligo. *Br. J. Dermatol.,* **1988**, *118*(2), 223-228.
        [http://dx.doi.org/10.1111/j.1365-2133.1988.tb01778.x] [PMID: 3348967]

[42]   Alkhateeb, A.; Fain, P.R.; Thody, A.; Bennett, D.C.; Spritz, R.A. Epidemiology of vitiligo and associated autoimmune diseases in Caucasian probands and their families. *Pigment Cell Res.,* **2003**, *16*(3), 208-214.
        [http://dx.doi.org/10.1034/j.1600-0749.2003.00032.x] [PMID: 12753387]

[43]   Laberge, G.; Mailloux, C.M.; Gowan, K.; Holland, P.; Bennett, D.C.; Fain, P.R.; Spritz, R.A. Early disease onset and increased risk of other autoimmune diseases in familial generalized vitiligo. *Pigment Cell Res.,* **2005**, *18*(4), 300-305.
        [http://dx.doi.org/10.1111/j.1600-0749.2005.00242.x] [PMID: 16029422]

[44]   Ando, I.; Chi, H.I.; Nakagawa, H.; Otsuka, F. Difference in clinical features and HLA antigens between familial and non-familial vitiligo of non-segmental type. *Br. J. Dermatol.,* **1993**, *129*(4), 408-410.
        [http://dx.doi.org/10.1111/j.1365-2133.1993.tb03167.x] [PMID: 8217754]

[45]   Singh, A.; Sharma, P.; Kar, H.K.; Sharma, V.K.; Tembhre, M.K.; Gupta, S.; Laddha, N.C.; Dwivedi, M.; Begum, R.; Gokhale, R.S.; Rani, R. HLA alleles and amino-acid signatures of the peptide-binding pockets of HLA molecules in vitiligo. *J. Invest. Dermatol.,* **2012**, *132*(1), 124-134.
        [http://dx.doi.org/10.1038/jid.2011.240] [PMID: 21833019]

[46]   Levandowski, C.B.; Mailloux, C.M.; Ferrara, T.M.; Gowan, K.; Ben, S.; Jin, Y.; McFann, K.K.;

Holland, P.J.; Fain, P.R.; Dinarello, C.A.; Spritz, R.A. NLRP1 haplotypes associated with vitiligo and autoimmunity increase interleukin-1β processing via the NLRP1 inflammasome. *Proc. Natl. Acad. Sci. USA,* **2013**, *110*(8), 2952-2956.
[http://dx.doi.org/10.1073/pnas.1222808110] [PMID: 23382179]

[47]   Kemp, E.H.; Waterman, E.A.; Hawes, B.E.; O'Neill, K.; Gottumukkala, R.V.; Gawkrodger, D.J.; Weetman, A.P.; Watson, P.F. The melanin-concentrating hormone receptor 1, a novel target of autoantibody responses in vitiligo. *J. Clin. Invest.,* **2002**, *109*(7), 923-930.
[http://dx.doi.org/10.1172/JCI0214643] [PMID: 11927619]

[48]   Schallreuter, K.U.; Bahadoran, P.; Picardo, M.; Slominski, A.; Elassiuty, Y.E.; Kemp, E.H.; Giachino, C.; Liu, J.B.; Luiten, R.M.; Lambe, T.; Le Poole, I.C.; Dammak, I.; Onay, H.; Zmijewski, M.A.; Dell'Anna, M.L.; Zeegers, M.P.; Cornall, R.J.; Paus, R.; Ortonne, J.P.; Westerhof, W. Vitiligo pathogenesis: autoimmune disease, genetic defect, excessive reactive oxygen species, calcium imbalance, or what else? *Exp. Dermatol.,* **2008**, *17*(2), 139-140.
[http://dx.doi.org/10.1111/j.1600-0625.2007.00666.x] [PMID: 18205713]

[49]   van den Boorn, J.G.; Konijnenberg, D.; Dellemijn, T.A.; van der Veen, J.P.; Bos, J.D.; Melief, C.J.; Vyth-Dreese, F.A.; Luiten, R.M. Autoimmune destruction of skin melanocytes by perilesional T cells from vitiligo patients. *J. Invest. Dermatol.,* **2009**, *129*(9), 2220-2232.
[http://dx.doi.org/10.1038/jid.2009.32] [PMID: 19242513]

[50]   Shen, C.; Gao, J.; Sheng, Y.; Dou, J.; Zhou, F.; Zheng, X.; Ko, R.; Tang, X.; Zhu, C.; Yin, X.; Sun, L.; Cui, Y.; Zhang, X. Genetic Susceptibility to Vitiligo: GWAS Approaches for Identifying Vitiligo Susceptibility Genes and Loci. *Front. Genet.,* **2016**, *7*, 3.
[http://dx.doi.org/10.3389/fgene.2016.00003] [PMID: 26870082]

[51]   Zhou, L.; Li, K.; Shi, Y.L.; Hamzavi, I.; Gao, T.W.; Henderson, M.; Huggins, R.H.; Agbai, O.; Mahmoud, B.; Mi, X.; Lim, H.W.; Mi, Q.S. Systemic analyses of immunophenotypes of peripheral T cells in non-segmental vitiligo: Implication of defective natural killer T cells. *Pigment Cell Melanoma Res.,* **2012**, *25*(5), 602-611.
[http://dx.doi.org/10.1111/j.1755-148X.2012.01019.x] [PMID: 22591262]

[52]   Lerner, A.B. Vitiligo. *J. Invest. Dermatol.,* **1959**, *32*(2, Part 2), 285-310.
[http://dx.doi.org/10.1038/jid.1959.49] [PMID: 13641799]

[53]   Poojary, S.; Minni, K. Genetics of Vitiligo: An Insight. *Pigmentary Disorders,* **2015**, *2*, 178.
[http://dx.doi.org/10.4172/2376-0427.1000178]

[54]   Boissy, R.E.; Manga, P. On the etiology of contact/occupational vitiligo. *Pigment Cell Res.,* **2004**, *17*(3), 208-214.
[http://dx.doi.org/10.1111/j.1600-0749.2004.00130.x] [PMID: 15140065]

[55]   Puri, N.; Mojamdar, M.; Ramaiah, A. *In vitro* growth characteristics of melanocytes obtained from adult normal and vitiligo subjects. *J. Invest. Dermatol.,* **1987**, *88*(4), 434-438.
[http://dx.doi.org/10.1111/1523-1747.ep12469795] [PMID: 3559270]

[56]   Gauthier, Y.; Cario Andre, M.; Taïeb, A. A critical appraisal of vitiligo etiologic theories. Is melanocyte loss a melanocytorrhagy? *Pigment Cell Res.,* **2003**, *16*(4), 322-332.
[http://dx.doi.org/10.1034/j.1600-0749.2003.00070.x] [PMID: 12859615]

[57]   Gauthier, Y.; Cario-Andre, M.; Lepreux, S.; Pain, C.; Taïeb, A. Melanocyte detachment after skin friction in non lesional skin of patients with generalized vitiligo. *Br. J. Dermatol.,* **2003**, *148*(1), 95-101.
[http://dx.doi.org/10.1046/j.1365-2133.2003.05024.x] [PMID: 12534601]

[58]   Le Poole, I.C.; Das, P.K.; van den Wijngaard, R.M.; Bos, J.D.; Westerhof, W. Review of the etiopathomechanism of vitiligo: A convergence theory. *Exp. Dermatol.,* **1993**, *2*(4), 145-153.
[http://dx.doi.org/10.1111/j.1600-0625.1993.tb00023.x] [PMID: 8162332]

[59]   Westerhof, W.; Nieuweboer-Krobotova, L. Treatment of vitiligo with UV-B radiation *vs* topical psoralen plus UV-A. *Arch. Dermatol.,* **1997**, *133*(12), 1525-1528.

[http://dx.doi.org/10.1001/archderm.1997.03890480045006] [PMID: 9420536]

[60] Lim, H.W.; Grimes, P.E.; Agbai, O.; Hamzavi, I.; Henderson, M.; Haddican, M.; Linkner, R.V.; Lebwohl, M. Afamelanotide and narrowband UV-B phototherapy for the treatment of vitiligo: A randomized multicenter trial. *JAMA Dermatol.,* **2015**, *151*(1), 42-50.
[http://dx.doi.org/10.1001/jamadermatol.2014.1875] [PMID: 25230094]

[61] Kim, S.R.; Heaton, H.; Liu, L.Y.; King, B.A. Rapid Repigmentation of Vitiligo Using Tofacitinib Plus Low-Dose, Narrowband UV-B Phototherapy. *JAMA Dermatol.,* **2018**, *154*(3), 370-371.
[http://dx.doi.org/10.1001/jamadermatol.2017.5778] [PMID: 29387870]

[62] Lotti, T.; Berti, S.; Moretti, S. Vitiligo therapy. *Expert Opin. Pharmacother.,* **2009**, *10*(17), 2779-2785.
[http://dx.doi.org/10.1517/14656560903357509] [PMID: 19929701]

[63] Pacifico, A.; Leone, G. Photo(chemo)therapy for vitiligo. *Photodermatol. Photoimmunol. Photomed.,* **2011**, *27*(5), 261-277.
[http://dx.doi.org/10.1111/j.1600-0781.2011.00606.x] [PMID: 21950634]

[64] Park, K.K.; Liao, W.; Murase, J.E. A review of monochromatic excimer light in vitiligo. *Br. J. Dermatol.,* **2012**, *167*(3), 468-478.
[http://dx.doi.org/10.1111/j.1365-2133.2012.11008.x] [PMID: 22524428]

[65] Le Duff, F.; Fontas, E.; Giacchero, D.; Sillard, L.; Lacour, J.P.; Ortonne, J.P.; Passeron, T. 308-nm excimer lamp *vs.* 308-nm excimer laser for treating vitiligo: A randomized study. *Br. J. Dermatol.,* **2010**, *163*(1), 188-192.
[PMID: 20346025]

[66] Shi, Q.; Li, K.; Fu, J.; Wang, Y.; Ma, C.; Li, Q.; Li, C.; Gao, T. Comparison of the 308-nm excimer laser with the 308-nm excimer lamp in the treatment of vitiligo-a randomized bilateral comparison study. *Photodermatol. Photoimmunol. Photomed.,* **2013**, *29*(1), 27-33.
[http://dx.doi.org/10.1111/phpp.12015] [PMID: 23281694]

[67] Kwinter, J.; Pelletier, J.; Khambalia, A.; Pope, E. High-potency steroid use in children with vitiligo: A retrospective study. *J. Am. Acad. Dermatol.,* **2007**, *56*(2), 236-241.
[http://dx.doi.org/10.1016/j.jaad.2006.08.017] [PMID: 17224367]

[68] Njoo, M.D.; Spuls, P.I.; Bos, J.D.; Westerhof, W.; Bossuyt, P.M. Nonsurgical repigmentation therapies in vitiligo. Meta-analysis of the literature. *Arch. Dermatol.,* **1998**, *134*(12), 1532-1540.
[http://dx.doi.org/10.1001/archderm.134.12.1532] [PMID: 9875190]

[69] Falabella, R.; Barona, M.I. Update on skin repigmentation therapies in vitiligo. *Pigment Cell Melanoma Res.,* **2009**, *22*(1), 42-65.
[http://dx.doi.org/10.1111/j.1755-148X.2008.00528.x] [PMID: 19040503]

[70] Kostovic, K.; Pasic, A. New treatment modalities for vitiligo: Focus on topical immunomodulators. *Drugs,* **2005**, *65*(4), 447-459.
[http://dx.doi.org/10.2165/00003495-200565040-00002] [PMID: 15733009]

[71] Kapoor, R.; Phiske, M.M.; Jerajani, H.R. Evaluation of safety and efficacy of topical prostaglandin E2 in treatment of vitiligo. *Br. J. Dermatol.,* **2009**, *160*(4), 861-863.
[http://dx.doi.org/10.1111/j.1365-2133.2008.08923.x] [PMID: 19014395]

[72] Malakar, S.; Dhar, S. Treatment of stable and recalcitrant vitiligo by autologous miniature punch grafting: A prospective study of 1,000 patients. *Dermatology (Basel),* **1999**, *198*(2), 133-139.
[http://dx.doi.org/10.1159/000018089] [PMID: 10325459]

[73] Lahiri, K.; Malakar, S.; Sarma, N.; Banerjee, U. Repigmentation of vitiligo with punch grafting and narrow-band UV-B (311 nm)-a prospective study. *Int. J. Dermatol.,* **2006**, *45*(6), 649-655.
[http://dx.doi.org/10.1111/j.1365-4632.2005.02697.x] [PMID: 16796620]

[74] Saldanha, K.D.; Machado Filho, C.D.; Paschoal, F.M. Action of topical mometasone on the pigmented halos of micrografting in patients with vitiligo. *An. Bras. Dermatol.,* **2012**, *87*(5), 685-690.
[http://dx.doi.org/10.1590/S0365-05962012000500002] [PMID: 23044558]

[75]   Falabella, R. Surgical treatment of vitiligo: Why, when and how. *J. Eur. Acad. Dermatol. Venereol.,*
         2003, *17*(5), 518-520.
         [http://dx.doi.org/10.1046/j.1468-3083.2003.00718.x] [PMID: 12941084]

[76]   Agrawal, K.; Agrawal, A. Vitiligo: Repigmentation with dermabrasion and thin split-thickness skin
         graft. *Dermatol. Surg.,* **1995**, *21*(4), 295-300.
         [http://dx.doi.org/10.1111/j.1524-4725.1995.tb00176.x] [PMID: 7728478]

[77]   Parsad, D.; Gupta, S. Standard guidelines of care for vitiligo surgery. *Indian J. Dermatol. Venereol.
         Leprol.,* **2008**, *74* Suppl., S37-S45.
         [PMID: 18688102]

[78]   Czajkowski, R.; Pokrywczynska, M.; Placek, W.; Zegarska, B.; Tadrowski, T.; Drewa, T.
         Transplantation of cultured autologous melanocytes: Hope or danger? *Cell Transplant.,* **2010**, *19*(5),
         639-643.
         [http://dx.doi.org/10.3727/096368910X491798] [PMID: 20350353]

[79]   Felsten, L.M.; Alikhan, A.; Petronic-Rosic, V. Vitiligo: a comprehensive overview Part II: Treatment
         options and approach to treatment. *J. Am. Acad. Dermatol.,* **2011**, *65*(3), 493-514.
         [http://dx.doi.org/10.1016/j.jaad.2010.10.043] [PMID: 21839316]

[80]   Budania, A.; Parsad, D.; Kanwar, A.J.; Dogra, S. Comparison between autologous noncultured
         epidermal cell suspension and suction blister epidermal grafting in stable vitiligo: A randomized study.
         Br. J. Dermatol., **2012**, *167*(6), 1295-1301.
         [http://dx.doi.org/10.1111/bjd.12007] [PMID: 22897617]

[81]   Nahhas, A.F.; Mohammad, T.F.; Hamzavi, I.H. Vitiligo Surgery: Shuffling Melanocytes. *J. Investig.
         Dermatol. Symp. Proc.,* **2017**, *18*(2), S34-S37.
         [http://dx.doi.org/10.1016/j.jisp.2017.01.001] [PMID: 28941491]

[82]   Zhang, X.; Zhao, W.; Wang, Y.; Lu, J.; Chen, X. The chemical constituents and bioactivities of
         Psoralea corylifolia Linn: A Review. *Am. J. Chin. Med.,* **2016**, *44*(1), 35-60.
         [http://dx.doi.org/10.1142/S0192415X16500038] [PMID: 26916913]

[83]   Donata, S.; Kesavan, M.; Austin, S.; Mohan, K.S.; Rajagopalan, K.; Kuttan, R. Clinical trial of certain
         ayurvedic medicines indicated in vitiligo. *Anc. Sci. Life,* **1990**, *9*(4), 202-206.
         [PMID: 22557698]

[84]   Xu, J.G.; Shang, J. The activation of *Psoralea corylifolia* on tryosinase. *Chin. Tradit. Herbal Drugs,*
         1991, *4*, 168-169.

[85]   Liu, Z.L.; Xu, Y.F.; Tu, C.X.; Wu, K.K. Studies on the effect of ethanol extracts of 56 traditional
         Chinese drugs on the activity of tyrosinase. *Dalian Yike Daxue Xuebao,* **2000**, *22*(1), 7-10.

[86]   Ali, S.A.; Sultan, T.; Galgut, J.M.; Sharma, R.; Meitei, K.V.; Ali, A.S. *In vitro* responses of fish
         melanophores to lyophilized extracts of *Psoralea corylifolia* seeds and pure psoralen. *Pharm. Biol.,*
         2011, *49*(4), 422-427.
         [http://dx.doi.org/10.3109/13880209.2010.521164] [PMID: 21391886]

[87]   Hussain, I.; Hussain, N.; Manan, A.; Rashid, A.; Khan, B.; Bakhsh, S. Fabrication of anti-vitiligo
         ointment containing *Psoralea corylifolia*: in vitro and in vivo characterization. *Drug Des. Devel. Ther.,*
         2016, *10*(10), 3805-3816.
         [http://dx.doi.org/10.2147/DDDT.S114328] [PMID: 27920496]

[88]   Paarakh, P.M. Nigella sativaLinn. A comprehensive review. *IJNPR,* **2010**, *1*(4), 409-429.

[89]   Ali, S.A.; Meitei, K.V. *Nigella sativa* seed extract and its bioactive compound thymoquinone: The new
         melanogens causing hyperpigmentation in the wall lizard melanophores. *J. Pharm. Pharmacol.,* **2011**,
         63(5), 741-746.
         [http://dx.doi.org/10.1111/j.2042-7158.2011.01271.x] [PMID: 21492177]

[90]   Ghorbanibirgani, A.; Khalili, A.; Rokhafrooz, D. Comparing *Nigella sativa* oil and fish oil in treatment

of vitiligo. *Iran. Red Crescent Med. J.,* **2014**, *16*(6), e4515.
[http://dx.doi.org/10.5812/ircmj.4515] [PMID: 25068060]

[91]   Singh, P.; Guleri, R.; Singh, V.; Kaur, G.; Kataria, H.; Singh, B.; Kaur, G.; Kaul, S.C.; Wadhwa, R.; Pati, P.K. Biotechnological interventions in *Withania somnifera* (L.) Dunal. *Biotechnol. Genet. Eng. Rev.,* **2015**, *31*(1-2), 1-20.
[http://dx.doi.org/10.1080/02648725.2015.1020467] [PMID: 25787309]

[92]   Dar, P.A.; Singh, L.R.; Kamal, M.A.; Dar, T.A. Unique medicinal properties of *Withania somnifera*: Phytochemical constituents and protein component. *Curr. Pharm. Des.,* **2016**, *22*(5), 535-540.
[http://dx.doi.org/10.2174/1381612822666151125001751] [PMID: 26601969]

[93]   Ali, S.A.; Meitei, K.V. On the action and mechanism of withaferin-A from *Withania somnifera*, a novel and potent melanin dispersing agent in frog melanophores. *J. Recept. Signal Transduct. Res.,* **2011**, *31*(5), 359-366.
[http://dx.doi.org/10.3109/10799893.2011.602414] [PMID: 21848494]

[94]   Ali, S.A.; Meitei, K.V. *Withania somnifera* root extracts induce skin darkening in wall lizard melanophores *via* stimulation of cholinergic receptors. *Nat. Prod. Res.,* **2012**, *26*(17), 1645-1648.
[http://dx.doi.org/10.1080/14786419.2011.589053] [PMID: 21950559]

[95]   Manoharan, S.; Balakrishnan, S.; Menon, V.P.; Alias, L.M.; Reena, A.R. Chemopreventive efficacy of curcumin and piperine during 7,12-dimethylbenz[a]anthracene-induced hamster buccal pouch carcinogenesis. *Singapore Med. J.,* **2009**, *50*(2), 139-146.
[PMID: 19296028]

[96]   Sajid, M.; Ali, S.A. Mediation of cholino-piperine like receptors by extracts of Piper nigrum induces melanin dispersion in *Rana tigerina* tadpole melanophores. *J. Recept. Signal Transduct. Res.,* **2011**, *31*(4), 286-290.
[http://dx.doi.org/10.3109/10799893.2011.583254] [PMID: 21663558]

[97]   Parganiha, R.; Verma, S.; Chandrakar, S.; Pal, S.; Sawarkar, H.A.; Kashyap, P. *In vitro* anti- asthmatic activity of fruit extract of *Piper nigrum* (Piperaceae). *Inter J Herbal Drug Res,* **2011**, *1*, 15-18.

[98]   Ahmad, N.; Fazal, H.; Abbasi, B.H.; Farooq, S.; Ali, M. Biological role of *Piper nigrum* L. (Black pepper): A review. *Asian Pac. J. Trop. Biomed.,* **2012**, •••, S1945-S1953.
[http://dx.doi.org/10.1016/S2221-1691(12)60524-3]

[99]   Lin, Z.; Hoult, J.R.; Bennett, D.C.; Raman, A. Stimulation of mouse melanocyte proliferation by *Piper nigrum* fruit extract and its main alkaloid, piperine. *Planta Med.,* **1999**, *65*(7), 600-603.
[http://dx.doi.org/10.1055/s-1999-14031] [PMID: 10575373]

[100] Lin, Z.; Liao, Y.; Venkatasamy, R.; Hider, R.C.; Soumyanath, A. Amides from *Piper nigrum* L. with dissimilar effects on melanocyte proliferation *in-vitro*. *J. Pharm. Pharmacol.,* **2007**, *59*(4), 529-536.
[http://dx.doi.org/10.1211/jpp.59.4.0007] [PMID: 17430636]

[101] Vinod, K.R.; Santhosha, D.; Anbazhagan, S. Formulation and evaluation of piperine creama new herbal dimensional approach for vitiligo patients. *Int. J. Pharm. Pharm. Sci.,* **2011**, *3*(2), 2933.

[102] Badgujar, S.B.; Patel, V.V.; Bandivdekar, A.H.; Mahajan, R.T. Traditional uses, phytochemistry and pharmacology of *Ficus carica*: A review. *Pharm. Biol.,* **2014**, *52*(11), 1487-1503.
[http://dx.doi.org/10.3109/13880209.2014.892515] [PMID: 25017517]

[103] Mahjour, M.; Khoushabi, A.; Miri Ghale Novi, M.; Feyzabadi, Z. Food strategies of renal atrophy based on Avicenna and conventional medicine. *J. Tradit. Complement. Med.,* **2017**, *7*(4), 375-379.
[http://dx.doi.org/10.1016/j.jtcme.2016.12.004] [PMID: 29034182]

[104] Joseph, B.; Raj, J.S. Pharmacognostic and phytochemical properties of *Ficus carica* Linn –An overview. *Int. J. Pharm. Tech. Res.,* **2011**, *3*(1), 8-12.

[105] Meitei, K.V.; Ali, S.A. Fig leaf extract and its bioactive compound psoralen induces skin darkening effect in reptilian melanophores via cholinergic receptor stimulation. *In Vitro Cell. Dev. Biol. Anim.,* **2012**, *48*(6), 335-339.

[http://dx.doi.org/10.1007/s11626-012-9521-0] [PMID: 22706602]

[106] Farhadi, A.K.; Gavadifar, K.; Farha, A. Effects of *Berberise vulgaris* fruit extract on blood cholesterol and triglyceride in hyperlipidemic patients. *J Semnan Univ Med Sci,* **2008**, *9*, 211-216.

[107] Mokhber-Dezfuli, N.; Saeidnia, S.; Gohari, A.R.; Kurepaz-Mahmoodabadi, M. Phytochemistry and pharmacology of berberis species. *Pharmacogn. Rev.,* **2014**, *8*(15), 8-15.
[http://dx.doi.org/10.4103/0973-7847.125517] [PMID: 24600191]

[108] Abd El-Wahab, A.E.; Ghareeb, D.A.; Sarhan, E.E.; Abu-Serie, M.M.; El Demellawy, M.A. *In vitro* biological assessment of *Berberis vulgaris* and its active constituent, berberine: Antioxidants, anti-acetylcholinesterase, anti-diabetic and anticancer effects. *BMC Complement. Altern. Med.,* **2013**, *13*, 218.
[http://dx.doi.org/10.1186/1472-6882-13-218] [PMID: 24007270]

[109] Ali, S.A.; Naaz, I.; Choudhary, R.K. Berberine-induced pigment dispersion in *Bufo melanostictus* melanophores by stimulation of beta-2 adrenergic receptors. *J. Recept. Signal Transduct. Res.,* **2014**, *34*(1), 15-20.
[http://dx.doi.org/10.3109/10799893.2013.843193] [PMID: 24099619]

[110] Mehta, N.R.; Patel, E.P.; Patani, P.V.; Shah, B. *Nelumbonucifera* (Lotus): A review on ethanobotany, phytochemistry and pharmacology. *Indian J Pharm Biol Res,* **2013**, *1*(4), 152-167.
[http://dx.doi.org/10.30750/ijpbr.1.4.26]

[111] Jeon, S.; Kim, N.H.; Koo, B.S.; Kim, J.Y.; Lee, A.Y. Lotus (*Nelumbo nuficera*) flower essential oil increased melanogenesis in normal human melanocytes. *Exp. Mol. Med.,* **2009**, *41*(7), 517-525.
[http://dx.doi.org/10.3858/emm.2009.41.7.057] [PMID: 19322028]

[112] Chen, Y.; Wang, M.; Rosen, R.T.; Ho, C.T. 2,2-Diphenyl-1-picrylhydrazyl radical-scavenging active components from *Polygonum multiflorum* thunb. *J. Agric. Food Chem.,* **1999**, *47*(6), 2226-2228.
[http://dx.doi.org/10.1021/jf990092f] [PMID: 10794614]

[113] Lv, L.; Gu, X.; Tang, J.; Ho, C. Antioxidant activity of stilbene glycoside from *Polygonum multiflorum* Thunb *in vivo. Food Chem.,* **2007**, *104*, 1678-1681.
[http://dx.doi.org/10.1016/j.foodchem.2007.03.022]

[114] Wu, C.S.; Sun, R. [Research development and thinking of clinical study of *Polygonum multiflorum.*]. *Zhongguo Zhongyao Zazhi,* **2017**, *42*(2), 259-263.
[PMID: 28948728]

[115] Jiang, Z.; Xu, J.; Long, M.; Tu, Z.; Yang, G.; He, G. 2, 3, 5, 4′-tetrahydroxystilbene-2-O-b-ta-D-glucoside (THSG) induces melanogenesis in B16 cells by MAP kinase activation and tyrosinase upregulation. *Life Sci.,* **2009**, *85*(9-10), 345-350.
[http://dx.doi.org/10.1016/j.lfs.2009.05.022] [PMID: 19527735]

[116] Thanh, D.T.H.; Thanh, N.L.; Thang, N.D. Toxicological and melanin synthesis effects of *Polygonum multiflorum* root extracts on zebrafish embryos and human melanocytes. *Biomed. Res. Ther.,* **2016**, *3*(9), 808-818.
[http://dx.doi.org/10.7603/s40730-016-0042-4]

[117] Wu, Y.C.; Hsieh, C.L. Pharmacological effects of Radix *Angelica Sinensis* (Danggui) on cerebral infarction. *Chin. Med.,* **2011**, *6*(32), 32.
[http://dx.doi.org/10.1186/1749-8546-6-32] [PMID: 21867503]

[118] Raman, A.; Lin, Z.X.; Sviderskaya, E.; Kowalska, D. Investigation of the effect of *Angelica sinensis* root extract on the proliferation of melanocytes in culture. *J. Ethnopharmacol.,* **1996**, *54*(2-3), 165-170.
[http://dx.doi.org/10.1016/S0378-8741(96)01458-4] [PMID: 8953431]

[119] Deng, Y.; Yang, L. Effect of *Angelica sinensis* (Oliv.) on melanocytic proliferation, melanin synthesis and tyrosinase activity *in vitro. J. First Mil. Med. Univ.,* **2003**, *23*(3), 239-241.
[PMID: 12651240]

[120]   Monem El Mofty, A. A preliminary clinical report on the treatment of leucodermia with *Ammi majus* Linn. *J. Egypt. Med. Assoc.,* **1948**, *31*(8), 651-665.
[PMID: 18890453]

[121]   Kaminsky, A. Vitiligo: Its treatment with *Ammi majus. Dia Med.,* **1954**, *26*(10), 233-236.
[PMID: 13161656]

[122]   Oszast, Z.; Krasowska, H. First experimental application of *ammi majus* L. extract prepared in Poland, in the treatment of Vitiligo. *Przegl. Dermatol.,* **1957**, *7*(1), 1-14.
[PMID: 13465858]

[123]   Ossenkoppele, P.M.; van der Sluis, W.G.; van Vloten, W.A. Phototoxic dermatitis following the use of *Ammi majus* fruit for vitiligo. *Ned. Tijdschr. Geneeskd.,* **1991**, *135*(11), 478-480.
[PMID: 2023655]

[124]   Dhalwal, K.; Shinde, V.M.; Mahadik, K.R.; Namdeo, A.G. Rapid densitometric method for simultaneous analysis of umbelliferone, psoralen, and eugenol in herbal raw materials using HPTLC. *J. Sep. Sci.,* **2007**, *30*(13), 2053-2058.
[http://dx.doi.org/10.1002/jssc.200600418] [PMID: 17628870]

[125]   Middelkamp-Hup, M.A.; Bos, J.D.; Rius-Diaz, F.; Gonzalez, S.; Westerhof, W. Treatment of vitiligo vulgaris with narrow-band UVB and oral *Polypodium leucotomos* extract: A randomized double-blind placebo-controlled study. *J. Eur. Acad. Dermatol. Venereol.,* **2007**, *21*(7), 942-950.
[http://dx.doi.org/10.1111/j.1468-3083.2006.02132.x] [PMID: 17659004]

[126]   Conforti, F.; Marrelli, H.; Menichini, F.; Bonesi, M.; Statti, G.; Provenzano, E.; Menichini, F. Natural and synthetic furanocoumarins as treatment for vitiligo and psoriasis. *J Curr Drug Ther,* **2009**, *4*, 38-58.
[http://dx.doi.org/10.2174/157488509787081886]

[127]   Bhowmik, D.; Chiranjb, L.; Yadav, J.; Tripathi, K.K.; Kumar, S. Herbal Remedies of *Azadirachta indica* and its Medicinal Application. *J. Chem. Pharm. Res.,* **2010**, *2*, 62-72.

[128]   Del, R.J.A.; Ortuno, A.; Perez, I.; Bennett, R.G.; Real, D.; Correal, E. Furanocoumarin content in *Bituminaria bituminosa* varieties and Cullen Species. *Journal of Options Mediterraneennes,* **2010**, *92*, 67-70.

[129]   Kamble, S.Y.; Patil, S.R.; Sawant, P.S.; Sawant, S.; Pawar, S.G.; Singh, E.A. Studies on Plants Used in Traditional Medicine by Bhilla Tribe of Maharashtra. *IJTK,* **2010**, *9*, 591-598.

[130]   Singh, P.K.; Kumar, V.; Tiwari, R.K.; Sharma, A.; Rao, C.V.; Singh, R.H. Medico-Ethnobotony of Chatara Block of District Sonebhadra Uttar Pradesh India. *J Advances Biol Res,* **2010**, *4*, 65-80.

[131]   Soni, P.; Patidav, R.; Soni, V.; Soni, S. A Review on traditional and alternative treatment for skin disease: Vitiligo. *Int. J. Pharm. Biol. Arch.,* **2010**, *1*, 220-227.

[132]   Szczurko, O.; Shear, N.; Taddio, A.; Boon, H. Ginkgo biloba for the treatment of vitilgo vulgaris: An open label pilot clinical trial. *BMC Complement. Altern. Med.,* **2011**, *11*(21), 21.
[http://dx.doi.org/10.1186/1472-6882-1S1-21] [PMID: 21406109]

SUBJECT INDEX

A

Abrus precatorius 190, 194, 195
  antitumor activity of 194
  seeds 194, 195
Absinthium 54
Acetone 4, 58, 97, 98
Acetylcholine 262
Acid 51, 57, 46, 60, 61, 62, 64, 227, 228
  deoxyribonucleic 46
  nitrous 60, 61, 62, 64
  punicic 227, 228
  tannic 51, 57
Active chemical constituents 190, 191, 192, 193, 194
Activity 13, 14, 15, 31, 32, 58, 100, 123, 128, 129, 133, 135, 137, 152, 154, 156, 157, 158, 159, 161, 162, 165, 167, 169, 186, 195, 198, 200, 201, 217, 218, 221, 223, 224, 227, 230, 232
  anti-cancer 159
  anti-tumor 157, 167, 169, 201
Acute 163, 167, 170
  myelogenous leukaemia (AML) 163, 167
  promyelocytic leukaemia (APL) 170
Administration, oral 112, 130, 134, 151, 200
Aegle marmelos 204, 222
Aerobic cells 4
Aflatoxin B1 49, 52, 53, 54, 55, 65
Agents 205, 215, 224, 225, 235, 259
  chemotherapeutic 205, 224, 225
  therapeutic 215, 235, 259
Aggressive breast cancer 167
Aglycones 97, 101
AhR 156, 157
  active derivatives of indirubins 156
  ligands 156, 157
Ajwain 55
Alkaloids 13, 26, 28, 57, 191, 198, 199, 200, 215, 216, 224, 225, 263, 264
  Vinca 13, 215, 225
Allium sativum 190, 195, 217
Allium test 49

Allogeneic transplant 184
Allopathic medicines 247, 248
Aloe-emodin 195
Aloe vera 190, 195, 223
Alstonia scholaris 196
Alzheimer's disease 154
Amaranthaceae 57
  Plants 57
Amarus 199, 200
American cancer society 215
Ames test 46, 48, 49, 52, 54, 55, 56, 57, 58, 59, 62, 65, 66, 67, 68, 69, 74, 75, 79, 80
AML-derived cancer cell line 163
Ammi majus 248, 265, 266
Amooranin 188, 196
Anacardic acids 191, 196, 197, 201
Analgesics 14, 128, 129
Andrographis paniculata 191, 197
Andrographolides 191, 197
Anemia 126, 127, 129
Angelica sinensis 265, 266
Annonaceous acetogenin 197
Anorexia 14, 127, 131, 134, 135
Anthocyanins 54, 92, 93
Anti-angiogenic 157, 167, 234
  activity of indirubins 157
  effects 167, 234
Anticancer 10, 32, 57, 58, 181, 186, 187, 215, 217, 219, 222, 228
  efficacy 219
  mechanism 215, 228
  molecules 186
  properties 57, 58, 181, 187, 217, 219, 222
  strategy, effective 10
  therapies 32, 228
Antidepressants 128, 129
Anti-fatigue effects 131
Anti-migratory effects 156
Antimutagenic 49, 52, 53,54, 55, 57, 58, 59, 62, 79, 192, 216
  activity 52, 54, 55, 58, 79, 192, 216
  substances 49
Antimutagens 48, 54, 62, 65, 66, 77, 80, 202

Antioxidant(s) 1, 5, 6, 13, 14, 15, 25, 28, 32,
        57, 58, 59, 64, 93, 96, 97, 99, 101, 102,
        108, 109, 111, 192, 200, 202, 220, 221,
        228, 229, 234, 262, 264, 265
    activity 13, 15, 25, 57, 108, 109, 111, 221
    capacity 93, 101, 102
    effects 28
    Inhibition 27
    natural plants-derived 1
    plant-derived 13
Antioxidation 264, 265
Anti-proliferative effects 153, 156, 159, 160,
        166
Apiaceae 266
Apoptosis 7, 11, 15, 16, 17, 18, 20, 22, 28, 64,
        102, 103, 110, 111, 113, 130, 136, 149,
        158, 159, 160, 162, 166, 168, 190, 191,
        193, 194, 195, 196, 197, 202, 203, 215,
        216, 217, 218, 220, 221, 222, 224, 227,
        228, 229, 230, 233
    cell 196, 217, 220
    induced 228, 229
    inducing 64, 224
    markers 160, 224
    mediated 190, 193, 202
    pathways 20, 230, 233
    process 229, 230
    thymocyte 193, 202
Apple polyphenol (AP) 104, 105
    extract 105
Approach, genetic 183
Aqueous extract 15, 27, 57, 199, 263
Aqueous plant extract 57
Aquilaria agallocha 204
Aristas 186
Ascorbic acid (AA) 4, 6, 51, 59, 62, 63, 65,
        66, 67, 69, 70, 71, 76, 77, 79, 222
Asthma 26, 182, 198, 200, 224
Astragalus membranaceus 130, 131, 132
Atherosclerosis 15, 16, 162
Autoimmune hypothesis 255
Autophagy 12, 169, 227
    induction of 12
Autophagy activation 12
Ayurveda 181, 182, 185, 186, 187, 190, 194,
        196, 197, 198, 200, 203, 205, 247, 248,
        260, 261, 262

Ayurvedic 181, 182, 183, 186, 200, 201, 203,
        206
    formulations 181, 186, 201, 203, 206
    perspective 182, 183
    plants 183
    system of medicine 200, 201
Azadirachtin 16, 17, 18, 21, 22

B

Baoyuan Jiedu Decoction (BYJD) 132
Basal lamina 11
Benzyl 26
    glucosinolate (BG) 26
    isothiocyanate 26
Berberis aristata 191, 197
Berberis vulgaris 248, 264, 266
    root extract 264
Bioactive compounds 13, 27, 57, 100, 103,
        106, 108, 109, 215, 216, 224, 230, 235,
        236, 261
    natural 100, 106, 216
Bioavailability of polyphenols 101
Bituminaria bituminosa 266, 267
Bladder cancer cells 10, 190, 221
    human 10, 190
Blood vessels 11, 233, 234
Boerhaavia diffusa 203, 204
Brain cancer 223
Breast cancer 113, 114, 135, 156, 158, 184,
        201, 205, 217, 220, 222, 223, 224, 225,
        226, 228
    cells 113, 114, 156, 158, 220, 222
    human bone- homing 224
    MAK 205
    metastasis 224
    tissue 226
Brick gravels 201
Bullwort 265, 266
Busulfan 168, 169, 170

C

Calotropis gigantean 197
Cambrex BioScience 23
Camptothecin 186, 216, 225, 226

Nelumbo nucifera 264
Nervous systems 123, 137
Neural crest cells (NCC) 249
Neural hypothesis 256
Neuroblastoma cells, human 167, 168
Nigella sativa 191, 199, 248, 261, 262, 266
  oil 262
Nimbin 16
Nimbolide 16, 17, 18, 19, 21, 22
Nitric oxide synthase, inducible 224, 226
Nitrite 4, 46, 49, 60, 61, 62, 63, 65, 69, 70, 71,
    72, 73, 76, 77, 78, 79, 80
  molar ratio 77
Nitrogenous bases 7, 8
Nitro-indirubinoxime 167, 169
  5'fluoro-indirubinoxime 167
Nitrosation 60, 61, 63, 69
Nitrosocompounds 60
N-Nitrosocompounds 60, 62
N-Nitrosodiethylamine 191, 197, 199, 200
Non-cancerous conditions 162
Non-small cell lung cancer (NSCLC) 136, 231
Novel indirubin derivatives 162
Nuclear factor-kB 105, 148, 163, 164
Nucleotides 8
Nutraceuticals 58, 105, 106
Nutritional problem 127

O

Oil 54, 99, 108, 109, 112, 182, 199, 201, 262,
    264
  coconut 112, 201
  fish 262
Olomucine 187, 231
Oncogenesis 154, 157, 158
Oral cancer 192, 200, 224
  chemopreventive activity of piperine in 192,
    200
Organic solvent consumption 99, 100
Oroxylum indicum 204
Oxidases, enzyme polyphenol 64
Oxidative 1, 2, 6, 7, 10, 11, 12, 13, 15, 22, 25,
    28, 29, 30, 31, 57, 60, 102, 103, 195,
    216, 220, 235
  damage 7, 28, 57, 102, 103
  stress 1, 2, 6, 7, 10, 11, 12, 13, 15, 22, 25,
    28, 29, 30, 31, 60, 195, 216, 220, 235

Oxygen species, reactive 2, 167, 168, 219

P

Panax ginseng 130, 131, 133, 134, 222
Pancreatic cancer 113, 157, 219, 224
  human 157
Papaya extracts 27, 28, 32
Papaya seeds extract 29, 30, 31
Pathogenesis 161, 165, 181, 182
Pathogenesis of cancer-related fatigue 125
Perforin 18, 21
Phagocytic cells 3
Phaseolus adenanthus 203, 204
Phenolic acids 26, 28, 55, 56, 57, 64, 91, 92,
    93, 95, 98, 99, 101, 110, 217, 263
  compounds 26, 28, 55, 56, 98, 99, 101, 217,
    263
  known plant-derived 110
Phenolic content 95, 96, 98, 99
Phenotypes, malignant 183
Pheomelanin 250
Phosphoinositide 155
Phosphorylate 157, 158
Phosphorylation 12, 152, 153, 154, 155, 159,
    161, 163, 218, 232, 234
  reduced 153, 154, 161
Phototherapy 247, 257, 258, 267
Phyllanthus amarus 199, 200
Phytochemicals 15, 16, 26, 27, 54, 104, 206,
    215, 216, 220, 228, 229, 235, 236, 263
Phytopharmacology 181
Phytosoms 110
Phytotherapy 1, 2, 13, 14, 32
Picrorrhiza kurroa 192, 200
Pigment epithelium-derived factor (PEDF)
    160
P-Induced forestomach tumorigenesis 20
Piperine cream 263
Piper longum 192, 200, 203, 204, 205
Piper nigrum 203, 248, 263, 266
Plantaginaceae 56
Plant(s) 1, 13, 14, 26, 52, 53, 57, 92, 94, 129,
    181, 182, 186, 215, 225, 229, 236, 264,
    265
  alkaloids 225
  aquatic perennial 264
  decorative 53, 264